Bioactive Glass Materials for Biological Applications

Bioactive Glass Materials for Biological Applications envelopes the complexities, challenges, and advancement in developing a new class of bioactive materials for versatile applications. It outlines the materials involved, bioactivity against bioinert materials, phase change materials, biomolecular nature, synthetic biodegradable polymers, and bioactive glasses. The processing techniques of the bioactive glasses for versatile applications are also covered. A comprehensive focus is on the review of additive manufacturing routes suitable for biological applications with the ability to print various bioactive materials whilst carrying living cells.

Features:

- Introduces bioactive glass materials and their nature aimed towards biological applications.
- Covers how biological materials behave in vivo and in vitro for tailoring materials and sensitivity to the biological environment.
- Explores relevant additive manufacturing platforms.
- Reviews new chemistry and molecules for therapeutic and drug delivery applications alongside bone tissue and regenerative medicine.
- Spotlights the future scope of bioactive glass nanoparticles, their limitations, and research focus areas.

This book is aimed at graduate students and researchers in glasses and ceramics and biomaterials.

Bioactive Glass Materials for Biological Applications

**Edited by Gujjala Raghavendra,
P. Syam Prasad and Dheeraj Kumar Gara**

CRC Press
Taylor & Francis Group
Boca Raton London New York

CRC Press is an imprint of the
Taylor & Francis Group, an **informa** business

First edition published 2026
by CRC Press
2385 NW Executive Center Drive, Suite 320, Boca Raton FL 33431

and by CRC Press
4 Park Square, Milton Park, Abingdon, Oxon, OX14 4RN

CRC Press is an imprint of Taylor & Francis Group, LLC

ISBN: 9781032689852 (hbk)
ISBN: 9781041116066 (pbk)
ISBN: 9781003660781 (ebk)

DOI: 10.1201/9781003660781

Typeset in Times
by codeMantra

Contents

Preface

Drug delivery, regenerative medicine, and other niche areas such as bone tissue engineering have received significant attention in the scientific community, and more than five decades of work have been dedicated to the global research. Despite being, still there are challenges appraising these new areas due to the nature of the biological environment that makes them sophisticated to accept a new foreign material. To realize this, materials scientists have come up with practical solutions that display some possibilities towards meeting the golden standards of human environment. In lieu of this, materials referred to as bioactive glass materials have been found to be potential materials since they show up an intriguing characteristic of interacting with the host environment and thus enabling the growth factors to perform various growth-induced activities in the physiological environment.

However, they are backed by a few complexities to use them in a more potential way due to their nature and characteristics that are required to tailor or mimic the bioactivity at various scales. This book envelopes the various complexities and challenges, advancement in developing new class of bioactive materials for versatile applications that developed over a phase of last five decades, and a potential for the future towards developing these materials. This book technically outlines the materials involved with human environment and discussion on bioactivity against bioinert materials, phase change materials, biomolecules nature and synthetic biodegradable polymers, and bioactive glasses. The processing techniques of the bioactive glasses for versatile applications will be covered, and novel approaches that can actually allow integration of live cells for clinical in vivo will be discussed. This book also discusses the recent post-processing techniques such as additive manufacturing routes.

A comprehensive focus on the review of additive manufacturing routes that are suitable for biological applications will be put forth. At the same time, an emphasis will be made on 3D and 4D bioprinting that has the ability to print various bioactive materials whilst carrying living cells. Finally, a foresee on the outlook of the potential for developing these materials will be included that give readers to understand, identify, and investigate towards contribution to the development of bioactive glass materials for regenerative, bone tissue, drug delivery, and orthodontic applications.

About the Editors

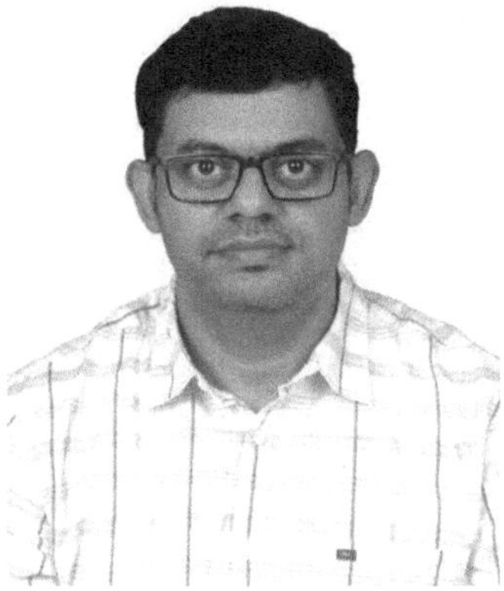

Gujjala Raghavendra is currently working as an Assistant Professor in the Department of Mechanical Engineering at the National Institute of Technology, Warangal, Telangana, India. He obtained his M.Tech and Ph.D. degrees from NIT Rourkela. His research interests include composite materials, functionally graded materials (FGMs), nanomaterials, and bioglasses. Under his supervision, seven Ph.D. degrees have been awarded, and twelve more are currently in progress. He has published over 130 articles in international and national journals and conferences, along with more than 12 book chapters. He has also edited books in the Lecture Notes in Mechanical Engineering series (Springer) and with CRC Press. Dr. Raghavendra serves as a reviewer for several national and international journals and currently manages three sponsored research projects. He has taught courses on composites, tribology, and material characterization at both undergraduate and postgraduate levels.

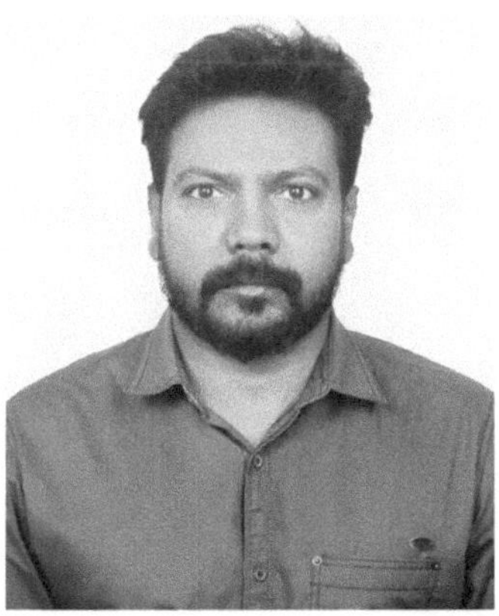

P. Syam Prasad is working as a Professor in the Department of Physics, National Institute of Technology, Warangal, Telangana, INDIA. He has received his MSc (Physics), MPhil (Glass Science), and PhD (Material Sciences and Engineering), respectively. He possesses more than 18 years of combined teaching and research experience in the field of physical sciences and glass science, in particular. His current research theme focuses on the development and characterization of glasses and glass ceramics for photonic, electronic, and biomedical applications. He has published nearly 50 articles in various reputed international and national journals and conferences. He has completed six and two ongoing R&D projects sanctioned by the Government of India. Currently, six PhD students are working under his supervision, and three students have completed their PhDs under his guidance. He has reviewed many papers in reputed research journals like *Scientific Reports*, *Spectroscopy Letters*, *Physics B: Condensed Matter Physics*, the *Journal of Alloys and Compounds*, the *Journal of American Ceramic Society*, the *Journal of Molecular Liquids*, *Ceramic International*, *Optical Materials*, and *Bioactive Materials*. He has presented his research in the USA, Portugal, Hungary, Egypt, Slovakia, Switzerland, Austria, and other countries in the world. His research interests include glasses and glass-ceramics for electronic, optical, and biomedical applications, nanostructured magnetic and semiconductor materials, magnetic and semiconductor thin films and devices.

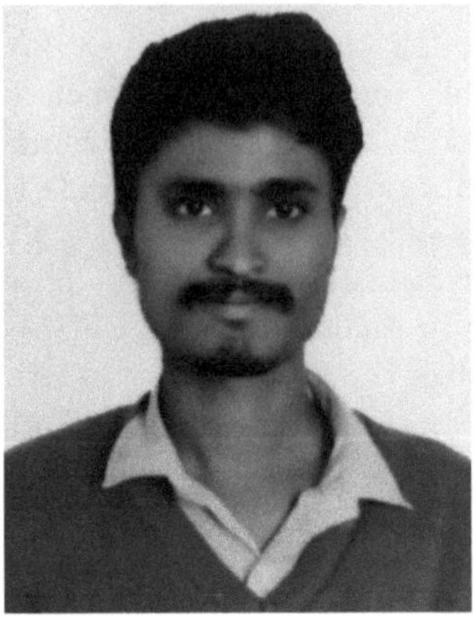

Dheeraj Kumar Gara is an Assistant Professor in the Department of Aerospace Engineering at Jain University and PhD scholar in Mechanical Engineering, National Institute of Technology, Warangal. His areas of interest lie in composite materials for aerospace and biomedical applications, energy storage devices, bioactive materials, functionally graded materials, shape memory alloys, and nanoparticles. He has published a decent number of journals in aerospace and biomedical domains and currently heads his lab on Biostimulus Materials Laboratory at Jain University, Bengaluru, India, dedicated for the development of 3D and 4D bioprinting platforms for printing tissues.

Contributors

Che Azurahanim Binti Che Abdullah
Faculty of Science, Department of Physics
Universiti Putra Malaysia
Seri Kembangan, Malaysia

V.N. Radha Manohar Aepuru
Department of Mechanical Engineering
Advanced Materials Laboratory
Universidad de Chile
Santiago, Chile

P. Abdul Azeem
Department of Physics
NIT Warangal
Telangana, India

Aswani Kumar Bandaru
Department of Mechanical/Biomedical Engineering
Munster Technological University
Cork, Ireland

Gebru Kiros Berhe
Professor, Department of Aerospace Engineering
College of Engineering
Ethiopian Defence University
Bishoftu, Ethiopia

M. Sharan Chandran
School of Mechanical Engineering
Vellore Institute of Technology
Vellore, India

Laxmikanth Cherupally
Energy and Materials Research Lab, Department of Physics
College of Natural and Mathematical Sciences
The University of Dodoma, Tanzania

P. Gopinath Chowdary
Department of Mechanical Engineering
NIT Warangal
Telangana, India

Somaiah Chowdary
Department of Mechanical Engineering
IIT Guwahati, Guwahati
Assam, India

Locherla Daloji
Department of Mechanical Engineering
NIT Warangal
Telangana, India

Teegala Divya
Faculty of Science and Technology (IcfaiTech), Department of Mathematics
ICFAI Foundation for Higher Education
Hyderabad, Telangana, India

Tan Fırat Eyüboğlu
Faculty of Dentistry, Department of Endodontics
Istanbul Medipol University
Istanbul, Türkiye

Dheeraj Kumar Gara
Department of Aerospace Engineering
Jain University
Bangalore, Karnataka, India
Department of Mechanical Engineering
NIT Warangal
Telangana, India

Krina Goda
Scholar, Department of Aerospace Engineering
Jain University
Bangalore, Karnataka, India

Kondaiah Gudimetla
Department of Mechanical Engineering
Pace Institute of Technology & Sciences
Ongole, India

Raghavendra Gujjala
Department of Mechanical Engineering
NIT Warangal
Telangana, India

Ramu Inala
Department of Mechanical Engineering
Vishnu Institute of Technology
Bhimavaram
Andhra Pradesh, India

S. Indran
Research Scientist, Department
of Materials and Production
Engineering
King Mongkut's University of
Technology
North Bangkok, Thailand

Satish Jain
Department of Mechanical Engineering
NIT Warangal
Telangana, India

Rakesh Kanakam
Department of Mechanical
Engineering
NIT Warangal
Telangana, India

Yugesh A. Kharche
Department of Mechanical
Engineering
Padmashri Dr. V.B. Kolte College of
Engineering
Malkapur, Maharashtra, India

Vishnu Vijay Kumar
International Institute of Aerospace
Engineering and Management
JAIN (Deemed-to-be-University)
Bangalore, Karnataka, India

Akanksha Mohanty
Department of Biomedical Engineering
NIT Rourkela
Odisha, India

Muhammad Akhsin Muflikhun
Mechanical and Industrial Engineering
Department
Gadjah Mada University
Yogyakarta, Indonesia

M. S. Narayanan
Department of Biotechnology
Indian Institute of Technology Madras
Tamil Nadu, India

P. Navaneethakrishnan
Department of Energy Science and
Engineering
Indian Institute of Technology Bombay
Mumbai, India

Shakuntala Ojha
Department of Mechanical Engineering
Pace Institute of Technology & Sciences
Ongole, India

Mutlu Özcan
Center for Dental Medicine
Clinic of Masticatory Disorders and
Dental Biomaterials
University of Zurich
Zurich, Switzerland

R. G. Asuwin Prabu
School of Bioscience and Technology
Vellore Institute of Technology
Vellore, India
Department of Applied Mechanics and
Biomedical Engineering
Indian Institute of Technology Madras
Tamil Nadu, India

P. Syam Prasad
Department of Physics
NIT Warangal
Telangana, India

P. Phani Prasanthi
Department of Mechanical Engineering
PVP Sidhartha Institute of Technology
Andhra Pradesh, India

K. G. Prashanth
Department of Mechanical and Industrial Engineering
Tallinn, Estonia

Shanmukha Raju
Department of Pharmacy
University College of Technology
Osmania University
Hyderabad, Telangana, India

Parthiban Ramaswamy
Erich Schmid Institute of Material Science of the Austrian Academy of Sciences
Leoben, Austria

H. Jeevan Rao
Department of Aerospace, AIAE
Amity University
Noida, India

P. Venkateswara Rao
Department of Physics
The University of West Indies
Mona Campus, Jamaica

Manuela Reben
Department of Glass Technology and Amorphous Coatings
Faculty of Materials Science and Ceramics
AGH University of Science and Technology
Krakow, Poland

S. Shiva
Department of Mechanical Engineering
Centre for Nanotechnology & Sustainability
National University of Singapore
Singapore
School of Bioscience and Technology
Vellore Institute of Technology
Vellore, India

Y. B. Sudhir Sastry
Department of Aerospace Engineering
IIAEM, Jain University
Bangalore, Karnataka, India

Santosh R. Shekokar
Department of Mechanical Engineering
Padmashri Dr. V.B. Kolte College of Engineering
Malkapur, Maharashtra, India

Nadeem Siddiqui
Department of Biotechnology
Koneru Lakshmaiah Education Foundation
Andhra Pradesh, India

Ishika Singh Solanki
Scholar, Department of Aerospace Engineering
Jain University
Bangalore, Karnataka, India

Shrishail B. Sollappur
International Institute of Aerospace Engineering and Management
Jain deemed-to-be-University, JGI Global Campus
Bangalore, Karnataka, India

Marcin Środa
Department of Glass Technology and Amorphous Coatings
Faculty of Materials Science and Ceramics
AGH University of Science and Technology
Krakow, Poland

Riessom Weldegiorgis
Institute of Research and Development
Director for Flight Dynamics and Control Center Bishoftu
Bishoftu, Ethiopia

1 Introduction to Bioactive Materials
Metals to Non-metals

Dheeraj K. Gara, Raghavendra Gujjala, P. Syam Prasad, Madaboosi. Srinivasan. Narayanan and Mutlu Özcan

1.1 METALS AS A BIOACTIVE MATERIAL

Basically, metals are used as biocompatible materials rather than bioactive materials due to their bulk nature that a human body cannot afford. Conventional metals such as aluminium, titanium, copper, mild steel, nickel and other transition block elements which are anticorrosive in nature can be used as implants in bulk form as a support system to enable the growth of the bone or sometimes as a permanent implant. This literature dates back to the early 18th century of using metals as implants; however, over more than a century, this practice was followed by the clinicians to treat mostly various bone-related issues such as cartilage damages, osteoporosis and arthritis. When titanium is considered, it is a popular material for bone implants due to its biocompatibility, strength and light weight. It is also corrosion resistant and has a low modulus of elasticity, which means it is flexible enough to move with the bone without causing pain or discomfort. It is used in joint replacement, fracture fixation, spinal fusion and dental implants. Likewise, aluminium was found to be one of the potential materials for biomedical applications due to its interesting properties such as biocompatibility, light weight and strength; i.e., high strength to weight ratio, corrosion resistance and Osseointegration potential make them more versatile. Unlike the titanium, the Osseo integration potential of the aluminium makes it potential for biological applications, since the process of Osseo integration involves the bonding of the bone tissue and promoting the growth through exchange of ions. Such materials are referred to as bioactive materials and lie in the interest of the current scientific community. However, excess amount of aluminium can result in adverse effects such as induced cytotoxicity due to degradation of excess aluminium ions and limited applications such as dental and orthopaedic applications where their properties are particularly beneficial.

Considering one more potential material from the transition group, nickel also has potential for use in biomedical applications as implants, but they were found to be very limited due to their allergic reaction observed in many of the individuals who are treated for the same. Hence, it is ensured that before using nickel as an implant,

DOI: 10.1201/9781003660781-1

a previous medical history of the allergy reaction towards metals is to be taken into consideration, whereas the most versatile material used in biomedical applications is stainless steel. Stainless steel is a versatile and commonly used material for biomedical applications due to its excellent corrosion resistance, biocompatibility and good mechanical properties. It is used in a wide range of medical devices that includes orthopaedic implants, such as hip and knee replacements, as well as dental implants. It is also used for some cardiovascular implants, such as stents and valves, and surgical instruments, such as scalpels, forceps and clamps. It is also used for a variety of other medical devices, such as needles, syringes and catheters, and sterilization equipment, such as autoclaves and ovens. It is also used for laboratory equipment and other medical equipment. The properties of the stainless steel include corrosion resistance, biocompatibility, strength and durability and ease to clean and sterilize. On the other side, other problems include wear and tear over time and inference for medical imaging procedures due to their strong magnetic properties.

Cobalt-chromium (Co-Cr) alloys are a class of materials that have gained significant traction in the field of biomedical applications due to their remarkable combination of properties. These alloys exhibit exceptional corrosion resistance, high strength and toughness, biocompatibility and wear resistance, making them ideal candidates for various medical implants and devices. Few properties of these alloys include corrosion resistance, high strength and toughness, biocompatibility and excellent wear resistance. They have foreseen few applications such as orthopaedic implants, dental implants, cardiovascular devices and surgical instruments. Alongside, they also have amenability towards inducing bioactivity in the form of Osseo integration and biodegradation.

Another interesting material tantalum is valued for its remarkable properties that make it an ideal material for various implants and devices. Tantalum is considered biocompatible, meaning it is well-tolerated by the human body and has a low risk of triggering adverse reactions or causing tissue damage. This property makes it suitable for long-term implantation without the risk of rejection or inflammatory responses. Tantalum also exhibits exceptional resistance to corrosion in various bodily fluids, making it a durable and long-lasting material for implants. Its inertness prevents the release of harmful ions into the body, further enhancing its biocompatibility. It also possesses high strength and stiffness, making it suitable for load-bearing implants, such as orthopaedic components. Its mechanical properties can be tailored through alloying and processing techniques to match the specific requirements of different applications. Tantalum has demonstrated the ability to bond with bone tissue, a process known as Osseo integration. This property promotes the stability and long-term success of bone implants, particularly in orthopaedic and dental applications. Tantalum is radiopaque, meaning it is visible under X-rays and other imaging modalities. This property allows for easy tracking of implants during surgery and follow-up assessments, aiding in patient care and monitoring implant performance. Based on various applications, these different materials are used in versatile locations in the human body as implants as shown in Figure 1.1.

Alongside these metals, we shall discuss most common metal ions used as a dopants in the bioactive glasses that are displayed in Figure 1.2. These are used in

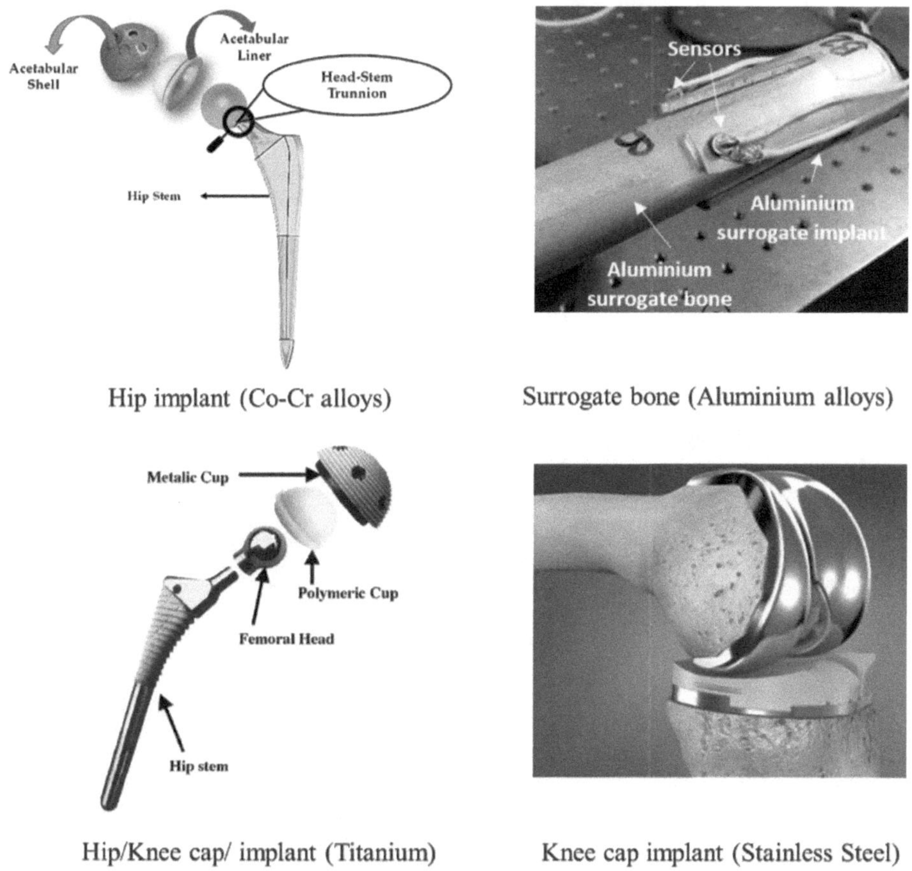

FIGURE 1.1 Various metals used as implants in bone tissues

analogues to the bioactive glasses. However, a comprehensive list of the metals and their applications towards biological applications can be inferred in Table 1.1.

1.2 BIOACTIVE GLASSES

The spongy centre of the bone consists of stem cells that progenitors into mesenchymal stem cells aiding in the repair, development and growth of the bone through the supply of osteogenic cells [42]. When a biomaterial is implanted in the site of the fracture or defect, it requires a delivery vehicle for the carrying of proteins to the bone marrow where mesenchymal cells promote bone regeneration. The most abundant protein in the bone is Type I Collagen, and interestingly, this is synthesized by osteoblasts. However, there is a lot of disambiguation in the scientific text, whether osteoblasts directly synthesize Type I Collagen or by forming precursors of osteocytes. From our earlier understanding, osteocytes perform traverse control of ions from minerals into bone via canaliculi, realizing that matured osteoblast differentiated from osteoblasts will synthesize the Type I Collagen protein. One more strong

TABLE 1.1
List of metal-based bioactive materials for versatile biological applications

Groups	Elements	Bioactivity	References
Alkali metals	Lithium	Angiogenesis and osteogenesis	[1–4]
	Sodium	Improved hydroxyapatite formation	
	Potassium	Delays the tendency of crystallization	
	Rubidium	Cell adhesion, proliferation and ALP activity.	
Alkaline earth metals	Magnesium	Antimicrobial activity, enhanced apatite layer formation	[5–8]
	Calcium	Major constituent mineral of the bone which forms apatite.	
	Strontium	Early osseointegration	
	Barium	Better biological radiation resistance/better opacifier	
Transition metals	Yttrium	Improves chemical durability	[9–24]
	Titanium	Lesser or no bioactivity	
	Zirconia	Increases antibacterial activity	
	Vanadium	Cerium ions improve the blood vessel formations and no antibacterial activity but lower angiogenesis	
	Niobium	Enhanced cell proliferation and stimulated osteogenic differentiation	
	Tantalum	Antibacterial and antifungal, non-toxic and simulated Osseo integration.	
	Chromium	No bioactivity	
	Molybdenum	Promotes the osteogenic gene expressions of collagen I secretion and bone sialoprotein in ADSCs.	
	Manganese	Antibacterial activity/improves adhesion and proliferation of osteoblastic-like cells (MC3T3E1)	
	Rhenium	Biocompatibility and osteoconductivity	
	Iron	Bone cancer nanotherapeutics	
	Cobalt	Enhances the hydroxyapatite layer formation	
	Nickel	Better density and mechanical properties can be increased	
	Copper	For antimicrobial properties to the bioglass	
	Silver	Antimicrobial property to the bioglass	
	Gold	Optimal cellular proliferation, decent angiogenesis, enhanced vimentin positive cells	
	Zinc and Cadmium	Able to stimulate osteoblast differentiation and mineralization by enhancing the osteogenic genes expression.	

(continued)

TABLE 1.1
(Continued)

Groups	Elements	Bioactivity	References
Post-transition metals	Aluminium	Accelerates the rate of osteoprogenitor cell differentiation and formation of osteoid nodules alongside inhibiting mineralization.	[25–27]
	Gallium	Absence of antibacterial activity/lower angiogenesis.	
	Bismuth	Antimicrobial activity, promotes osteogenic cell proliferation, differentiation and mineralization.	
Metalloids	Boron	An excellent substrate for cell adhesion, differentiation and proliferation and capable of promoting osteogenesis and neovascularization.	[28–31]
	Silica	Main constituent of bone, formation of hydroxyapatite.	
	Germanium	Treatment of cancer, arthritis and senile osteoporosis due to the therapeutic attributes such as immune enhancement, oxygen enrichment and heavy metal detoxification.	
	Tellurium	Antibacterial, antioxidant and radiation shielding properties.	
Reactive non-metals	Phosphorous	Main constituent in human body and enables ion transfer.	[32, 33]
	Selenium	Drug-delivery system for bone therapy, tissue regeneration, accelerates mineralization process.	
Lanthanides	Lanthanum	Enhanced osteoblast performance by promoting differentiation and proliferation, by raising protein expression.	[34–40]
	Cerium	Absence of antibacterial activity	
	Samarium	Improved osteoblastic cell response and higher cell proliferation	
	Europium	Can be used for labelling bone marrow stromal cells, enhanced osteogenic gene expression	
	Gadolinium	Promotes osteogenic differentiation of human bone marrow-derived mesenchymal stem cells.	
	Terbium	Radiation shielding characteristic	
	Erbium	Radiation shielding characteristic	

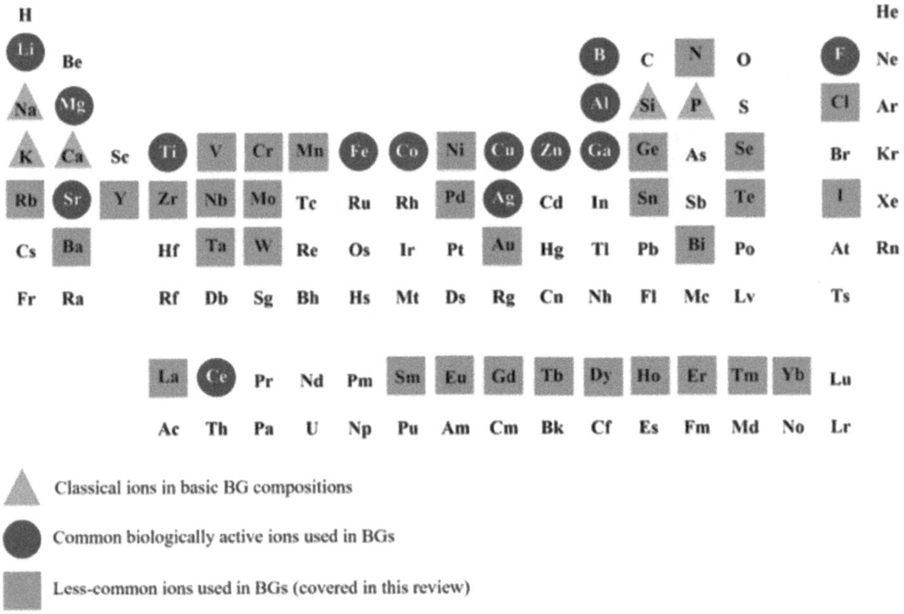

FIGURE 1.2 Biologically active ions used for biological applications [41]

understanding is that the protein concentration is lower in interstitial fluid present in bone marrow and thus osteocytes participate in mineralization and osteoblasts participate in bone strengthening. An understanding of ion behaviour in osteocytes and osteoblasts can be realized from Figure 1.3.

The biomechanics of the bone is controlled and monitored at a micro and sometimes at mesoporous scale through altering mineral and protein nutrient ions. It is clinically evident that transition metals due to their advantage of electronic configurations are best suitable for the protein ions, whereas alkali earth metals for mineral ions [43, 44]. The implants made of these materials in the current scientific community are referred to as bioactive glasses. Bioglass 45S5 is the first of its kind in bioactive glass which received wide attention in terms of clinical compliance. Classic Bioglass [45] constitutes the composition of 45 wt% SiO_2, 24.5 wt%CaO, 24.5 wt%Na_2O and 6 wt%P_2O_5.

This bioglass is implanted at the fracture sight, where ion transport is disconnected and growth factors' accumulation will be very slow or sometimes may not be possible if the intensity of crack magnitude is severe. Immediately the sodium and calcium ions on the glass surface rapidly begin exchange of ions with the hydrogen ions present in the physiological body fluid particularly intracellular. This intracellular fluid has more charged macromolecules and high alkali ion concentrations that are referred to as cytosol [46]. Cytosol is involved in various cell signalling, pertaining to the current context; calcium and sodium signalling are few amongst others and enable exchange of ions with hydrogen carriers to the bioglass comprising of calcium and sodium. This ion exchange takes place until silane groups condense to the silica gel layer which forms the bridge between the fracture mode as displayed in Figure 1.3.

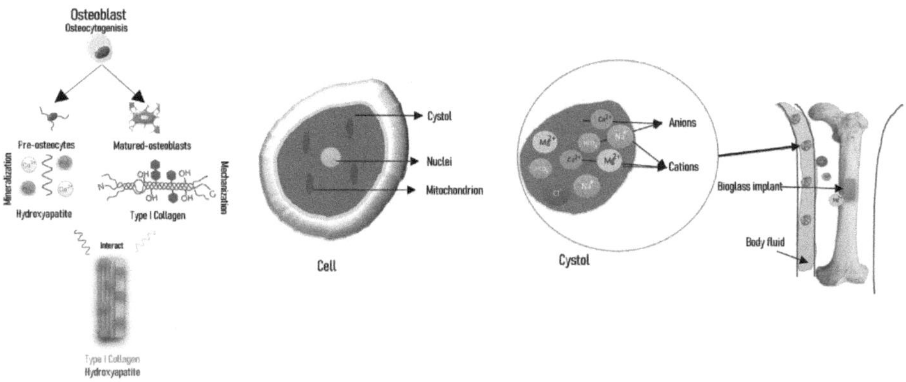

FIGURE 1.3 ECM-BG coalescence for tissue regeneration

Now calcium and phosphate (either from body fluid or from simulated body fluid (SBF)) ions pleat at the silica gel and assimilate carbonate and hydroxyl ions from the extracellular fluid that forms a layer modifying the silica network with rich carbonated hydroxyapatite (HA). This phase, in coalescence, works with the native tissue for the regeneration through exchange of ions and hence BAGs are referred to as bio-coalescent materials. Most commonly observed phosphorus apatite mineral configuration is hydroxyl apatite, however few other apatite configurations such as fluorapatite and chlorapatite are also cited in the literature for tissue regeneration applications. From the literature, it can be pursued that hydroxyl apatite shows greater ability to form apatite compared to that of fluorapatite but has lower osteocalcin synthesis [47]. Nevertheless, chlorapatite received contemplation in literature, but it hasn't shown much potential for clinical compliance. One must realize that sodium used in the current bioglass assimilates with chlorine thus forming a salt, sodium chloride, which actually tunes the bone resorption rate relative to bone formation rate. Since the percentage of chlorine present is very minute, the chlorapatite is ignored, but at an ionic scale its impact is decipherable. Hence, a bioglass combination with the addition of fluorine and chlorine is also of equal importance where biomimicking is desired. There is no such work cited in the literature as in contrast to the bone tissue engineering applications in this combination and hence an understanding in this context can show some significant potential. We shall now discourse on the development of materials that exhibit bioactivity, biocompatibility and biomimicking. It is understood by nature that the human body poses a large number of materials in appropriate compositions with respect to the majority of elements within the body. The term biocompatibility in context to the bone tissue engineering refers to cytotoxicity and genotoxicity. Metals that are used as a constituent in processing the bioglass should be biocompatible and bioactive in nature. Table 1.2 displays various classic bioglass configurations with different dopants as metals, and their characteristic enhancements in terms of mechanical and biological parameters are emphasized [47–57].

TABLE 1.2
Bioglass with various dopants for versatile applications pertaining to biological environment

S. No	Constituent composition (wt%)	Processing technique	Characteristics	Applications	Limitations
1	Bioglass 45S5 SiO_2-45%, CaO-24.5% Na_2O-24.5, P_2O_5-6%	Melt Quench followed by Ball Milling and sinter	Low pathological calcification	Soft tissues	Ca-P induction is unclear, low bone formation
2	SiO_2-60%, CaO-34.0% Ag_2O-2%%, P_2O_5-4%	Sol-gel method	Bactericidal properties, controlled porosity	Sterile skin	Composition of Ag on visco-elastic trends and thermal properties.
3	SiO_2-45%, CaO-24.5% Na_2O-24.5, P_2O_5-6%, CNT-0.12, 0.20 gm	Electrophoretic deposition	Able to produce nanostructured internal surface that enables osteoblast cell attachment and proliferation	Soft and hard tissues	Ordered formation of nanostructured HA layer
4	SiO_2-45%, CaO-24.5% K_2O-24.4, P_2O_5-2.6% Boron oxide-2 wt%	Melt derived	Rate of bone formation can be drastically increased than Bioglass45S5	Intramedullary canal (Bone marrow)	Ca:P ratio is drastically increasing which is not desired and needs to be controlled
5	SiO_2-46.1%, CaO-26.9% K_2O-24.4, P_2O_5-2.6%	Melt derived	Enhanced mechanical properties (Strength)	Cancellous bone	Uniform porosity cannot be achieved
6	SiO_2-80%, CaO-15% Na_2O-0, P_2O_5-5%	Sol-gel method	Exhibited interconnected macroporous structure, mesoporous pore walls	Cancellous bone	Decrease in the surface area
	SiO_2-80%, CaO-10% ZrO_2-5, P_2O_5-5%				

	SiO_2-80%, CaO-10% MgO-5, P_2O_5-5%				
	SiO_2-80%, CaO-10% SrO-5, P_2O_5-5%				
7	SiO_2-45.8%, CaO-27.7% Na_2O-24.2, P_2O_5-2.2%	Melt Quench	CaO/P_2O_5 has no effect on glass transition temperature for constant Na_2O composition.	Cortical bone/hard tissues	Lowest bulk and Young's modulus
	SiO_2-46.1%, CaO-26.9% Na_2O-24.3, P_2O_5-2.6%		Higher content of Na_2O has lowest glass transition temperature.		Increase in CaO reduces the glass transition temperature
	SiO_2-47.1%, CaO-24.0% Na_2O-24.8, P_2O_5-4.0% SiO_2-48.4%, CaO-19.9%		Lower biodegradation rate due to higher silica content		Change in P_2O_5 will not have influence on glass transition temperature
	Na_2O-25.5, P_2O_5-5.9%				Low glass transition
	SiO_2-56.5%, CaO-21.4% Na_2O-19.4, P_2O_5-2.6%				High glass transition
	SiO_2-57.3%, CaO-19.5% Na_2O-19.7, P_2O_5-3.5%				Matching P_2O_5 and Na_2O will not have any impact on glass transition temperature
	SiO_2-58.4%, CaO-16.5% Na_2O-20.1, P_2O_5-4.95%				Enhanced bulk and Young's modulus
	SiO_2-59.8%, CaO-13.1% Na_2O-20.5, P_2O_5-6.5%				Higher content of SiO_2 is not preferable.

(continued)

TABLE 1.2
(Continued)

S. No	Constituent composition (wt%)	Processing technique	Characteristics	Applications	Limitations
8	SiO_2-45%, CaO-13.1% Na_2O-24.5, P_2O_5-24.5%, ZrO_2-0 SiO_2-42%, CaO-13.1% Na_2O-24.5, P_2O_5-24.5% ZrO_2-3% SiO_2-39%, CaO-13.1% Na_2O-24.5, P_2O_5-24.5%, ZrO_2-6% SiO_2-35%, CaO-13.1% Na_2O-24.5, P_2O_5-24.5%, ZrO_2-10%	Melt Quench	Increase in ZrO_2 content increases the apatite formation. Without compromising the bioactivity and mechanical properties, 3 wt% is the most suitable composition.	Load-bearing applications, predominantly cortical tissue.	Porosity and Young's modulus can be decreased as the content of ZrO_2 is enhanced. Whereas the compressive strength and hardness increased.
9	SiO_2-46.1%, CaO-26.9% Na_2O-24.4, P_2O_5-2.6%, SiO_2-46.1%, CaO-26.9% Na_2O-24.4, P_2O_5-0%, Nb_2O_5-2.6% SiO_2-46.1%, CaO-26.9% Na_2O-24.4, P_2O_5-1.3%, Nb_2O_5-1.3%	Melt Quench	Nb is a non-toxic, allergy-free metal, excellent biocompatibility, osteoconductivity and excellent chemical stability	Soft tissues	Low Nb composition enhances apatite formation and higher the composition is its adverse effect. Highest cell viability is observed. Highest E_{corr}/mV with sol-gel process when compared to melt quench.

S. No	Constituent composition (wt%)	Processing technique	Characteristics	Applications	Limitations
10	SiO_2-35.4%, CaO-43.7%, SrO-6.2% CaF_2-0.4, P_2O_5-7.1%, MgO-7.1%	Melt Quench	Mesenchymal stem cells from the human body were able to attach, expand and differentiate on the materials.	Soft and hard tissues	Increase in strontium resulted in loss of porosity. The flexural strength is also decreased with the increase in the strontium content. Solution pH was significantly increased with the increase in the content of the strontium.
	SiO_2-35.4%, CaO-37.4%, SrO-12.5% CaF_2-0.4, P_2O_5-7.1%, MgO-7.1%				
	SiO_2-35.4%, CaO-31.2%, SrO-18.7% CaF_2-0.4, P_2O_5-7.1%, MgO-7.1%				
	SiO_2-35.4%, CaO-25.0%, SrO-24.9% CaF_2-0.4, P_2O_5-7.1%, MgO-7.1%				

1.3 NATURE-INSPIRED MATERIALS

The colloidal stability of the nanoparticles not only for metals but also for polymers has also been well researched in the literature and is inclined towards biological applications. Recently, there has been substantial attention in the peer community towards specific areas such as bone tissue engineering, regenerative medicine and drug delivery [58–61]. Along with stability, the other additional characteristics such as biocompatibility, non-cytotoxicity, biodegradation and biomineralization are crucial for biological applications [62]. Lab-scale research has been conducted for more than 20 years, and as a result, bioactive materials have been created. However, there are still pursuable key lacunae in the scientific text due to the lack of controllability and observability. Controllability and observability are duals, and hence achieving one of them intuitively addresses the other. Over the last decade, interesting works have been appraising a new area referred to as biomimetics [63]. Biomimicking refers to the adaptability of foreign materials to the physiological environment through interatomic interactions. We shall discuss interface interactions between the foreign implants and the physiological environment followed by the role of nanoparticle characteristics.

In context to bone tissue engineering applications, consider the bone, which constitutes elements such as calcium as the majority, silica as minor constituent, and phosphorus as a physiological solution of the body. When cartilage damage, osteoporosis or arthritis is diagnosed, the preliminary medication is implanting surgery. Historically, these implants were made out of metals and are permanent implants that are considered to be permanently based on the age factor and growth behaviour of an individual. Whereas in the case of the biodegradable implant when comes in contact with the bone and physiological body conditions, ion exchange and modification of the network takes place, as a result, biomineralization takes place in parallel to biodegradation and growth [64, 65]. Here interface science deals with the network connectivity, porosity and shape and size of the nanoparticles that direct cell proliferation and growth vectorization [66]. From the literature, it was identified that having a mesoporous structure will have better biomineralization, and hence cell proliferation can take place uniformly. The uniform porosity in combination with mesoporous within the nanoparticle allows enhanced biomineralization since dietary supplements such as protein and mineral phase easily coagulate and disperse throughout the cavities of the mesoporous network. At the same time, network connectivity is also one of the major concerns since the delivery vehicles of the dietary supplements, i.e., minerals and proteins must be able to mechanically strengthen the bone which can happen only if the network is properly connected [67], otherwise the stability of the system may be degraded and cell proliferation along the direction of desired growth will deviate.

In most biological systems, the role of nanoparticles is to assist in delivering the drug to the site of diagnosis or trigger antimicrobial or antigen-presenting cells (APC) and luminescence for easy monitoring. The most commonly used bioactive material is Bioglass 45S which is proven to be in clinical compliance. The configuration of the Bioglass 45S comprises calcium-silica-phosphate in various constituents [68]. Over the last two decades, nanomaterials have come into existence due to their excellent mechanobiological properties suitable for biological applications [69–71]. However, these materials cannot be directly used in the raw form due to their intractability to the physiological body environment which is full of ions and functional groups which are uniformly structured. Hence, these nanomaterials must be functionalized such that they form bridging between the various functional groups to enable bioactivity. One interesting aspect is that the composition of these nanomaterials or nanoparticles is too low to be used in a biological environment as they may induce toxicity and are prone to be dangerous to life or organ failure. Hence, their exposure is very limited and needs to be carefully monitored.

It can be inferred from the literature that the nanoparticles, mostly metal based, require a host material where they can be aggregated as desired to perform their task such as to enhance bioactivity or induce antimicrobial activity. Sometimes to enhance the mechanical properties and biomimic through mechanosensing properties. Table 1.3 displays the nature-inspired biosynthesis, and inherent materials that are used for biological applications are emphasized. The role of each of these metals and polymers together on the natural inspiration for biomimicking is discussed.

TABLE 1.3
Bioactive glass nanoparticles for Nature-inspired biosynthesis towards bone tissue engineering applications

S. No	Bioglass nanoparticles	Nature-inspired material	Biomimicking	Application	References
1	$46.13SiO_2$-$24.35Na_2O$-$26.91CaO$-$2.6P_2O_5$	Type I Collagen from fish scale	Enhancing the osteoblast marker genes	Bone tissue engineering	[72]
2	Acrylite	–	Mimic native extracellular matrix (ECM)	Tissue engineering	[73]
3	Methacrylate	–	Proteoglycan and collagen	Tissue engineering	[74]
4	Synthetic peptides	–	Growth factors and angiogenesis	Tissue engineering	[75]
5	–	Collagen from ocean waste	Mechano sensing interactions	–	[76]
6	–	Gelatin from animal body parts	Simulation of cellular attachment	–	[77]
7	–	Chitosan from shellfish	Trigger immune system	–	[78]
8	–	Silk fibroin from silk produced by various insects	Cell proliferation	Skin tissue engineering	[78]

(continued)

TABLE 1.3
(Continued)

S. No	Bioglass nanoparticles	Nature-inspired material	Biomimicking	Application	References
9	Hydroxyapatite	–	Osteoinduction	Bone tissue engineering	[79]
10	Tricalcium phosphate	–	Osteoinduction	Bone tissue engineering	[80]
11	–	Poly lactic-co-glycolic acid from sugarcane and sour milk followed by fruits	Osteogenesis	Versatile biological applications	[81]
12	–	Poly lactic acid	Mechanosensing interactions	Bone tissue engineering	[82]
13	–	Polyglycolic acid	Mechanosensing interactions	Bone tissue engineering	[83]
14	–	Lignin from plants	Mechanobiological support	Versatile biological applications	[84]

In the aforementioned Table 1.3, they are the most widely used bioactive materials derived from natural materials to inhibit their characteristics in real-time *in vivo* biological applications. However, metal nanoparticles as discussed earlier in Table 1.2 are also used in combination with the above-said material configuration making them suitable for biological applications. The biological characteristics also depend on the interface between the substrate material, nanoparticles and bone tissue. Hence, interface science plays a crucial role in mineralizing the bone and enhancing cell adhesion and proliferation. A more detailed discussion with the help of microstructural and spectroscopic evidence will be emphasized in the later session. We have been discussing various aspects of nanoparticles and their role in heat transfer and their biological applications, but by the nature of nanoparticles due to their small size and large surface area, they possess greater functionalization and thus enhanced characteristics.

1.4 CLOSING REMARKS

We have discoursed on a detailed introduction to metals and non-metals and their transition from being bio-metals to bioactive materials. We have also discoursed on the new class of materials that are in clinical compliances and featured materials such as bioinspired materials for the next generation applications such as drug delivery, regenerative medicine, wound healing, therapeutic and bone tissue engineering. However, most of the research in these niche areas has been disseminated in the scientific community but still there is lack of understanding of the dynamic behaviour of the biological environments. Hence as an introductory chapter, we have disseminated how transition from being biomaterials to bioactive materials has emerged.

REFERENCES

1. Durand, L.A.H., Vargas, G.E., Gomez-Gramajo, F., Vera-Mesones, R., Miguez-Pacheco, V., Boccaccini, A.R. and Gorustovich, A., 2019. Lithium-containing bioactive glasses for bone regeneration. In: G. Kaur (Ed.), *Biomedical, therapeutic and clinical applications of bioactive glasses*, Woodhead Publishing, pp.201–217.
2. Chen, X., Chen, X., Brauer, D.S., Wilson, R.M., Law, R.V., Hill, R.G. and Karpukhina, N., 2017. Sodium is not essential for high bioactivity of glasses. *International Journal of Applied Glass Science*, *8*(4), pp.428–437.
3. Cannillo, V. and Sola, A., 2009. Potassium-based composition for a bioactive glass. *Ceramics International*, *35*(8), pp.3389–3393.
4. Tan, Y.N., Chen, W.J., Wei, W., Huang, Q.L. and Xiang, H.E., 2021. Rubidium-modified bioactive glass-ceramics with hydroxyapatite crystals for bone regeneration. *Transactions of Nonferrous Metals Society of China*, *31*(2), pp.521–532.
5. Singh, A.K., Pramanik, K. and Biswas, A., 2019. MgO enables enhanced bioactivity and antimicrobial activity of nano bioglass for bone tissue engineering application. *Materials Technology*, *34*(13), pp.818–826.
6. Liu, H., Yazici, H., Ergun, C., Webster, T.J. and Bermek, H., 2008. An in vitro evaluation of the Ca/P ratio for the cytocompatibility of nano-to-micron particulate calcium phosphates for bone regeneration. *Acta Biomaterialia*, *4*(5), pp.1472–1479.
7. Poh, P.S., Hutmacher, D.W., Stevens, M.M. and Woodruff, M.A., 2013. Fabrication and in vitro characterization of bioactive glass composite scaffolds for bone regeneration. *Biofabrication*, *5*(4), p.045005.
8. Singh, J., Kumar, V., Vermani, Y.K., Al-Buriahi, M.S., Alzahrani, J.S. and Singh, T., 2021. Fabrication and characterization of barium based bioactive glasses in terms of physical, structural, mechanical and radiation shielding properties. *Ceramics International*, *47*(15), pp.21730–21743.
9. Hadush Tesfay, A., Chou, Y.J., Tan, C.Y., Fufa Bakare, F., Tsou, N.T., Huang, E.W. and Shih, S.J., 2019. Control of dopant distribution in yttrium-doped bioactive glass for selective internal radiotherapy applications using spray pyrolysis. *Materials*, *12*(6), p.986.
10. Smith, S., ElKashty, O., Tamimi, F., Tran, S.D. and Cerruti, M., 2021. Titanium-containing silicate-based sol–gel bioactive glass: development, characterization, and applications. *Langmuir*, *37*(49), pp.14243–14253.
11. Faria, D.M.M., de Castro Henriques, B.A.P., De Souza, A.C.B., da Silva, F.S.C.P. and Carvalho, Ó.S.N., 2022. Laser-assisted manufacturing of 45S5 bioglass-coated zirconia structured surfaces targeting medical implants: adhesive, wettability, mechanical, and bioactivity evaluation. *The International Journal of Advanced Manufacturing Technology*, *119*(3), pp.1595–1612.
12. Li, J., Li, J., Wei, Y., Xu, N., Li, J., Pu, X., Wang, J., Huang, Z., Liao, X. and Yin, G., 2021. Ion release behavior of vanadium-doped mesoporous bioactive glass particles and the effect of the released ions on osteogenic differentiation of BMSCs via the FAK/MAPK signaling pathway. *Journal of Materials Chemistry B*, *9*(37), pp.7848–7865.
13. de Siqueira, L., Campos, T.M., Camargo, S.E., Thim, G.P. and Triches, E.S., 2021. Structural, crystallization and cytocompatibility evaluation of the 45S5 bioglass-derived glass-ceramic containing niobium. *Journal of Non-Crystalline Solids*, *555*, p.120629.

14. Pádua, A.S., Gavinho, S.R., Graça, M.P.F., Sá-Nogueira, I. and Silva, J.C., 2022. Tantalum doped bioactive glass: towards a pro-regenerative and antibacterial response. *Materials Proceedings*, *8*(1), p.51.
15. Decker, S., Kunisch, E., Moghaddam, A., Renkawitz, T. and Westhauser, F., 2021. Molybdenum trioxide enhances viability, osteogenic differentiation and extracellular matrix formation of human bone marrow-derived mesenchymal stromal cells. *Journal of Trace Elements in Medicine and Biology*, *68*, p.126827.
16. Wen, C., Bai, N., Luo, L., Ye, J., Zhan, X., Zhang, Y. and Sa, B., 2021. Structural behavior and in vitro bioactivity evaluation of hydroxyapatite-like bioactive glass based on the SiO_2-CaO-P_2O_5 system. *Ceramics International*, *47*(13), pp.18094–18104.
17. Matsuno, H., Yokoyama, A., Watari, F., Uo, M. and Kawasaki, T., 2001. Biocompatibility and osteogenesis of refractory metal implants, titanium, hafnium, niobium, tantalum and rhenium. *Biomaterials*, *22*(11), pp.1253–1262.
18. Shankhwar, N. and Srinivasan, A., 2016. Evaluation of sol–gel based magnetic 45S5 bioglass and bioglass–ceramics containing iron oxide. *Materials Science and Engineering: C*, *62*, pp.190–196.
19. Bafandeh, M.R., Gharahkhani, R. and Fathi, M.H., 2016. Fabrication, characterization and osteoblast response of cobalt-based alloy/nano bioactive glass composites. *Journal of Advanced Materials and Processing*, *4*(3), pp.3–13.
20. Vyas, V.K., Kumar, A.S., Singh, S.P. and Pyare, R., 2016. Effect of nickel oxide substitution on bioactivity and mechanical properties of bioactive glass. *Bulletin of Materials Science*, *39*(5), pp.1355–1361.
21. Wang, Y., Zhang, W. and Yao, Q., 2021. Copper-based biomaterials for bone and cartilage tissue engineering. *Journal of Orthopaedic Translation*, *29*, pp.60–71.
22. Balamurugan, A., Balossier, G., Laurent-Maquin, D., Pina, S., Rebelo, A.H.S., Faure, J. and Ferreira, J.M.F., 2008. An in vitro biological and anti-bacterial study on a sol–gel derived silver-incorporated bioglass system. *Dental Materials*, *24*(10), pp.1343–1351.
23. Dreanca, A., Muresan-Pop, M., Taulescu, M., Tóth, Z.R., Bogdan, S., Pestean, C., Oren, S., Toma, C., Popescu, A., Páll, E. and Sevastre, B., 2021. Bioactive glass-biopolymers-gold nanoparticle based composites for tissue engineering applications. *Materials Science and Engineering: C*, *123*, p.112006.
24. Paramita, P., Ramachandran, M., Narashiman, S., Nagarajan, S., Sukumar, D.K., Chung, T.W. and Ambigapathi, M., 2021. Sol–gel based synthesis and biological properties of zinc integrated nano bioglass ceramics for bone tissue regeneration. *Journal of Materials Science: Materials in Medicine*, *32*(1), pp.1–11.
25. Tripathi, H., Kumar, A.S. and Singh, S.P., 2016. Preparation and characterization of Li_2O–CaO–Al_2O_3–P_2O_5–SiO_2 glasses as bioactive material. *Bulletin of Materials Science*, *39*(2), pp.365–376.
26. Deliormanlı, A.M., Vatansever, H.S., Yesil, H. and Özdal-Kurt, F., 2016. In vivo evaluation of cerium, gallium and vanadium-doped borate-based bioactive glass scaffolds using rat subcutaneous implantation model. *Ceramics International*, *42*(10), pp.11574–11583.
27. Khatua, C., Bodhak, S., Kundu, B. and Balla, V.K., 2018. In vitro bioactivity and bone mineralization of bismuth ferrite reinforced bioactive glass composites. *Materialia*, *4*, pp.361–366.
28. Furlan, R.G., Correr, W.R., Russi, A.F.C., da Costa Iemma, M.R., Trovatti, E. and Pecoraro, É., 2018. Preparation and characterization of boron-based bioglass by sol–gel process. *Journal of Sol-Gel Science and Technology*, *88*(1), pp.181–191.
29. Arcos, D. and Vallet-Regí, M., 2010. Sol–gel silica-based biomaterials and bone tissue regeneration. *Acta Biomaterialia*, *6*(8), pp.2874–2888.

30. Mokhtari, S., Krull, E.A., Sanders, L.M., Coughlan, A., Mellott, N.P., Gong, Y., Borges, R. and Wren, A.W., 2019. Investigating the effect of germanium on the structure of SiO_2-ZnO-CaO-SrO-P_2O_5 glasses and the subsequent influence on glass polyalkenoate cement formation, solubility and bioactivity. *Materials Science and Engineering: C*, *103*, p.109843.
31. Vernè, E., Miola, M. and Renzi, E., 2019. Synthesis and characterization of innovative silica-based bioactive glass doped with tellurium.
32. O'Neill, E., Awale, G., Daneshmandi, L., Umerah, O. and Lo, K.W.H., 2018. The roles of ions on bone regeneration. *Drug Discovery Today*, *23*(4), pp.879–890.
33. Hu, M., Fang, J., Zhang, Y., Wang, X., Zhong, W. and Zhou, Z., 2020. Design and evaluation a kind of functional biomaterial for bone tissue engineering: selenium/mesoporous bioactive glass nanospheres. *Journal of Colloid and Interface Science*, *579*, pp.654–666.
34. Zhu, D., Lu, B., Yang, Q., Yu, H., Liu, P., Yin, J., Chen, Y., Huang, Y., Ke, Q., Zhang, C. and Guo, Y., 2021. Lanthanum-doped mesoporous bioglasses/chitosan composite scaffolds enhance synchronous osteogenesis and angiogenesis for augmented osseous regeneration. *Chemical Engineering Journal*, *405*, p.127077.
35. Morais, D.S., Fernandes, S., Gomes, P.S., Fernandes, M.H., Sampaio, P., Ferraz, M.P., Santos, J.D., Lopes, M.A. and Hussain, N.S., 2015. Novel cerium doped glass-reinforced hydroxyapatite with antibacterial and osteoconductive properties for bone tissue regeneration. *Biomedical Materials*, *10*(5), p.055008.
36. Morais, D.S., Coelho, J., Ferraz, M.P., Gomes, P.S., Fernandes, M.H., Hussain, N.S., Santos, J.D. and Lopes, M.A., 2014. Samarium doped glass-reinforced hydroxyapatite with enhanced osteoblastic performance and antibacterial properties for bone tissue regeneration. *Journal of Materials Chemistry B*, *2*(35), pp.5872–5881.
37. Li, F., Wang, M., Pi, G. and Lei, B., 2018. Europium doped monodispersed bioactive glass nanoparticles regulate the osteogenic differentiation of human marrow mesenchymal stem cells. *Journal of Biomedical Nanotechnology*, *14*(4), pp.756–764.
38. Zhu, D.Y., Lu, B., Yin, J.H., Ke, Q.F., Xu, H., Zhang, C.Q., Guo, Y.P. and Gao, Y.S., 2019. Gadolinium-doped bioglass scaffolds promote osteogenic differentiation of hBMSC via the Akt/GSK3β pathway and facilitate bone repair in vivo. *International Journal of Nanomedicine*, *14*, p.1085.
39. Wang, X., Zhang, Y., Lin, C. and Zhong, W., 2017. Sol-gel derived terbium-containing mesoporous bioactive glasses nanospheres: in vitro hydroxyapatite formation and drug delivery. *Colloids and Surfaces B: Biointerfaces*, *160*, pp.406–415.
40. Deliormanli, A.M., Issa, S.A., Al-Buriahi, M.S., Rahman, B., Zakaly, H.M. and Tekin, H.O., 2021. Erbium (III)-and Terbium (III)-containing silicate-based bioactive glass powders: physical, structural and nuclear radiation shielding characteristics. *Applied Physics A*, *127*(6), pp.1–18.
41. Pantulap, U., Arango-Ospina, M. and Boccaccini, A.R., 2022. Bioactive glasses incorporating less-common ions to improve biological and physical properties. *Journal of Materials Science: Materials in Medicine*, *33*(1), pp.1–41.
42. Friedman, M.S., Long, M.W. and Hankenson, K.D., 2006. Osteogenic differentiation of human mesenchymal stem cells is regulated by bone morphogenetic protein-6. *Journal of Cellular Biochemistry*, *98*(3), pp.538–554.
43. Dudev, T. and Lim, C., 2014. Competition among metal ions for protein binding sites: determinants of metal ion selectivity in proteins. *Chemical Reviews*, *114*(1), pp.538–556.
44. Gao, J., Feng, L., Chen, B., Fu, B. and Zhu, M., 2022. The role of rare earth elements in bone tissue engineering scaffolds–a review. *Composites Part B: Engineering*, *235*, p.109758.
45. Hench, L.L., 2006. The story of Bioglass®. *Journal of Materials Science: Materials in Medicine*, *17*(11), pp.967–978.

46. Zhu, M., Zhang, R., Mao, Z., Fang, J. and Ren, F., 2022. Topographical biointerface regulating cellular functions for bone tissue engineering. *Biosurface and Biotribology*, *8*(3), pp.165–187.
47. Maximov, M., Maximov, O.C., Craciun, L., Ficai, D., Ficai, A. and Andronescu, E., 2021. Bioactive glass—an extensive study of the preparation and coating methods. *Coatings*, *11*(11), p.1386.
48. Blaker, J.J., Nazhat, S.N. and Boccaccini, A.R., 2004. Development and characterisation of silver-doped bioactive glass-coated sutures for tissue engineering and wound healing applications. *Biomaterials*, *25*(7–8), pp.1319–1329.
49. Boccaccini, A.R., Chicatun, F., Cho, J., Bretcanu, O., Roether, J.A., Novak, S. and Chen, Q.Z., 2007. Carbon nanotube coatings on bioglass-based tissue engineering scaffolds. *Advanced Functional Materials*, *17*(15), pp.2815–2822.
50. Gorustovich, A.A., López, J.M.P., Guglielmotti, M.B. and Cabrini, R.L., 2006. Biological performance of boron-modified bioactive glass particles implanted in rat tibia bone marrow. *Biomedical Materials*, *1*(3), p.100.
51. Bellucci, D., Cannillo, V., Ciardelli, G., Gentile, P. and Sola, A., 2010. Potassium based bioactive glass for bone tissue engineering. *Ceramics International*, *36*(8), pp.2449–2453.
52. Zhu, Y., Li, X., Yang, J., Wang, S., Gao, H. and Hanagata, N., 2011. Composition–structure–property relationships of the $CaO–M_xO_y–SiO_2–P_2O_5$ (M= Zr, Mg, Sr) mesoporous bioactive glass (MBG) scaffolds. *Journal of Materials Chemistry*, *21*(25), pp.9208–9218.
53. Lin, C.C., Chen, S.F., Leung, K.S. and Shen, P., 2012. Effects of CaO/P_2O_5 ratio on the structure and elastic properties of $SiO_2–CaO–Na_2O– P_2O_5$ bioglasses. *Journal of Materials Science: Materials in Medicine*, *23*(2), pp.245–258.
54. Mondal, D., So-Ra, S. and Lee, B.T., 2013. Fabrication and characterization of $ZrO_2–CaO–P_2O_5–Na_2O–SiO_2$ bioactive glass ceramics. *Journal of Materials Science*, *48*(5), pp.1863–1872.
55. Souza, L., Lopes, J.H., Encarnação, D., Mazali, I.O., Martin, R.A., Camilli, J.A. and Bertran, C.A., 2018. Comprehensive in vitro and in vivo studies of novel melt-derived Nb-substituted 45S5 bioglass reveal its enhanced bioactive properties for bone healing. *Scientific Reports*, *8*(1), pp.1–15.
56. Safavi, M.S., Walsh, F.C., Visai, L. and Khalil-Allafi, J., 2022. Progress in niobium oxide-containing coatings for biomedical applications: a critical review. *ACS Omega*, *7*(11), pp.9088–9107.
57. Vickers, W., 2013. *The effect of strontium substitution on apatite-wollastonite glass-ceramics*. University of Leeds.
58. Deirram, N., Zhang, C., Kermaniyan, S.S., Johnston, A.P.R. and Such, G.K., 2019. pH-responsive polymer nanoparticles for drug delivery. *Macromolecular Rapid Communications*, *40*(10), p.1800917.
59. Bharadwaz, A. and Jayasuriya, A.C., 2020. Recent trends in the application of widely used natural and synthetic polymer nanocomposites in bone tissue regeneration. *Materials Science & Engineering C-Materials for Biological Applications*, *110*, p.110698.
60. Smith, I.O., Liu, X., Smith, L.A. and Ma, P.X., 2009. Nanostructured polymer scaffolds for tissue engineering and regenerative medicine. *Nanomedicine and Nanobiotechnology*, *1*(2), pp.226–236.
61. Samal, S.K. and Dubruel, P., 2014. *Cationic polymers in regenerative medicine*. Royal Society of Chemistry.
62. Pitt, C. and Schindler, A., 2019. *Biodegradation of polymers, controlled drug delivery*. CRC Press, pp.53–80.
63. Gruber, P., Bruckner, D., Hellmich, C., Schmiedmayer, H.-B., Stachelberger, H., Gebeshuber, I.C., 2011. *Biomimetics–materials, structures and processes: examples, ideas and case studies*. Springer Science & Business Media.

64. Potter, W., Kalil, R.E. and Kao, W.J., 2008. Biomimetic material systems for neural progenitor cell-based therapy. *Frontiers in Bioscience*, *13*(3), pp.806–821.
65. Liao, S., Chan, C.K. and Ramakrishna, S., 2008. Stem cells and biomimetic materials strategies for tissue engineering. *Materials Science and Engineering: C*, *28*(8), pp.1189–1202.
66. Ouasti, S., Donno, R., Cellesi, F., Sherratt, M.J., Terenghi, G. and Tirelli, N., 2011. Network connectivity, mechanical properties and cell adhesion for hyaluronic acid/PEG hydrogels. *Biomaterials*, *32*(27), pp.6456–6470.
67. Kumar, A., Murugavel, S., Aditya, A. and Boccaccini, A.R., 2017. Mesoporous 45S5 bioactive glass: synthesis, in vitro dissolution and biomineralization behavior. *Journal of Materials Chemistry B*, *5*(44), pp.8786–8798.
68. Vissers, C.A., Harvestine, J.N. and Leach, J.K., 2015. Pore size regulates mesenchymal stem cell response to bioglass-loaded composite scaffolds. *International Journal of Bioprinting*, *3*(44), pp.8650–8658.
69. Kashani, A.S. and Packirisamy, M., 2021. Cancer-nano-interaction: from cellular uptake to mechanobiological responses. *International Journal of Molecular Sciences*, *22*(17), p.9587.
70. Tay, C.Y., Setyawati, M.I., Xie, J., Parak, W.J. and Leong, D.T., 2014. Back to basics: exploiting the innate physico-chemical characteristics of nanomaterials for biomedical applications. *Advanced Functional Materials*, *24*(38), pp.5936–5955.
71. Wu, C., Shen, Y., Chen, M., Wang, K., Li, Y. and Cheng, Y, 2018. Recent advances in magnetic-nanomaterial-based mechanotransduction for cell fate regulation. *Advanced Materials*, *30*(17), p.1705673.
72. Chen, L., Cheng, G., Meng, S. and Ding, Y., 2022. Collagen membrane derived from fish scales for application in bone tissue engineering. *Polymers (Basel)*, *14*(13), p.2532.
73. West, J.L. and Hubbell, J.A., 1999. Polymeric biomaterials with degradation sites for proteases involved in cell migration. *Macromolecules*, *32*(1), pp.241–244.
74. Elisseeff, J., McIntosh, W., Anseth, K., Riley, S., Ragan, P. and Langer, R., 2000. Photoencapsulation of chondrocytes in poly (ethylene oxide)-based semi-interpenetrating networks. *Journal of Biomedical Materials Research*, *51*(2), pp.164–171.
75. Sreejalekshmi, K.G. and Nair, P.D., 2011. Biomimeticity in tissue engineering scaffolds through synthetic peptide modifications—altering chemistry for enhanced biological response. *Journal of Biomedical Materials Research Part A*, *96*(2), pp.477–491.
76. Govindharaj, M., Roopavath, U.K. and Rath, S.N., 2019. Valorization of discarded Marine Eel fish skin for collagen extraction as a 3D printable blue biomaterial for tissue engineering. *Journal of Cleaner Production*, *230*, pp.412–419.
77. Teotia, A.K., Gupta, A., Raina, D.B., Lidgren, L. and Kumar, A., 2016. Gelatin-modified bone substitute with bioactive molecules enhance cellular interactions and bone regeneration. *ACS Applied Materials & Interfaces*, *8*(17), pp.10775–10787.
78. Hayes, M., Carney, B., Slater, J. and Brück, W., 2008. Mining marine shellfish wastes for bioactive molecules: chitin and chitosan – part B: applications. *Biotechnology Journal*, *3*(7), pp.878–889.
79. Pollini, M. and Paladini, F., 2020. Bioinspired materials for wound healing application: the potential of silk fibroin. *Materials (Basel)*, *13*(15), p.3361.
80. Ramaswamy, Y., Roohani, I., No, Y.J., Madafiglio, G., Chang, F., Zhao, F., Lu, Z. and Zreiqat, H., 2021. Nature-inspired topographies on hydroxyapatite surfaces regulate stem cells behaviour. *Bioactive Materials*, *6*(4), pp.1107–1117.
81. Bian, W., Li, D., Lian, Q., Li, X., Zhang, W., Wang, K. and Jin, Z., 2012. Fabrication of a bio-inspired beta-Tricalcium phosphate/collagen scaffold based on ceramic stereolithography and gel casting for osteochondral tissue engineering. *Rapid Prototyping Journal*, *18*(1), pp.68–80.

82. Ilyas, R., Sapuan, S., Harussani, M., Hakimi, M., Haziq, M., Atikah, M., Asyraf, M., Ishak, M., Razman, M. and Nurazzi, N., 2021. Polylactic acid (PLA) biocomposite: processing, additive manufacturing and advanced applications. *Polymers*, *13*(8), p.1326.
83. Lui, F., Wang, Y., Mobbs, R. and Sorrell, C., 2022. Nature-inspired discontinuous calcium coatings on polyglycolic acid for orthopaedic applications. *Journal of Materials Science*, *57*, pp.1–10.
84. Gan, D., Xing, W., Jiang, L., Fang, J., Zhao, C., Ren, F., Fang, L., Wang, K. and Lu, X., 2019. Plant-inspired adhesive and tough hydrogel based on Ag-Lignin nanoparticles-triggered dynamic redox catechol chemistry. *Nature Communications*, *10*(1), p.1487.

2 Bioactive Glasses for Biological Applications

Ramu Inala, Raghavendra Gujjala, Shanmukha Raju, Rakesh Kanakam, and Marcin Środa

2.1 BIOACTIVE GLASSES

Bioactive glass is a unique class of materials that holds immense promise in various biomedical applications due to its remarkable ability to interact with biological tissues and promote healing and regeneration. Composed primarily of silica (SiO_2), calcium oxide (CaO), and phosphorus pentoxide (P_2O_5), among other elements, bioactive glass differs significantly from traditional inert glasses due to its ability to form a strong bond with living tissues [1]. This property arises from the formation of a biologically active hydroxyapatite (HA) layer on its surface when in contact with bodily fluids. This concept of bioactive glass was first introduced by Dr. Larry Hench in the 1960s. Dr. Hench and his team at the University of Florida were exploring materials that could be used to repair and replace hard tissues in the body. They discovered that certain compositions of glasses, when implanted in the body, could stimulate bone growth and integrate seamlessly with surrounding tissues. This groundbreaking discovery paved the way for the development of bioactive glasses for various biomedical applications [2–4].

One of the key characteristics of bioactive glass is its ability to initiate a series of biological responses upon contact with bodily fluids. When implanted into the body, bioactive glass undergoes a process called surface reactions, where ions from the glass are released into the surrounding environment, triggering the formation of a layer of HA [5]. HA is a mineral that is chemically similar to the mineral component of natural bone, providing an ideal substrate for the attachment and growth of bone cells. This biologically active layer not only promotes bone growth but also facilitates the integration of the glass with surrounding tissues, leading to enhanced biocompatibility [6, 7].

In biomedical applications, bioactive glasses have shown significant promise as implant materials for bone repair and regeneration [8]. They are commonly used in orthopedic surgeries, dental procedures, and wound healing applications. In orthopedics, bioactive glasses are utilized in the form of bone graft substitutes, implants, and coatings for orthopedic implants [9]. Their ability to stimulate osteogenesis, the formation of new bone tissue, makes them ideal candidates for treating bone defects and fractures. Furthermore, bioactive glasses can be tailored to release therapeutic ions

DOI: 10.1201/9781003660781-2

such as calcium, phosphorus, and silicon, which further enhances their regenerative properties and antimicrobial effects [10]. Apart from bone tissue engineering, bioactive glasses have found applications in other areas of biomedicine as well. They are used in drug delivery systems, where they can serve as carriers for various therapeutic agents [11]. The porous structure of bioactive glasses allows for the controlled release of drugs, making them suitable for targeted therapies. Additionally, bioactive glasses are employed in biosensing platforms for detecting biomolecules and monitoring biological processes [12].

The versatility of bioactive glasses extends beyond their use as standalone materials. They are often incorporated into composite materials, such as polymers and ceramics, to create multifunctional constructs with enhanced mechanical strength and bioactivity. These composite materials are used in the fabrication of tissue scaffolds, implants, and medical devices [13]. The ability to customize the composition, porosity, and degradation kinetics of bioactive glass composites allows for the development of patient-specific implants tailored to individual needs.

2.1.1 Bioactive Glasses for Bone Tissue Engineering Applications

Bioactive glasses have garnered significant attention in tissue engineering and regenerative medicine due to their unique properties that promote tissue regeneration and integration with the host biological environment. Various types of bioactive glasses have been developed, each with distinct compositions and characteristics tailored for specific tissue regeneration applications.

2.1.1.1 Silicate-Based Bioactive Glasses

Silicate-based bioactive glasses are among the most extensively studied and utilized materials in tissue regeneration. Composed primarily of silica (SiO_2), calcium oxide (CaO), and sodium oxide (Na_2O), silicate-based glasses have shown remarkable bioactivity and biocompatibility. They stimulate the formation of HA on their surface upon exposure to bodily fluids, facilitating bone regeneration [14]. Additionally, silicate-based glasses can be doped with therapeutic ions such as boron [15], strontium [16], or zinc [17] to enhance their biological properties and modulate cellular responses.

2.1.1.2 Phosphate-Based Bioactive Glasses

Phosphate-based bioactive glasses offer unique advantages for bone tissue engineering due to their higher dissolution rates compared to silicate-based glasses. These glasses are composed of phosphorus pentoxide (P_2O_5), calcium oxide (CaO), and other oxides. Their higher dissolution rates promote the release of biologically active ions, such as calcium and phosphate, which stimulate osteogenic activity and bone formation. Phosphate-based bioactive glasses have shown promise in promoting rapid bone regeneration and are particularly useful in treating critical-sized bone defects [18]. Few other dopants were also reported such as titania [19], Zinc [20], and titanium [21] for enhanced antimicrobial and osteogenic promotion.

2.1.1.3 Borate-Based Bioactive Glasses

Borate-based bioactive glasses have gained attention for their excellent bioactivity and glass-forming ability. Borate glasses typically contain boric oxide (B_2O_3) as a primary component, along with calcium and other oxides. These glasses exhibit fast degradation rates and ion release kinetics, making them suitable for applications where rapid tissue regeneration is desired. Borate-based bioactive glasses have shown promise in promoting angiogenesis, the formation of blood vessels, which is crucial for supplying nutrients and oxygen to regenerating tissues [22].

2.1.1.4 Bioactive Glass-Ceramics

Bioactive glass-ceramics are hybrid materials that combine the bioactivity of glasses with the mechanical strength of ceramics. These materials are typically produced by controlled heat treatment of bioactive glass powders, leading to the formation of crystalline phases within the glass matrix. Bioactive glass-ceramics exhibit enhanced mechanical properties, making them suitable for load-bearing applications in bone tissue engineering. They promote bone ingrowth and osseointegration while maintaining excellent biocompatibility [23].

2.1.1.5 Composite Bioactive Materials

Composite materials combining bioactive glasses with polymers or other ceramics offer synergistic advantages for tissue regeneration applications. By incorporating bioactive glasses into polymer matrices, researchers can tailor the mechanical properties, degradation kinetics, and bioactivity of the resulting composites. These materials can be fabricated into scaffolds, implants, or coatings for medical devices, providing versatile platforms for tissue regeneration in various anatomical sites [24].

2.1.2 Bioactive Glasses Sustained Drug Release Applications

Bioactive glasses have emerged as promising candidates for sustained drug release applications, offering a versatile platform for controlled delivery of therapeutic agents in various medical contexts. Their unique properties, including tunable degradation kinetics, high surface area, and ability to incorporate drugs, make them suitable for prolonged and localized release of bioactive molecules. Here, we foresee into the mechanisms and applications of bioactive glasses in sustained drug release.

2.1.2.1 Mechanisms of Drug Release

Bioactive glasses facilitate sustained drug release through several mechanisms. Upon implantation or exposure to physiological fluids, bioactive glasses undergo dissolution, releasing ions into the surrounding environment. This process creates pores and channels within the glass matrix, which can be loaded with drugs or therapeutic agents. As the glass degrades, the encapsulated drugs are released gradually, either through diffusion or dissolution of drug particles from the glass pores. The degradation rate of the glass can be tailored to match the desired release profile of the drug, ensuring sustained and controlled delivery over an extended period [25, 26].

2.1.2.2 Tailoring Drug Release Profiles

One of the key advantages of bioactive glasses in sustained drug release is their tunable degradation kinetics. By modifying the composition, structure, and porosity of the glass, researchers can precisely control the rate of glass degradation and drug release. For example, altering the ratio of silica to calcium oxide in the glass composition can influence its degradation rate, thereby modulating the release kinetics of encapsulated drugs. Additionally, the pore size and morphology of the glass matrix can be adjusted to regulate the diffusion of drugs and achieve specific release profiles tailored to the therapeutic needs of the application [27, 28].

2.1.2.3 Applications in Biomedical Therapeutics

Bioactive glasses find wide-ranging applications in biomedical therapeutics, where sustained drug release is desired for the treatment of various diseases and conditions. In orthopedics, bioactive glass-based implants and scaffolds can be loaded with growth factors, antibiotics, or anti-inflammatory drugs to promote bone regeneration and prevent infections. Similarly, in dentistry, bioactive glass-based materials are used for dental fillings, coatings, and implants, delivering antimicrobial agents or remineralizing agents to combat tooth decay and promote tissue repair [29]. Moreover, bioactive glasses are employed in drug-eluting stents for cardiovascular interventions, where they release antiproliferative drugs to prevent restenosis and maintain vessel patency [30].

2.1.2.4 Advantages over Conventional Drug Delivery Systems

Compared to conventional drug delivery systems, such as polymeric matrices or nanoparticles, bioactive glasses offer several advantages for sustained drug release applications. Firstly, their inherent biocompatibility and bioactivity minimize adverse reactions and tissue inflammation, making them suitable for implantable devices. Secondly, bioactive glasses provide a stable and durable matrix for drug encapsulation, ensuring long-term storage and release of therapeutic agents. Additionally, their ability to promote tissue regeneration and integration with the host tissue further enhances the therapeutic efficacy of the released drugs.

2.1.2.5 Encapsulation of Drugs

Bioactive glasses possess a high surface area and porous structure, making them ideal carriers for encapsulating a wide range of drugs, including small molecules, proteins, and nucleic acids. Drugs can be incorporated into bioactive glasses through various methods, such as physical adsorption, chemical bonding, or co-precipitation during the synthesis process. The porous nature of bioactive glasses allows for efficient loading of drugs within the glass matrix, ensuring uniform distribution and high drug-loading capacities.

2.1.3 Bioactive glasses for therapeutic applications

Bioactive glasses have shown promise in cancer therapy due to their unique properties, which enable controlled drug delivery, modulation of the tumor microenvironment, and targeted destruction of cancer cells. Here, we discuss in detail various bioactive glasses used in cancer therapy, their compositions, mechanisms of action, and therapeutic applications [31].

2.1.3.1 Silicate-Based Bioactive Glasses

Silicate-based bioactive glasses have been investigated for localized therapies, such as implantable devices or injectable formulations, for targeted drug delivery to tumors [32].

They can also be functionalized with chemotherapeutic drugs or photodynamic agents to enhance their anticancer efficacy [33].

2.1.3.2 Phosphate-Based Bioactive Glasses

Phosphate-based bioactive glasses are used in localized therapies for bone tumors and metastases, where rapid drug release and effective tumor targeting are crucial. They can also be incorporated into implants or scaffolds for combination therapies, such as surgical resection followed by localized drug delivery [34].

2.1.3.3 Borate-Based Bioactive Glasses

Borate-based bioactive glasses have been investigated for localized therapies, particularly for the treatment of brain tumors and other central nervous system cancers. They can also be functionalized with therapeutic agents for combination therapies or used as carriers for drug delivery to inaccessible tumor sites [35].

2.1.3.4 Composite-Based Bioactive Glasses

Composite bioactive glasses have been explored for a wide range of cancer therapies, including localized drug delivery, combination therapies, and tissue engineering approaches for cancer treatment. They offer versatility in design and can be customized to meet the specific needs of different types of cancer [36].

2.1.3.5 Silver-Based Bioactive Glasses

Silver-doped bioactive glasses are used in various therapeutic applications, including wound healing, dental materials, and orthopedic implants. They can be incorporated into dressings, coatings, or scaffolds to provide sustained antimicrobial activity and promote tissue regeneration. Silver ions have potent antimicrobial properties, making silver-doped bioactive glasses effective against a wide range of pathogens, including bacteria, viruses, and fungi. The release of silver ions from the glass matrix inhibits microbial growth and biofilm formation, making these materials valuable for preventing infections in medical implants, wound dressings, and surgical instruments [37, 38].

2.1.3.6 Copper-Based Bioactive Glasses

Copper-doped bioactive glasses are used in wound healing applications, where they can promote faster healing and reduce the risk of infection. They are also being investigated for orthopedic implants and dental materials, where they can enhance osseointegration and prevent peri-implant infections. Copper ions exhibit antimicrobial properties and have been shown to promote angiogenesis, the formation of new blood vessels, and tissue regeneration. Copper-doped bioactive glasses release copper ions into the surrounding environment, which inhibit microbial growth and stimulate vascularization and tissue repair processes [39, 40].

2.1.3.7 Zinc-Based Bioactive Glasses

Zinc-doped bioactive glasses are used in wound dressings, where they can accelerate wound healing and reduce the risk of infection. They are also being explored for bone tissue engineering applications, where they can enhance bone regeneration and integration with the host tissue. Zinc ions have antimicrobial properties and play essential roles in wound healing, immune function, and tissue repair. Zinc-doped bioactive glasses release zinc ions, which contribute to the antimicrobial activity of the material and promote tissue regeneration processes such as cell proliferation and collagen synthesis [41].

Metal-doped bioactive glasses with strontium ions, for example, have been investigated for their potential in treating osteoporosis and promoting bone formation. Cobalt-doped bioactive glasses may be used for controlled drug delivery or as coatings for medical implants to prevent bacterial infections. These metal ions can impart various therapeutic properties to the bioactive glass, including antimicrobial activity, anti-inflammatory effects, and enhancement of bone regeneration.

2.2 BIOCOMPATIBILITY OF THE BIOACTIVE GLASSES

Bioactive glasses have garnered significant attention in biomedical applications due to their unique ability to form a strong bond with living tissues, a property termed as bioactivity. This bioactivity stems from the ability of these glasses to undergo surface reactions when exposed to physiological fluids, leading to the formation of a hydroxycarbonate apatite (HCA) layer, similar in composition to the mineral phase of bone tissue. This HCA layer promotes the integration of the bioactive glass with surrounding tissues, making them promising materials for various biomedical applications such as bone regeneration, wound healing, and tissue engineering.

One of the key factors contributing to the biocompatibility of bioactive glasses is their chemical composition. Typically, bioactive glasses are composed of silica (SiO_2), calcium oxide (CaO), sodium oxide (Na_2O), and phosphorus pentoxide (P_2O_5). The presence of these components plays a crucial role in the formation of the HCA layer. When the bioactive glass comes into contact with physiological fluids, such as blood plasma or simulated body fluid (SBF), ions from the glass surface are released into the surrounding environment. This ion exchange process leads to the formation of a silica-rich layer on the glass surface, which subsequently reacts with calcium and phosphate ions present in the physiological fluid to form the HCA layer [42]. The formation of the HCA layer is essential for the bioactivity of the glass, as it facilitates the bonding between the implant and the surrounding tissue. This bonding is crucial for the long-term stability and integration of the implant within the body. Moreover, the presence of silica in the bioactive glass composition is known to promote the formation of a silica gel layer on the glass surface, which acts as a precursor for the formation of the HCA layer. This gel layer not only enhances the bioactivity of the glass but also provides a protective barrier against undesirable reactions with the surrounding biological environment.

In addition to their chemical composition, the physical properties of bioactive glasses also play a significant role in their biocompatibility. The porosity and surface roughness of the glass can influence cell adhesion, proliferation, and differentiation [43]. Porous bioactive glasses, for example, have been shown to promote bone ingrowth and vascularization, making them ideal candidates for bone regeneration applications. Furthermore, the mechanical properties of the glass, such as its strength and modulus of elasticity, should match those of the surrounding tissue to prevent stress shielding and implant failure.

Another important aspect of the biocompatibility of bioactive glasses is their degradation behavior. Unlike inert materials such as titanium or stainless steel, bioactive glasses degrade over time, gradually releasing ions into the surrounding tissue. This degradation process is essential for the remodeling of the implant site, as it provides space for new bone formation and integration. However, the rate of degradation should be carefully controlled to ensure that it does not lead to premature implant failure or adverse tissue reactions. Various factors, including the composition, porosity, and surface area of the glass, can influence its degradation kinetics. The biocompatibility of bioactive glasses is also influenced by their surface chemistry and topography. Surface modifications, such as the incorporation of bioactive ions or functional groups, can enhance cell attachment and proliferation, as well as modulate the release of therapeutic ions from the glass matrix [44]. Furthermore, the introduction of nanostructured topographies, such as nanoparticles or nanofibers, can mimic the natural extracellular matrix and promote cell-matrix interactions.

In terms of biological response, numerous in vitro and in vivo studies have demonstrated the biocompatibility of bioactive glasses. In vitro studies typically involve culturing cells, such as osteoblasts or mesenchymal stem cells, on the surface of the glass and evaluating their viability, proliferation, and differentiation. These studies have consistently shown that bioactive glasses support cell attachment and spreading, as well as the production of extracellular matrix proteins such as collagen and osteocalcin [45]. Moreover, in vivo studies using animal models have demonstrated the ability of bioactive glasses to integrate with surrounding tissues and promote bone regeneration in defects or fractures. Despite their promising biocompatibility, bioactive glasses may elicit immune responses or adverse reactions in some individuals. Factors such as the size, shape, and surface charge of the glass particles can influence their interaction with immune cells and cytokines, potentially leading to inflammation or fibrous encapsulation. Moreover, impurities or defects in the glass structure can affect its biocompatibility and degradation behavior. Therefore, careful characterization and quality control are essential to ensure the safety and efficacy of bioactive glass-based implants.

In inference, bioactive glasses exhibit excellent biocompatibility due to their ability to form a strong bond with living tissues through the formation of an HCA layer. This bioactivity is governed by the chemical composition, physical properties, degradation behavior, surface chemistry, and topography of the glass. While numerous studies have demonstrated the biocompatibility of bioactive glasses in vitro and in vivo, further research is needed to optimize their properties and performance for specific biomedical applications. With continued advancements in materials science and biomedical engineering, bioactive glasses hold great promise for the development of next-generation biomaterials for tissue regeneration and repair.

2.3 CYTOTOXICITY OF BIOACTIVE GLASSES

Cytotoxicity investigations play a crucial role in assessing the biocompatibility of bioactive glasses, as they determine the potential adverse effects of these materials on living cells. Various studies have been conducted to evaluate the cytotoxicity of different bioactive glasses using standardized in vitro assays and cell culture models. These investigations aim to understand the interaction between bioactive glasses and mammalian cells, including their effects on cell viability, proliferation, morphology, and function. In this discussion, we will explore some key findings from scientific literature regarding cytotoxicity investigations of various bioactive glasses.

2.3.1 Standardized In Vitro Assays

One of the commonly used assays to assess the cytotoxicity of bioactive glasses is the MTT (3-(4,5-dimethylthiazol-2-yl)-2,5-diphenyltetrazolium bromide) assay. This colorimetric assay measures the metabolic activity of cells, with a reduction in MTT indicating a decrease in cell viability. Many studies have utilized the MTT assay to evaluate the cytotoxic effects of bioactive glasses on different cell types, including osteoblasts, fibroblasts, and mesenchymal stem cells (MSCs) [46].

2.3.2 Effects on Cell Viability

Several studies have reported that bioactive glasses exhibit minimal cytotoxicity and support cell viability and proliferation. For example, a study by [47] investigated the cytotoxicity of various bioactive glasses (45S5, 52S4, and 55S4) on human osteoblast-like cells (HOBs) using the MTT assay. The results showed that all three glass compositions promoted cell proliferation over a 14-day period, with no significant difference compared to the control group.

2.3.3 Influence of Glass Composition

The composition of bioactive glasses can significantly influence their cytotoxicity profile. Studies have shown that altering the composition of bioactive glasses, such as varying the ratio of silica (SiO_2), calcium oxide (CaO), and phosphorus pentoxide (P_2O_5), can affect their cytocompatibility. For instance, a study by [48] investigated the cytotoxicity of bioactive glasses with different compositions (SiO_2-CaO-P_2O_5 system) on human osteoblast-like cells (MG63). The results indicated that glasses with higher silica content exhibited lower cytotoxicity compared to glasses with higher calcium and phosphorus content.

2.3.4 Surface Modification and Cytocompatibility

Surface modification techniques can be employed to further enhance the cytocompatibility of bioactive glasses. For example, bioactive glasses can be functionalized with bioactive molecules, such as growth factors or peptides, to promote cell attachment and proliferation. Additionally, surface treatments, such as plasma spraying or sol-gel coating, can modify the surface chemistry and topography of bioactive glasses, thereby influencing their interaction with cells. These surface modifications have been shown to improve the cytocompatibility of bioactive glasses and enhance their performance in biomedical applications [49].

2.3.5 Influence of Degradation Products

The degradation products released from bioactive glasses can also impact cell behavior and cytotoxicity. Studies have shown that the release of ions, such as silicon (Si), calcium (Ca), and phosphate (PO4), from bioactive glasses can stimulate cell proliferation and differentiation. However, excessive ion release may lead to cytotoxic effects and impair cell function. Therefore, controlling the degradation rate of bioactive glasses is essential to ensure optimal cytocompatibility [50].

2.3.6 Long-Term Cytotoxicity Assessment

In addition to short-term cytotoxicity assays, long-term cytotoxicity assessments are important to evaluate the biocompatibility of bioactive glasses over extended periods. Long-term studies can provide insights into the sustained effects of bioactive glasses on cell behavior, including cell proliferation, differentiation, and mineralization. Moreover, long-term cytotoxicity assessments are crucial for predicting the performance of bioactive glasses in vivo and assessing their potential for clinical applications.

Investigations into the luminescence characteristics of various bioactive glasses have provided valuable insights into their structural properties and potential applications in biomedical imaging and sensing. Luminescence, the emission of light by a material, can arise from different mechanisms, including fluorescence, phosphorescence, and photoluminescence. In the context of bioactive glasses, luminescence studies often focus on understanding the origins of luminescence, the effects of glass composition and structure, and the potential biomedical applications of luminescent bioactive glasses [51].

2.4 LUMINESCENCE CHARACTERISTICS

2.4.1 Origins of Luminescence

The luminescence observed in bioactive glasses can originate from intrinsic defects within the glass structure or from dopant ions intentionally introduced during the fabrication process. Intrinsic luminescence typically arises from defects such as oxygen vacancies, which can trap charge carriers and lead to the emission of light when these carriers recombine. Dopant ions, on the other hand, can introduce energy levels within the band gap of the glass, allowing for the absorption and emission of light at specific wavelengths [52].

2.4.1.1 Effects of Glass Composition

The composition of bioactive glasses plays a significant role in determining their luminescence characteristics. Studies have shown that variations in the relative concentrations of silica (SiO_2), calcium oxide (CaO), and other additives can influence the luminescence properties of the glass. For example, the introduction of rare-earth ions, such as europium (Eu) or neodymium (Nd), into the glass matrix can result in characteristic emission spectra due to electronic transitions within the dopant ions [53].

2.4.2 Structural Features and Luminescence

The structural features of bioactive glasses, including their phase composition, crystallinity, and morphology, can also affect their luminescence behavior [54]. Amorphous bioactive glasses typically exhibit broad emission bands attributed to defects within the glass network, whereas crystalline phases may exhibit sharp emission peaks associated with specific energy transitions. Additionally, the presence of nanoscale features, such as nanoparticles or nanocrystalline domains, can enhance light-matter interactions and lead to modified luminescence properties.

2.4.3 Biomedical Applications

Luminescent bioactive glasses have shown promise for various biomedical applications, including bioimaging, biosensing, and drug delivery. The ability to tailor the luminescence properties of these glasses through compositional modifications and dopant ion incorporation makes them attractive candidates for advanced biomedical technologies. For example, bioactive glasses doped with lanthanide ions have been explored as luminescent markers for cell tracking and imaging in regenerative medicine and tissue engineering applications.

2.4.4 Characterization Techniques

Several techniques are commonly employed to characterize the luminescence properties of bioactive glasses, including photoluminescence spectroscopy, time-resolved luminescence measurements, and electron microscopy. Photoluminescence spectroscopy provides information about the emission spectra and intensity of luminescent materials, allowing researchers to identify the dominant emission peaks and assess their dependence on experimental parameters such as excitation wavelength and temperature. Time-resolved luminescence measurements can reveal information about the lifetimes of luminescent states, which can be indicative of the underlying luminescence mechanisms and the presence of energy transfer processes. Electron microscopy techniques, such as scanning electron microscopy (SEM) and transmission electron microscopy (TEM), can provide insights into the morphology and nanostructure of luminescent bioactive glasses, facilitating correlations between structural features and luminescence behavior.

2.5 FUNCTIONAL CHARACTERISTICS OF THE BIOACTIVE GLASSES

Functional characteristics of bioactive glasses encompass a broad spectrum of properties that render them suitable for a multitude of biomedical applications. These characteristics are intricately linked to the composition, structure, and surface properties of the glasses, and they play a pivotal role in determining their performance in specific biomedical contexts. Scientific literature extensively documents various functional characteristics of bioactive glasses, ranging from their ability to promote tissue regeneration to their capacity for controlled drug delivery. Below, we infer some key functional characteristics of bioactive glasses as reported in scientific literature.

2.5.1 Bioactivity and Biomineralization

One of the defining functional characteristics of bioactive glasses is their ability to induce biomineralization, a process in which the glass surface interacts with physiological fluids to form a biologically active HA layer. This HA layer mimics the mineral phase of natural bone and facilitates the integration of the glass with surrounding tissues. Studies have shown that bioactive glasses with compositions rich in calcium and phosphorus ions exhibit enhanced bioactivity, promoting the formation of a robust HA layer upon immersion in SBF or in vivo. The kinetics of biomineralization can be modulated by altering the composition, surface area, and porosity of the glass, offering control over the rate of tissue regeneration and osseointegration [55].

2.5.2 Osteoconductivity and Bone Regeneration

Bioactive glasses possess osteoconductive properties, meaning they provide a favorable environment for bone cell attachment, proliferation, and differentiation. The bioactive nature of these glasses promotes the recruitment of osteogenic cells and the deposition of new bone tissue, leading to accelerated bone regeneration. Numerous in vitro and in vivo studies have demonstrated the osteoconductive potential of bioactive glasses in various bone defect models, including fractures, non-unions, and periodontal defects. The interconnected pore structure of bioactive glasses facilitates the infiltration of blood vessels and bone-forming cells, promoting rapid tissue ingrowth and vascularization [56].

2.5.3 Antibacterial Activity

Recent research has highlighted the intrinsic antibacterial properties of certain bioactive glasses, particularly those containing silver (Ag) or copper (Cu) ions. These ions are known for their broad-spectrum antimicrobial activity against a wide range of bacterial pathogens, including antibiotic-resistant strains. Incorporating silver or copper ions into the glass matrix can effectively inhibit bacterial colonization and biofilm formation, thereby reducing the risk of implant-associated infections. Moreover, the release of antibacterial ions from bioactive glasses can be controlled to achieve sustained antimicrobial activity while minimizing cytotoxic effects on host cells [57].

2.5.4 Controlled Drug Delivery

Bioactive glasses can serve as versatile carriers for controlled drug delivery, offering a platform for localized and sustained release of therapeutic agents. By incorporating bioactive glasses into drug delivery systems, researchers can achieve targeted delivery of drugs to specific tissues or organs, minimizing systemic side effects and improving therapeutic outcomes. The porous structure and large surface area of bioactive glasses facilitate the loading and release of drugs, while the bioactive nature of the glasses promotes tissue regeneration at the implant site. Various drug molecules, including antibiotics, growth factors, and anti-inflammatory agents, have been successfully encapsulated within bioactive glass matrices for applications in bone regeneration, wound healing, and cancer therapy [58].

2.5.5 Angiogenic Potential

Angiogenesis, the formation of new blood vessels from pre-existing vasculature, is critical for tissue repair and regeneration. Bioactive glasses have been shown to possess angiogenic properties, promoting the proliferation and migration of endothelial cells and the formation of functional blood vessels. The release of angiogenic factors from bioactive glasses, such as vascular endothelial growth factor (VEGF) and fibroblast growth factor (FGF), can stimulate angiogenesis and improve tissue perfusion. This angiogenic potential makes bioactive glasses promising materials for enhancing vascularization in tissue-engineered constructs and promoting the integration of implants with host vasculature [59].

2.6 OUTLOOK

In conclusion, bioactive glasses exhibit a diverse array of functional characteristics that make them highly attractive for biomedical applications. From their ability to induce biomineralization and promote tissue regeneration to their antimicrobial activity and controlled drug delivery capabilities, bioactive glasses offer unique advantages for addressing various healthcare challenges. Ongoing research efforts continue to advance our understanding of the underlying mechanisms governing the functional properties of bioactive glasses and their potential applications in regenerative medicine, drug delivery, and tissue engineering. With continued innovation and interdisciplinary collaboration, bioactive glasses hold tremendous promise for improving patient outcomes and revolutionizing biomedical therapies.

REFERENCES

1. Li, R., Clark, A.E. and Hench, L.L., 1991. An investigation of bioactive glass powders by sol-gel processing. *Journal of Applied Biomaterials*, *2*(4), pp.231–239.
2. Gough, J.E., Notingher, I. and Hench, L.L., 2004. Osteoblast attachment and mineralized nodule formation on rough and smooth 45S5 bioactive glass monoliths. *Journal of Biomedical Materials Research Part A*, *68*(4), pp.640–650.
3. Hench, L.L. and Wilson, J., 2007, September. Biocompatibility of silicates for medical use. In *Ciba Foundation Symposium 121-Silicon Biochemistry: Silicon Biochemistry: Ciba Foundation Symposium 121* (pp.231–253). Chichester: John Wiley & Sons, Ltd.
4. Lobel, K.D. and Hench, L.L., 1996. In-vitro protein interactions with a bioactive gel-glass. *Journal of Sol-Gel Science and Technology*, *7*, pp.69–76.

5. Kaur, G., Pandey, O.P., Singh, K., Homa, D., Scott, B. and Pickrell, G., 2014. A review of bioactive glasses: their structure, properties, fabrication and apatite formation. *Journal of Biomedical Materials Research Part A: An Official Journal of The Society for Biomaterials, The Japanese Society for Biomaterials, and The Australian Society for Biomaterials and the Korean Society for Biomaterials*, *102*(1), pp.254–274.
6. Abdollahi, S., Ma, A.C.C. and Cerruti, M., 2013. Surface transformations of bioglass 45S5 during scaffold synthesis for bone tissue engineering. *Langmuir*, *29*(5), pp.1466–1474.
7. Bellucci, D., Sola, A. and Cannillo, V., 2016. Hydroxyapatite and tricalcium phosphate composites with bioactive glass as second phase: state of the art and current applications. *Journal of Biomedical Materials Research Part A*, *104*(4), pp.1030–1056.
8. Hench, L.L., Roki, N. and Fenn, M.B., 2014. Bioactive glasses: importance of structure and properties in bone regeneration. *Journal of Molecular Structure*, *1073*, pp.24–30.
9. Huang, C., Yu, M., Li, H., Wan, X., Ding, Z., Zeng, W. and Zhou, Z., 2021. Research progress of bioactive glass and its application in orthopedics. *Advanced Materials Interfaces*, *8*(22), p.2100606.
10. Fernandes, J.S., Gentile, P., Pires, R.A., Reis, R.L. and Hatton, P.V., 2017. Multifunctional bioactive glass and glass-ceramic biomaterials with antibacterial properties for repair and regeneration of bone tissue. *Acta biomaterialia*, *59*, pp.2–11.
11. Xia, W. and Chang, J., 2006. Well-ordered mesoporous bioactive glasses (MBG): a promising bioactive drug delivery system. *Journal of Controlled Release*, *110*(3), pp.522–530.
12. Won, Y.H., Jang, H.S., Kim, S.M., Stach, E., Ganesana, M., Andreescu, S. and Stanciu, L.A., 2010. Biomagnetic glasses: preparation, characterization, and biosensor applications. *Langmuir*, *26*(6), pp.4320–4326.
13. Bellucci, D., Sola, A., Anesi, A., Salvatori, R., Chiarini, L. and Cannillo, V., 2015. Bioactive glass/hydroxyapatite composites: mechanical properties and biological evaluation. *Materials Science and Engineering: C*, *51*, pp.196–205.
14. Al-Harbi, N., Mohammed, H., Al-Hadeethi, Y., Bakry, A.S., Umar, A., Hussein, M.A., Abbassy, M.A., Vaidya, K.G., Al Berakdar, G., Mkawi, E.M. and Nune, M., 2021. Silica-based bioactive glasses and their applications in hard tissue regeneration: a review. *Pharmaceuticals*, *14*(2), p.75.
15. Balasubramanian, P., Büttner, T., Pacheco, V.M. and Boccaccini, A.R., 2018. Boron-containing bioactive glasses in bone and soft tissue engineering. *Journal of the European Ceramic Society*, *38*(3), pp.855–869.
16. Kargozar, S., Montazerian, M., Fiume, E. and Baino, F., 2019. Multiple and promising applications of strontium (Sr)-containing bioactive glasses in bone tissue engineering. *Frontiers in Bioengineering and Biotechnology*, *7*, p.161.
17. Neščáková, Z., Zheng, K., Liverani, L., Nawaz, Q., Galusková, D., Kaňková, H., Michálek, M., Galusek, D. and Boccaccini, A.R., 2019. Multifunctional zinc ion doped sol–gel derived mesoporous bioactive glass nanoparticles for biomedical applications. *Bioactive Materials*, *4*, pp.312–321.
18. Abou Neel, E.A., Pickup, D.M., Valappil, S.P., Newport, R.J. and Knowles, J.C., 2009. Bioactive functional materials: a perspective on phosphate-based glasses. *Journal of Materials Chemistry*, *19*(6), pp.690–701.
19. Abou Neel, E.A., Chrzanowski, W. and Knowles, J.C., 2014. Biological performance of titania containing phosphate-based glasses for bone tissue engineering applications. *Materials Science and Engineering: C*, *35*, pp.307–313.
20. Qaysi, M.A., Petrie, A., Shah, R. and Knowles, J.C., 2016. Degradation of zinc containing phosphate-based glass as a material for orthopedic tissue engineering. *Journal of Materials Science: Materials in Medicine*, *27*, pp.1–11.

21. Kiani, A., Lakhkar, N.J., Salih, V., Smith, M.E., Hanna, J.V., Newport, R.J., Pickup, D.M. and Knowles, J.C., 2012. Titanium-containing bioactive phosphate glasses. *Philosophical Transactions of the Royal Society A: Mathematical, Physical and Engineering Sciences*, *370*(1963), pp.1352–1375.
22. Jung, S.B., 2010. Borate based bioactive glass scaffolds for hard and soft tissue engineering. Doctoral Dissertations. Missouri University of Science and Technology.
23. Gerhardt, L.C. and Boccaccini, A.R., 2010. Bioactive glass and glass-ceramic scaffolds for bone tissue engineering. *Materials*, *3*(7), pp.3867–3910.
24. Boccaccini, A.R. and Blaker, J.J., 2005. Bioactive composite materials for tissue engineering scaffolds. *Expert Review of Medical Devices*, *2*(3), pp.303–317.
25. Xu, Y., Hu, Y., Feng, P., Yang, W. and Shuai, C., 2019. Drug loading/release and bioactivity research of a mesoporous bioactive glass/polymer scaffold. *Ceramics International*, *45*(14), pp.18003–18013.
26. Hum, J. and Boccaccini, A.R., 2012. Bioactive glasses as carriers for bioactive molecules and therapeutic drugs: a review. *Journal of Materials Science: Materials in Medicine*, *23*, pp.2317–2333.
27. Anand, A., Das, P., Nandi, S.K. and Kundu, B., 2020. Development of antibiotic loaded mesoporous bioactive glass and its drug release kinetics. *Ceramics International*, *46*(4), pp.5477–5483.
28. Kouhi, M., Morshed, M., Varshosaz, J. and Fathi, M.H., 2013. Poly (ε-caprolactone) incorporated bioactive glass nanoparticles and simvastatin nanocomposite nanofibers: preparation, characterization and in vitro drug release for bone regeneration applications. *Chemical Engineering Journal*, *228*, pp.1057–1065.
29. Mocquot, C., Attik, N., Pradelle-Plasse, N., Grosgogeat, B. and Colon, P., 2020. Bioactivity assessment of bioactive glasses for dental applications: a critical review. *Dental Materials*, *36*(9), pp.1116–1143.
30. Scafa Udrişte, A., Niculescu, A.G., Grumezescu, A.M. and Bădilă, E., 2021. Cardiovascular stents: a review of past, current, and emerging devices. *Materials*, *14*(10), p.2498.
31. Baino, F., Novajra, G., Miguez-Pacheco, V., Boccaccini, A.R. and Vitale-Brovarone, C., 2016. Bioactive glasses: special applications outside the skeletal system. *Journal of Non-Crystalline Solids*, *432*, pp.15–30.
32. Moeini, A., Hassanzadeh Chinijani, T., Malek Khachatourian, A., Vinicius Lia Fook, M., Baino, F. and Montazerian, M., 2023. A critical review of bioactive glasses and glass–ceramics in cancer therapy. *International Journal of Applied Glass Science*, *14*(1), pp.69–87.
33. Borges, R., Pelosine, A.M., de Souza, A.C.S., Machado Jr, J., Justo, G.Z., Gamarra, L.F. and Marchi, J., 2022. Bioactive glasses as carriers of cancer-targeted drugs: challenges and opportunities in bone cancer treatment. *Materials*, *15*(24), p.9082.
34. Kargozar, S., Mozafari, M., Hamzehlou, S., Kim, H.W. and Baino, F., 2019. Mesoporous bioactive glasses (MBGs) in cancer therapy: full of hope and promise. *Materials Letters*, *251*, pp.241–246.
35. Kargozar, S., Mozafari, M., Ghenaatgar-Kasbi, M. and Baino, F., 2020. Bioactive glasses and glass/polymer composites for neuroregeneration: should we be hopeful? *Applied Sciences*, *10*(10), p.3421.
36. Keenan, T.J., Placek, L.M., Coughlan, A., Bowers, G.M., Hall, M.M. and Wren, A.W., 2016. Structural characterization and anti-cancerous potential of gallium bioactive glass/hydrogel composites. *Carbohydrate Polymers*, *153*, pp.482–491.
37. Blaker, J.J., Nazhat, S.N. and Boccaccini, A.R., 2004. Development and characterisation of silver-doped bioactive glass-coated sutures for tissue engineering and wound healing applications. *Biomaterials*, *25*(7–8), pp.1319–1329.

38. Mehrabi, T., Mesgar, A.S. and Mohammadi, Z., 2020. Bioactive glasses: a promising therapeutic ion release strategy for enhancing wound healing. *ACS Biomaterials Science & Engineering*, *6*(10), pp.5399–5430.
39. Alasvand, N., Behnamghader, A., Milan, P.B. and Mozafari, M., 2023. Synthesis and characterization of novel copper-doped modified bioactive glasses as advanced blood-contacting biomaterials. *Materials Today Chemistry*, *29*, p.101465.
40. Han, J., Hassani Besheli, N., Deng, D., Van Oirschot, B.A., Leeuwenburgh, S.C. and Yang, F., 2022. Tailoring copper-doped bioactive glass/chitosan coatings with angiogenic and antibacterial properties. *Tissue Engineering Part C: Methods*, *28*(7), pp.314–324.
41. Kim, D., Shim, Y.S., An, S.Y. and Lee, M.J., 2021. Role of zinc-doped bioactive glass encapsulated with microspherical gelatin in localized supplementation for tissue regeneration: a contemporary review. *Molecules*, *26*(7), p.1823.
42. Oyane, A., Kim, H.M., Furuya, T., Kokubo, T., Miyazaki, T. and Nakamura, T., 2003. Preparation and assessment of revised simulated body fluids. *Journal of Biomedical Materials Research Part A: An Official Journal of The Society for Biomaterials, The Japanese Society for Biomaterials, and The Australian Society for Biomaterials and the Korean Society for Biomaterials*, *65*(2), pp.188–195.
43. Bacakova, L., Filova, E., Parizek, M., Ruml, T. and Svorcik, V., 2011. Modulation of cell adhesion, proliferation and differentiation on materials designed for body implants. *Biotechnology Advances*, *29*(6), pp.739–767.
44. Kargozar, S., Kermani, F., Mollazadeh Beidokhti, S., Hamzehlou, S., Verné, E., Ferraris, S. and Baino, F., 2019. Functionalization and surface modifications of bioactive glasses (BGs): tailoring of the biological response working on the outermost surface layer. *Materials*, *12*(22), p.3696.
45. Sarker, B., Hum, J., Nazhat, S.N. and Boccaccini, A.R., 2015. Combining collagen and bioactive glasses for bone tissue engineering: a review. *Advanced Healthcare Materials*, *4*(2), pp.176–194.
46. Silver, I.A., Deas, J. and Erecińska, M., 2001. Interactions of bioactive glasses with osteoblasts in vitro: effects of 45S5 Bioglass®, and 58S and 77S bioactive glasses on metabolism, intracellular ion concentrations and cell viability. *Biomaterials*, *22*(2), pp.175–185.
47. Xynos, I.D., Hukkanen, M.V.J., Batten, J.J., Buttery, L.D., Hench, L.L. and Polak, J.M., 2000. Bioglass® 45S5 stimulates osteoblast turnover and enhances bone formation in vitro: implications and applications for bone tissue engineering. *Calcified Tissue International*, *67*, pp.321–329.
48. Sola, A., Bellucci, D., Cannillo, V. and Cattini, A., 2011. Bioactive glass coatings: a review. *Surface Engineering*, *27*(8), pp.560–572.
49. De Oliveira, A.A.R., De Souza, D.A., Dias, L.L.S., De Carvalho, S.M., Mansur, H.S. and de Magalhães Pereira, M., 2013. Synthesis, characterization and cytocompatibility of spherical bioactive glass nanoparticles for potential hard tissue engineering applications. *Biomedical Materials*, *8*(2), p.025011.
50. Fernandes, H.R., Gaddam, A., Rebelo, A., Brazete, D., Stan, G.E. and Ferreira, J.M., 2018. Bioactive glasses and glass-ceramics for healthcare applications in bone regeneration and tissue engineering. *Materials*, *11*(12), p.2530.
51. Rismanchian, M., Khodaeian, N., Bahramian, L., Fathi, M. and Sadeghi-Aliabadi, H., 2013. In-vitro comparison of cytotoxicity of two bioactive glasses in micropowder and nanopowder forms. *Iranian Journal of Pharmaceutical Research: IJPR*, *12*(3), p.437.
52. Zhang, C. and Lin, J., 2012. Defect-related luminescent materials: synthesis, emission properties and applications. *Chemical Society Reviews*, *41*(23), pp.7938–7961.

53. Jose, A., Krishnapriya, T., Jose, T.A., Joseph, C., Unnikrishnan, N.V. and Biju, P.R., 2021. Effective sensitization of Eu^{3+} ions on Eu^{3+}/Nd^{3+} co-doped multicomponent borosilicate glasses for visible and NIR luminescence applications. *Ceramics International*, *47*(5), pp.6790–6799.
54. Liu, D., Wang, M., Gong, L., Zhao, J., Zhu, M. and Wang, X., 2021. Photoluminescence properties of Eu^{3+} doped ZrO_2 with different morphologies and crystal structures. *Journal of Alloys and Compounds*, *864*, p.158781.
55. Kumar, A., Murugavel, S., Aditya, A. and Boccaccini, A.R., 2017. Mesoporous 45S5 bioactive glass: synthesis, in vitro dissolution and biomineralization behavior. *Journal of Materials Chemistry B*, *5*(44), pp.8786–8798.
56. El-Rashidy, A.A., Roether, J.A., Harhaus, L., Kneser, U. and Boccaccini, A.R., 2017. Regenerating bone with bioactive glass scaffolds: a review of in vivo studies in bone defect models. *Acta Biomaterialia*, *62*, pp.1–28.
57. Zhao, S., Zhang, J., Zhu, M., Zhang, Y., Liu, Z., Ma, Y., Zhu, Y. and Zhang, C., 2015. Effects of functional groups on the structure, physicochemical and biological properties of mesoporous bioactive glass scaffolds. *Journal of Materials Chemistry B*, *3*(8), pp.1612–1623.
58. Zhao, L., Yan, X., Zhou, X., Zhou, L., Wang, H., Tang, J. and Yu, C., 2008. Mesoporous bioactive glasses for controlled drug release. *Microporous and Mesoporous Materials*, *109*(1–3), pp.210–215.
59. Arkudas, A., Balzer, A., Buehrer, G., Arnold, I., Hoppe, A., Detsch, R., Newby, P., Fey, T., Greil, P., Horch, R.E. and Boccaccini, A.R., 2013. Evaluation of angiogenesis of bioactive glass in the arteriovenous loop model. *Tissue Engineering Part C: Methods*, *19*(6), pp.479–486.

3 Role of Nanomaterials in Bioactive Glasses

Manuela Reben, S. Indran, Somaiah Chowdary, Shakuntala Ojha, and Nadeem Siddiqui

3.1 NANOMATERIALS FOR BIOLOGICAL APPLICATIONS

Nanomaterials, with their unique physical, chemical, and biological properties, have emerged as transformative tools in biomedical research and healthcare. By leveraging the diverse elements of the periodic table, researchers have developed a wide array of nanomaterials tailored for specific biological applications. This introduction sets the stage for exploring the potential of periodic table-based elements in nanomaterials and their myriad applications in biomedicine. The periodic table, a fundamental framework in chemistry, organizes elements based on their atomic number, electronic configuration, and chemical properties. Each element possesses distinct characteristics that can be harnessed to design nanomaterials with tailored functionalities for biological applications. This introduction provides an overview of the key categories of nanomaterials derived from periodic table-based elements and highlights their significance in addressing challenges in diagnostics, therapeutics, and regenerative medicine.

Carbon-based nanomaterials represent one of the most versatile classes of nanomaterials, with applications spanning drug delivery, biosensing, and tissue engineering. Carbon nanotubes (CNTs), graphene, and fullerenes are prominent examples of carbon-based nanomaterials. CNTs, cylindrical carbon structures with remarkable mechanical strength and electrical conductivity, have garnered significant attention in drug delivery due to their high aspect ratio and ability to penetrate cellular membranes. Graphene, a two-dimensional carbon allotrope, exhibits exceptional electrical conductivity, high surface area, and mechanical strength, making it suitable for biosensing platforms and biomedical devices. Fullerenes, spherical carbon molecules with unique antioxidant properties, hold promise in photodynamic therapy, drug delivery, and bioimaging applications.

Metal-based nanomaterials offer diverse functionalities in biomedicine, owing to their optical, magnetic, and catalytic properties. Noble metal nanoparticles (NPs), including gold and silver NPs, are renowned for their surface plasmon resonance properties, which are exploited in biosensing, imaging, and photothermal therapy. Transition metal NPs, such as iron and cobalt NPs, exhibit tunable magnetic properties and find applications in magnetic resonance imaging (MRI), drug delivery, and

DOI: 10.1201/9781003660781-3

hyperthermia-based cancer therapy. Metal oxide NPs, including titanium dioxide and zinc oxide NPs, possess photocatalytic activity and are utilized in photodynamic therapy, antimicrobial coatings, and biosensing platforms.

Semiconductor nanomaterials offer precise control over optical and electronic properties, enabling sensitive detection and imaging in biological systems. Quantum dots (QDs), semiconductor nanocrystals with size-dependent optical properties, are employed in bioimaging, biosensing, and drug delivery due to their narrow emission spectra and photostability. Nanowires, one-dimensional semiconductor structures, show promise in neural interfacing, drug delivery, and tissue regeneration, leveraging their high surface-to-volume ratio and electrical conductivity. Other inorganic nanomaterials, including silica NPs, magnetic NPs, and metal-organic frameworks (MOFs), provide versatile platforms for biological applications. Silica NPs, with their biocompatibility and facile surface modification, are explored in drug delivery, biosensing, and imaging contrast enhancement. Magnetic NPs, such as iron oxide NPs, offer opportunities in MRI, targeted drug delivery, and magnetic hyperthermia-based cancer therapy. MOFs, porous crystalline materials composed of metal ions or clusters linked by organic ligands, show promise in drug delivery, imaging, and biosensing applications.

In biomedicine, nanomaterials derived from elements across the periodic table find diverse applications in diagnostics, therapeutics, and regenerative medicine. In drug delivery, nanomaterials offer precise control over drug release kinetics, enabling targeted delivery, sustained release, and improved therapeutic outcomes. Biosensing platforms based on nanomaterials provide rapid, sensitive, and selective detection of biomolecules, facilitating early disease diagnosis and monitoring. In imaging, nanomaterials offer high-resolution and contrast-enhanced modalities for visualizing biological structures and processes with unprecedented detail. Moreover, nanomaterials hold promise in regenerative medicine, tissue engineering, and personalized medicine, offering tailored solutions for repairing and replacing damaged tissues and organs. Despite the promising potential of nanomaterials in biological applications, several challenges need to be addressed for their successful translation into clinical practice. These challenges include biocompatibility, toxicity, scalability, and regulatory hurdles. Future research directions should focus on addressing these challenges while further exploring the synergistic interactions between nanomaterials and biological systems to unlock new avenues for biomedical innovation. Periodic table-based elements serve as building blocks for a wide array of nanomaterials with diverse functionalities and applications in biomedicine. Carbon-based nanomaterials, metal-based nanomaterials, semiconductor nanomaterials, and other inorganic nanomaterials offer unique properties and structural versatility for addressing critical challenges in diagnostics, therapeutics, and regenerative medicine. Continued research and innovation in this field are essential for realizing the full potential of nanomaterials in improving human health and well-being of individual needs.

3.2 NANOMATERIALS DOPED TO BIOACTIVE GLASSES

3.2.1 Alkali Metal-Based Bioactive Glasses

Alkali metal-based materials have foreseen decent attention in the scientific community; following are few materials that are currently in application.

A work from [1] explores the biodegradation, blood compatibility, and cytocompatibility of a bioactive lithium silicate glass-ceramic in vitro. It investigates the material's degradation behavior, its interaction with blood components, and its impact on cell viability. Results suggest promising biodegradability, minimal adverse effects on blood components, and favorable cytocompatibility, indicating its potential for biomedical applications. Another interesting work from [2] examines the hydroxycarbonate apatite formation, cytotoxicity, and antibacterial properties of rubidium-doped mesoporous bioactive glass NPs. It investigates their ability to promote the formation of hydroxycarbonate apatite, their impact on cell viability, and their antibacterial efficacy. Results suggest successful hydroxycarbonate apatite formation, minimal cytotoxicity, and significant antibacterial properties, indicating their potential for biomedical applications in bone regeneration and infection control.

A work from [3] investigated the structural, thermal, and physical properties of cesium-doped molybdenum-copper-lead glass. It investigates how the addition of cesium influences the glass's molecular structure, thermal behavior, and physical characteristics. Results reveal alterations in the glass's structure and thermal properties due to cesium doping, including changes in glass transition temperature and thermal expansion coefficient. The study provides insights into the effects of cesium on glass properties, which could inform the development of new glass formulations tailored for specific applications such as nuclear waste immobilization or optical devices.

3.3 ALKALINE EARTH METALS

Yet another interesting work from [4] investigated the reversibility of castration resistance status following treatment with Radium-223 dichloride. It presents clinical evidence and reviews existing literature on this topic. Findings suggest a potential for reversion of castration resistance status in some patients posttreatment with Radium-223, indicating a therapeutic effect on advanced prostate cancer. The study underscores the importance of further research to elucidate the mechanisms underlying this phenomenon and to optimize treatment strategies. Understanding the reversibility of castration resistance could lead to improved management and outcomes for prostate cancer patients receiving Radium-223 therapy.

The fabrication and characterization of barium-based bioactive glasses, focusing on their physical, structural, mechanical, and radiation shielding properties was investigated in the work from [5]. It investigates how variations in composition affect these properties, with a specific emphasis on their potential as radiation-shielding materials in biomedical applications. Results reveal promising characteristics such as bioactivity, mechanical strength, and effective radiation attenuation. The study highlights the versatility of barium-based bioactive glasses and their potential for use in medical devices or protective equipment where both structural integrity and radiation protection are essential considerations.

An investigation on the enhancement of remineralization and antibacterial properties in sol-gel glass ionomer cement through modification with fluoride-containing strontium-based bioactive glass or strontium-containing fluorapatite was reported in [6]. It explores how these modifications affect the cement's ability to remineralize tooth structures and inhibit bacterial growth. Results demonstrate improved remineralization capabilities and enhanced antibacterial properties compared to unmodified cement. The study underscores the potential of these modified materials for dental applications, suggesting their efficacy in promoting oral health by strengthening tooth structures and combating bacterial infections. Further research could refine these formulations for clinical use in restorative dentistry.

An interesting work from [7] elaborated on the influence of Na_2CO_3/Al_2O_3 ratio on calcium fluoroaluminosilicate-based bioactive glass-ceramics derived from waste materials. It investigates how varying this ratio impacts the properties of the resulting glass-ceramics, focusing on their bioactivity and suitability for biomedical applications. Results indicate that changes in the Na_2CO_3/Al_2O_3 ratio affect the crystalline phases, microstructure, and bioactivity of the glass-ceramics. Optimal ratios result in enhanced bioactivity and mechanical properties, making them potentially valuable materials for bone tissue engineering and other biomedical uses. Understanding these relationships contributes to the development of sustainable and effective bioactive materials from waste resources.

A work from [8] investigated the impact of time-dependent Al_2O_3 dissolution during melting on the structure-bioactivity correlation of Mg-containing silica-based bioactive glasses. It examines how variations in the dissolution rate of Al_2O_3 affect the glass structure and its bioactive properties over time. Results reveal that the extent of Al_2O_3 dissolution influences the formation of bioactive phases and alters the glass structure, ultimately affecting its bioactivity. Understanding this relationship is crucial for tailoring the properties of Mg-containing silica-based bioactive glasses for biomedical applications, offering insights into optimizing their composition and processing parameters to enhance their performance and bioactivity.

3.4 TRANSITION METALS

The potential of scandium-doped phosphate glasses for treating dental caries by assessing their antibacterial, remineralizing, and matrix metalloproteinase-inhibiting properties was assessed in [9]. It investigates how the incorporation of scandium affects these properties and evaluates the glasses' effectiveness in combating dental decay. Results indicate promising antibacterial activity against cariogenic bacteria, enhanced remineralization of enamel, and inhibition of matrix metalloproteinases implicated in tooth degradation. The study highlights the potential of scandium-doped phosphate glasses as multifunctional materials for addressing dental caries, suggesting their utility in developing innovative strategies for caries prevention and treatment. The behavior of yttrium-containing bioactive glasses in simulated body fluid (SBF) is investigated in [10]. It investigates the glasses' ability to induce hydroxyapatite (HA) formation and their overall bioactivity in a physiological environment. Results reveal that yttrium incorporation influences the glass's reactivity and HA formation kinetics in SBF. The study sheds light on the role of yttrium in modifying the bioactivity of glasses, which is crucial for their potential biomedical applications such as bone regeneration. Understanding their behavior in SBF aids in optimizing the composition of yttrium-containing bioactive glasses for enhanced bioactivity and performance in biomedical settings.

The potential of a new bioactive glass coating on titanium implants for orthopedic applications by assessing its anti-biofilm activity was inferred in the work [11]. It explores how the coating influences bacterial colonization and biofilm formation on implant surfaces. Results demonstrate the coating's significant anti-biofilm properties, effectively inhibiting bacterial attachment and biofilm formation. This suggests its potential for reducing implant-associated infections, a common complication in orthopedic surgeries. The study highlights the importance of bioactive coatings in enhancing the performance and safety of orthopedic implants, offering a promising avenue for improving patient outcomes and reducing the risk of postoperative complications.

An interesting work from [12] investigated the synergistic effect of zirconium and magnesium on the structural and biological characteristics of sol-gel-derived silicate-based bioactive glass. It examines how varying the concentrations of these elements influences the glass's composition, structure, and bioactivity. Results reveal that the combination of zirconium and magnesium enhances the glass's bioactivity, promoting HA formation and cell proliferation. This synergistic effect suggests potential applications in bone tissue engineering and regenerative medicine. Understanding the interplay between these elements contributes to the development of tailored bioactive glass formulations with optimized properties for biomedical applications. A work from [13] proposed a novel approach by incorporating hafnium phthalocyanine into a CaO-SiO_2-P_2O_5 nanobioglass system. It investigates the impact of this activation on the properties of the bioglass, focusing on its structural, mechanical, and bioactive characteristics. Results demonstrate that the addition of hafnium phthalocyanine enhances the bioglass's bioactivity and mechanical strength. This novel activation method shows promise for improving the performance and efficacy of bioglass materials in biomedical applications such as bone regeneration and tissue engineering. Understanding the synergistic effects between hafnium phthalocyanine and bioglass constituents provides valuable insights for developing advanced biomaterials with enhanced functionalities.

The synthesis and characterization of bioactive glass incorporating cerium and lanthanum were addressed in work [14]. It investigates the impact of these rare earth elements on the glass's composition, structure, and bioactivity. Results highlight the successful incorporation of cerium and lanthanum into the glass matrix, leading to alterations in its structural and chemical properties. The bioactive glass demonstrates promising bioactivity, suggesting its potential for biomedical applications such as bone regeneration. Understanding the effects of cerium and lanthanum incorporation enriches the knowledge base for developing bioactive materials tailored for specific biomedical needs, contributing to advancements in regenerative medicine and tissue engineering. A work from [15] investigated borate speciation and structural changes induced by vanadium ion doping in borate bioglass. It explores how the introduction of vanadium affects the glass's borate network and overall structure. Results reveal alterations in borate speciation and glass structure due to vanadium doping, with potential implications for the glass's bioactivity and mechanical properties. Understanding these changes sheds light on the interactions between vanadium ions and borate glass matrices, informing the development of bioactive materials with tailored properties for biomedical applications such as bone regeneration and tissue engineering.

Co–Cr–Mo-based composite reinforced with bioactive glass was investigated in the work from [16]. It explores the impact of incorporating bioactive glass particles into the composite on its mechanical properties and bioactivity. Results suggest enhanced mechanical strength and bioactivity of the composite due to the presence of bioactive glass. This indicates potential applications in orthopedic implants, where both mechanical stability and bioactivity are crucial. Understanding the synergistic effects between the composite matrix and bioactive glass particles offers insights into developing advanced biomaterials for orthopedic applications, aiming for improved implant performance and biocompatibility.

Two-dimensional molybdenum disulfide (MoS_2)/polymer-coated bioactive glass scaffolds for tissue engineering were studied in [17]. It examines the fabrication process and evaluates the scaffold's structural, mechanical, bioactive, and radiation interaction properties. Results indicate that the incorporation of MoS_2 and polymer coating enhances the scaffold's mechanical strength, bioactivity, and radiation shielding properties. This suggests its potential for tissue engineering applications where robust mechanical properties, bioactivity, and radiation protection are desired. Understanding the synergistic effects between MoS_2, polymer coating, and bioactive glass provides valuable insights for developing advanced scaffolds with improved performance and functionality for tissue engineering and regenerative medicine.

A work from [18] developed composite scaffolds for bone tissue engineering containing tungsten disulfide NPs within PCL and PLGA coatings on bioactive glass. It explores the fabrication process and evaluates the scaffolds' structural, mechanical, and bioactive properties. Results demonstrate improved mechanical strength and bioactivity due to the presence of tungsten disulfide NPs and polymer coatings. This suggests their potential for bone tissue engineering applications, where enhanced mechanical properties and bioactivity are crucial. Understanding the synergistic effects between tungsten disulfide, polymer coatings, and bioactive glass offers insights for developing advanced scaffolds with optimized performance for bone regeneration and repair.

Synthesis and characterization of manganese-containing mesoporous bioactive glass NPs intended for biomedical applications were investigated in [19]. It examines the fabrication process and evaluates the NPs' structural, chemical, and biological properties. Results demonstrate successful incorporation of manganese into the NPs, which exhibit desirable characteristics such as mesoporous structure and bioactivity. This suggests their potential for various biomedical applications, including drug delivery and tissue regeneration. Understanding the properties of manganese-containing bioactive glass NPs contributes to the development of advanced biomaterials with tailored functionalities for improving healthcare outcomes. On the other hand, investigations on the influence of cobalt incorporation and precursor selection on the structure and bioactivity of sol-gel-derived bioactive glass have been reported in the works of [20]. It examines the synthesis process and characterizes the structural and bioactive properties of the glasses. Results reveal varying effects on glass structure and bioactivity depending on cobalt incorporation and precursor choice. The study sheds light on optimizing cobalt-doped bioactive glasses for biomedical applications, considering their potential for enhancing bone regeneration and antibacterial properties. Understanding these factors contributes to the development of tailored bioactive glasses with optimized properties for diverse biomedical uses.

The work from [21] presents iridium oxide NP-protein corona neural interfaces, showcasing enhanced electroactivity and bioactivity. These interfaces enable both physical and chemical neuronal activation through electric manipulation. By exploiting the protein corona formation, the interfaces demonstrate heightened electrochemical performance, promoting efficient neural stimulation. The study underscores the significance of iridium oxide NPs in facilitating precise and controllable neuronal activation, advancing possibilities for neuroengineering applications. Understanding the interplay between NPs and protein corona enriches the development of sophisticated neural interfaces, offering potential avenues for refined therapeutic interventions and neurological research. Another intriguing work evaluated the impact of nickel oxide substitution on the in vitro bioactivity and mechanical properties of bioactive glass-ceramics [22]. It examines the synthesis process and characterizes the material's bioactivity and mechanical strength through in vitro experiments. Results suggest that nickel oxide substitution influences the material's bioactivity positively, facilitating HA formation. However, it also affects the mechanical properties, potentially compromising its strength. The study underscores the importance of balancing bioactivity with mechanical performance in biomaterial design. Understanding the effects of nickel oxide substitution provides insights for optimizing bioactive glass-ceramics for biomedical applications, aiming for enhanced performance and biocompatibility.

Another interesting article from [23], discoursed the multifaceted applications of copper-containing bioactive glasses and glass-ceramics, spanning from tissue regeneration to cancer therapeutic strategies. It investigates the synthesis, characterization, and biomedical functionalities of these materials, emphasizing their roles in promoting tissue regeneration and exerting anticancer effects. Results highlight the diverse mechanisms through which copper influences cellular responses, including angiogenesis stimulation and cancer cell apoptosis induction. The study underscores the versatility of copper-containing biomaterials for biomedical applications, offering promising avenues for both regenerative medicine and cancer therapy. Understanding these materials' dual roles provides valuable insights into developing innovative approaches for addressing diverse healthcare challenges. Other yet interesting aspects of the influence of various silver species on the structure of bioactive silicate glasses were investigated in [24]. It examines how different forms of silver affect the composition and properties of the glasses through structural characterization techniques. Results reveal distinct alterations in the glass structure depending on the type and concentration of silver species present. This suggests that silver incorporation leads to modifications in the network structure and potentially influences the glasses' bioactivity. Understanding the effects of different silver species on glass structure provides insights for tailoring bioactive glasses with optimized properties for diverse biomedical applications, including antimicrobial and tissue engineering purposes.

The work presents a solid-state synthesis method for producing gold-containing bioactive glasses, offering alternative biomaterials for bone implantations [25]. It investigates the synthesis process and characterizes the structural and bioactive properties of the glasses. Results demonstrate successful incorporation of gold into the glass matrix, influencing its composition and bioactivity. The study highlights the potential of gold-containing bioactive glasses as biomaterials for bone implants, suggesting their suitability for enhancing bone regeneration and implant biocompatibility. Understanding the synthesis and properties of these glasses contributes to the development of innovative biomaterials for orthopedic applications, addressing the demand for effective and biocompatible bone implants.

3.5 LANTHANIDE-BASED MATERIALS

An interesting article from [26] investigated the effects of incorporating cerium-doped bioactive glass into an alginate/gelatin scaffold for bone tissue engineering through in vitro characterizations. It explores how the inclusion of cerium-doped bioactive glass influences the scaffold's properties and its suitability for bone regeneration. Results indicate enhanced mechanical properties and bioactivity of the scaffold, attributed to the presence of cerium ions. This suggests potential applications in bone tissue engineering. Understanding the interactions between cerium-doped bioactive glass and scaffold materials provides valuable insights for optimizing scaffold design and advancing regenerative medicine approaches for bone repair. Samarium-doped glass-reinforced HA for bone tissue regeneration was investigated in the work from [27]. It explores the synthesis and characterization of the material, focusing on its osteoblastic performance and antibacterial properties. Results reveal enhanced osteoblastic activity and antibacterial efficacy due to samarium doping. This suggests its potential for promoting bone regeneration while mitigating bacterial infections. The study highlights the significance of incorporating samarium into HA-based materials for improved biomedical applications, offering promise for enhancing bone tissue regeneration and reducing the risk of postoperative infections. Understanding these properties contributes to the development of advanced biomaterials for orthopedic and dental surgeries.

An interesting article on erbium (III) and terbium (III) containing silicate-based bioactive glass powders was examined for their physical, structural, and nuclear radiation shielding characteristics [28]. It explores the synthesis process and characterizes the powders' properties through various analyses. Results reveal alterations in the physical and structural properties due to erbium and terbium incorporation, along with enhanced nuclear radiation shielding capabilities. This suggests the potential of these glasses for radiation protection applications in addition to their bioactive properties. Understanding the properties of erbium and terbium-containing bioactive glasses provides insights for developing versatile materials with applications in both biomedical and radiation shielding fields [29].

3.6 OUTLOOK ON STABILITY OF NPS

NPs hold immense promise for biological applications due to their unique properties, but their stability is crucial for ensuring their efficacy and safety in diverse biomedical contexts. Stability encompasses several aspects, including structural integrity, colloidal stability, chemical stability, and biological compatibility. Structural integrity refers to the ability of NPs to maintain their shape and size over time, which is critical for controlling their behavior and interactions in biological systems. Colloidal stability refers to the ability of NPs to remain dispersed in solution without aggregation or precipitation, ensuring uniform distribution and effective delivery. Chemical stability pertains to the resistance of NPs to degradation or chemical changes under physiological conditions, which is essential for maintaining their therapeutic activity and minimizing adverse effects. Lastly, biological compatibility refers to the ability of NPs to interact with biological molecules, cells, and tissues without inducing cytotoxicity or immunogenicity, ensuring their biocompatibility and safety for biomedical applications. Understanding and optimizing the stability of NPs is fundamental for advancing their use in drug delivery, imaging, diagnostics, regenerative medicine, and other biomedical applications, ultimately contributing to improved healthcare outcomes.

REFERENCES

1. de Magalhães Gomes, G.H., Guimarães, G.O., Rodas, A.C.D., Milesi, M.T.B., Costa, F.N., Alves, M.F.R.P., Santos, C. and Daguano, J.K.M.B., 2024. In vitro biodegradation, blood, and cytocompatibility studies of a bioactive lithium silicate glass-ceramic. *Materials Chemistry and Physics*, *314*, p.128828.
2. Pantulap, U., Unalan, I., Zheng, K. and Boccaccini, A.R., 2024. Hydroxycarbonate apatite formation, cytotoxicity, and antibacterial properties of rubidium-doped mesoporous bioactive glass nanoparticles. *Journal of Porous Materials*, *31*, pp.1–12.
3. Zagrai, M., Macavei, G.S., Popa, A., Barbu-Tudoran, L., Gavrea, R.C., Mereu, A.R. and Soran, M.L., 2023. Structural, thermal and physical properties of cesium doped molybdenum-copper-lead glass. *Journal of Non-Crystalline Solids*, *619*, p.122577.
4. Ricci, M., Frantellizzi, V., Bulzonetti, N. and De Vincentis, G., 2019. Reversibility of castration resistance status after Radium-223 dichloride treatment: clinical evidence and review of the literature. *International Journal of Radiation Biology*, *95*(5), pp.554–561.
5. Singh, J., Kumar, V., Vermani, Y.K., Al-Buriahi, M.S., Alzahrani, J.S. and Singh, T., 2021. Fabrication and characterization of barium based bioactive glasses in terms of physical, structural, mechanical and radiation shielding properties. *Ceramics International*, *47*(15), pp.21730–21743.
6. Thongsri, O., Thaitalay, P., Srisuwan, S., Khophai, S., Suksaweang, S., Rojviriya, C., Panpisutd, P., Patntirapong, S., Gough, J. and Rattanachan, S.T., 2024. Enhanced remineralisation ability and antibacterial properties of sol-gel glass ionomer cement modified by fluoride containing strontium-based bioactive glass or strontium-containing fluorapatite. *Dental Materials*, *40*(4), pp.716–727
7. Ismail, N.Q.A., Sa'at, N.K., Zaid, M.H.M., Zainuddin, N. and Mayzan, M.Z.H., 2024. Effect of Na_2CO_3/Al_2O_3 ratio on the calcium fluoroaluminosilicate-based bioactive glass-ceramics derived from waste materials. *Materials Chemistry and Physics*, *312*, p.128556.
8. Başak, O., Hruška, B., Buňová, L., Muñoz, F., Michálek, M. and Chromčíková, M., 2024. The influence of time dependent Al_2O_3 dissolution during melting on the structure-bioactivity correlation of Mg containing silica-based bioactive glasses. *Journal of Non-Crystalline Solids*, *629*, p.122873.
9. Valappil, S.P., Abou Neel, E.A., Pickup, D.M., Burden, E., Sahdev, R., Miles, E.J., Cooper, L., Ansari, T.I., Hanna, J.V. and Higham, S.M., 2022. Antibacterial, remineralising and matrix metalloproteinase inhibiting scandium-doped phosphate glasses for treatment of dental caries. *Dental Materials*, *38*(1), pp.94–107.
10. Cacaina, D., Ylänen, H., Hupa, M. and Simon, S., 2006. Study of yttrium containing bioactive glasses behaviour in simulated body fluid. *Journal of Materials Science: Materials in Medicine*, *17*, pp.709–716.

11. Marques, D.M., Oliveira, V.D.C., Souza, M.T., Zanotto, E.D., Issa, J.P.M. and Watanabe, E., 2020. Biomaterials for orthopedics: anti-biofilm activity of a new bioactive glass coating on titanium implants. *Biofouling*, *36*(2), pp.234–244.
12. Moghanian, A., Tajer, M.H.M., Zohourfazeli, M., Miri, Z. and Yazdi, M., 2021. Sol-gel derived silicate-based bioactive glass: studies of synergetic effect of zirconium and magnesium on structural and biological characteristics. *Journal of Non-crystalline Solids*, *554*, p.120613.
13. Gerasymchuk, Y., Wedzynska, A. and Lukowiak, A., 2022. Novel $CaO–SiO_2–P_2O_5$ nanobioglass activated with hafnium phthalocyanine. *Nanomaterials*, *12*(10), p.1719.
14. Ershad, M., Vyas, V.K., Prasad, S., Ali, A. and Pyare, R., 2017. Synthesis and characterization of cerium-and lanthanum containing bioactive glass. *Key Engineering Materials*, *751*, pp.617–628.
15. Elbasuoni, E.G., Abdelghany, A.M., Moustafa, Y.M. and El-Damrawi, G., 2024. Borate speciation and structural studies of vanadium ion doping in borate bioglass. *Applied Physics A*, *130*(2), pp.1–9.
16. Mostajeran, H., Baheiraei, N. and Bagheri, H., 2024. Effects of cerium-doped bioactive glass incorporation on an alginate/gelatin scaffold for bone tissue engineering: in vitro characterizations. *International Journal of Biological Macromolecules*, *255*, p.128094.
17. Oksiuta, Z., Dabrowski, J.R. and Olszyna, A., 2009. Co–Cr–Mo-based composite reinforced with bioactive glass. *Journal of Materials Processing Technology*, *209*(2), pp.978–985.
18. Deliormanli, A.M., Ensoylu, M., ALMisned, G. and Tekin, H.O., 2023. Two-dimensional molybdenum disulfide/polymer-coated bioactive glass scaffolds for tissue engineering: fabrication, structural, mechanical, bioactivity, and radiation interaction properties. *Ceramics International*, *49*(14), pp.22861–22874.
19. Ensoylu, M., Deliormanlı, A.M. and Atmaca, H., 2021. Tungsten disulfide nanoparticle-containing PCL and PLGA-coated bioactive glass composite scaffolds for bone tissue engineering applications. *Journal of Materials Science*, *56*(33), pp.18650–18667.
20. Nawaz, Q., Rehman, M.A.U., Burkovski, A., Schmidt, J., Beltrán, A.M., Shahid, A., Alber, N.K., Peukert, W. and Boccaccini, A.R., 2018. Synthesis and characterization of manganese containing mesoporous bioactive glass nanoparticles for biomedical applications. *Journal of Materials Science: Materials in Medicine*, *29*, pp.1–13.
21. Kermani, F., Vojdani-Saghir, A., Beidokhti, S.M., Nazarnezhad, S., Mollaei, Z., Hamzehlou, S., El-Fiqi, A., Baino, F. and Kargozar, S., 2022. Iron (Fe)-doped mesoporous 45S5 bioactive glasses: implications for cancer therapy. *Translational Oncology*, *20*, p.101397.
22. Barrioni, B.R., Norris, E., Jones, J.R. and Pereira, M.D.M., 2018. The influence of cobalt incorporation and cobalt precursor selection on the structure and bioactivity of sol–gel-derived bioactive glass. *Journal of Sol-Gel Science and Technology*, *88*, pp.309–321.
23. Chan, F.E., Syu, H.M., Wang, T.Y., Tang, Z.T., Huang, C.N., Lee, J.F., Burnouf, T., Hu, S.H., Chen, P.C. and Huang, W.C., 2021. Iridium oxide nanoparticle–protein corona neural interfaces with enhanced electroactivity and bioactivity enable electrically manipulatable physical and chemical neuronal activation. *Advanced Materials Interfaces*, *8*(16), p.2100694.
24. Morais, D.S., Coelho, J., Ferraz, M.P., Gomes, P.S., Fernandes, M.H., Hussain, N.S., Santos, J.D. and Lopes, M.A., 2014. Samarium doped glass-reinforced hydroxyapatite with enhanced osteoblastic performance and antibacterial properties for bone tissue regeneration. *Journal of Materials Chemistry B*, *2*(35), pp.5872–5881.
25. Vyas, V.K., Kumar, A.S., Ali, A., Prasad, S., Srivastava, P., Mallick, S.P., Ershad, M., Singh, S.P. and Pyare, R., 2016. Assessment of nickel oxide substituted bioactive glass-ceramic on in vitro bioactivity and mechanical properties. *Boletín de la sociedad española de cerámica y vidrio*, *55*(6), pp.228–238.

26. Kargozar, S., Mozafari, M., Ghodrat, S., Fiume, E. and Baino, F., 2021. Copper-containing bioactive glasses and glass-ceramics: from tissue regeneration to cancer therapeutic strategies. *Materials Science and Engineering: C*, *121*, p.111741.
27. Tóth, Z.R., Feraru, A., Debreczeni, D., Todea, M., Popescu, R.A., Gyulavári, T., Sesarman, A., Negrea, G., Vodnar, D.C., Hernadi, K. and Pap, Z., 2022. Influence of different silver species on the structure of bioactive silicate glasses. *Journal of Non-Crystalline Solids*, *583*, p.121498.
28. Aina, V., Cerrato, G., Martra, G., Bergandi, L., Costamagna, C., Ghigo, D., Malavasi, G., Lusvardi, G. and Menabue, L., 2013. Gold-containing bioactive glasses: a solid-state synthesis to produce alternative biomaterials for bone implantations. *Journal of The Royal Society Interface*, *10*(82), p.20121040.
29. Deliormanli, A.M., Issa, S.A., Al-Buriahi, M.S., Rahman, B., Zakaly, H.M. and Tekin, H.O., 2021. Erbium (III)-and Terbium (III)-containing silicate-based bioactive glass powders: physical, structural and nuclear radiation shielding characteristics. *Applied Physics A*, *127*(6), p.463.

4 Nature, Processing, and Characterization of Glass-Ceramics for Biological Applications

Ishika Singh Solanki, Dheeraj Kumar Gara, V. N. Radha Manohar Aepuru, Aswani Kumar Bandaru, and Akanksha Mohanty

4.1 INTRODUCTION

Glass-ceramics have gained substantial interest within the biomedical field due to their exceptional properties, such as biocompatibility, bioactivity, and mechanical strength [1]. These materials, which possess both glassy and crystalline phases, are particularly suitable for a variety of biological applications [2] as depicted in Figure 4.1. This chapter aims to provide a thorough exploration of the nature, processing methods, and characterization techniques of glass-ceramics, specifically in the context of their use in biomedical applications. Understanding the nature of glass-ceramics involves examining their composition and structure, which are crucial in determining their bioactive behavior and mechanical properties. The incorporation of specific oxides like silicon dioxide (SiO_2), calcium oxide (CaO), and phosphorus pentoxide (P_2O_5) is pivotal in imparting properties such as bioactivity and controlled degradation, essential for applications like bone regeneration and drug delivery [3].

The processing methods of glass-ceramics significantly influence their final properties and performance. Traditional techniques such as melt-quenching and advanced methods like the sol-gel process and sintering are explored in this chapter. Each technique offers unique advantages and allows for precise control over the microstructure and composition of the glass-ceramics, thereby tailoring their properties for specific applications. Furthermore, tailoring the properties of glass-ceramics is critical for their effective use in various biological applications. This chapter discusses how these materials can be engineered for use in tissue engineering, drug delivery, and biosensing. For instance, in tissue engineering, glass-ceramics can be designed to promote cell growth and tissue regeneration, while in drug delivery, their controlled degradation can facilitate sustained release of therapeutic agents.

DOI: 10.1201/9781003660781-4

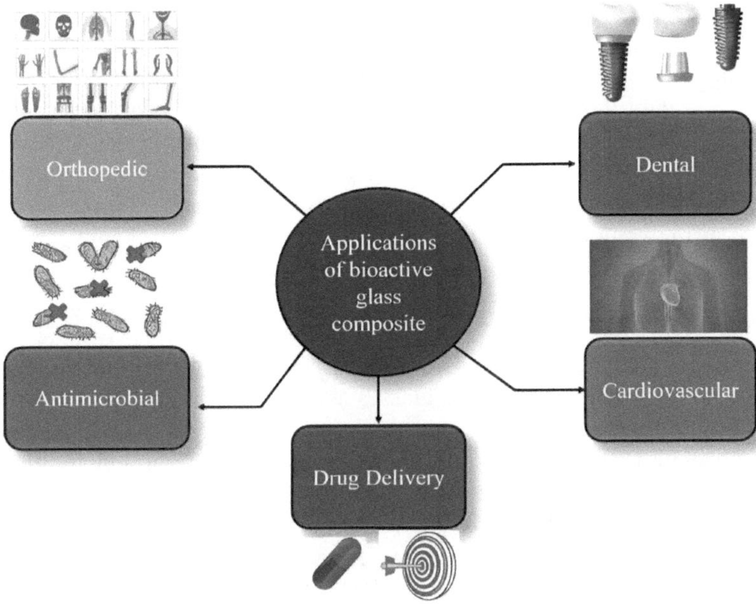

FIGURE 4.1 Biomedical application of glass-ceramic [4]

Characterization techniques such as X-ray diffraction (XRD), scanning electron microscopy (SEM), transmission electron microscopy (TEM), and atomic force microscopy (AFM) are essential for evaluating the properties and performance of glass-ceramics. These techniques provide detailed insights into the phase composition, surface morphology, and mechanical properties of the materials.

4.2 NATURE OF GLASS-CERAMICS FOR BIOLOGICAL APPLICATIONS

4.2.1 Composition and Structure

The composition of glass-ceramics is pivotal in determining their suitability for biomedical applications. These materials generally consist of a combination of oxides, with SiO_2 (silica) often serving as the primary component due to its ability to form a stable glass network. The inclusion of oxides such as CaO (calcium oxide), P_2O_2 (phosphorus pentoxide), and Na_2O (sodium oxide) is critical for imparting bioactivity and controlled degradation, which are essential features for biomedical use [1, 5].

Silica (SiO_2) provides a robust glass network that supports the integration of other oxides. The addition of calcium oxide (CaO) enhances the bioactivity of the glass-ceramic, promoting the formation of a hydroxyapatite (HA) layer when in contact with bodily fluids. This layer mimics the mineral phase of bone, facilitating bonding with surrounding bone tissue. Phosphorus pentoxide (P_2O_2) contributes to the glass's bioactivity and helps in regulating the material's degradation rate, which is crucial for applications where gradual resorption is desired. Sodium oxide (Na_2O)

serves as a flux, lowering the melting temperature and aiding in the formation of the glass [6].

The structural integrity of glass-ceramics is defined by their dual-phase nature, comprising an amorphous glassy matrix interspersed with crystalline phases. This microstructure can be tailored to optimize mechanical strength, degradation rates, and bioactivity. The crystalline phases within the glass matrix can be controlled through the selection of specific compositions and heat treatment processes, allowing for the customization of properties to suit different biomedical applications [7].

4.2.2 Role of Specific Oxides

The role of specific oxides in glass-ceramics is fundamental to their functionality in biological environments. Bioactive glasses and glass-ceramics are typically composed of a mixture of oxides. The most common components include silicon dioxide (SiO_2), calcium oxide (CaO), phosphorus pentoxide (P_2O_5), and sodium oxide (Na_2O). Each oxide plays a distinct role in determining the properties of the material:

- Silicon Dioxide (SiO_2): SiO_2 is the primary network former in bioactive glasses and glass-ceramics. It forms the backbone of the glass structure and is crucial for the formation of a stable glass network. SiO_2 content significantly influences the material's bioactivity, as it promotes the formation of a HA layer when the material comes into contact with bodily fluids. This HA layer is essential for bone bonding [6].
- Calcium Oxide (CaO): CaO is a key component for bioactivity. It participates in the formation of HA and enhances the material's ability to bond with bone tissue. The Ca^{2+} ions released from the glass-ceramic can stimulate osteoblast activity, promoting bone regeneration.
- Phosphorus Pentoxide (P_2O_5): P_2O_5 is another crucial component that contributes to the formation of the HA layer. Phosphate groups are involved in the nucleation and growth of HA, which is vital for the integration of the glass-ceramic with bone [8].
- Sodium Oxide (Na_2O): Na_2O acts as a network modifier, disrupting the glass network to create non-bridging oxygens. This modification lowers the melting temperature and enhances the bioactivity of the glass-ceramic. However, the content of Na_2O must be carefully controlled, as excessive amounts can lead to rapid dissolution rates, compromising the material's stability [8, 9].

4.3 PROCESSING METHODS

The processing methods employed for glass-ceramics significantly influence their microstructure and properties, which are crucial for their performance in biomedical applications. This section delves into the detailed methodologies and nuances of three primary processing techniques: conventional melting-quenching, sol-gel process, and sintering methods. Each method is discussed in the context of how it impacts the material's structure and suitability for specific biological applications.

4.3.1 Conventional Melting-Quenching

The melting-quenching technique is a traditional method widely used to produce glass-ceramics. This process involves melting the raw materials at high temperatures, typically in the range of 1,300–1,500°C, followed by rapid cooling (quenching) to form a glass. The resultant glass can then be subjected to controlled crystallization through subsequent heat treatments [11] (Figure 4.2).

Process Details:

- Raw Material Selection and Preparation: High-purity raw materials, such as silica (SiO_2), calcium carbonate ($CaCO_3$), and phosphorus pentoxide (P_2O_5), are carefully weighed and mixed. Impurities must be minimized to ensure the bioactivity and mechanical integrity of the final product.
- Melting: The mixture is placed in a platinum crucible and heated in a furnace. The temperature and duration of melting are critical parameters that influence the homogeneity and composition of the glass.
- Quenching: Rapid cooling is achieved by pouring the molten glass onto a cold metal plate or into cold water. This step is crucial to prevent crystallization and maintain an amorphous structure.
- Heat Treatment: The amorphous glass is then reheated to a specific temperature below its melting point, where controlled crystallization occurs. This step allows for the formation of desired crystalline phases within the glass matrix.

4.3.1.1 Impact on Microstructure and Properties

The melting-quenching method produces glass-ceramics with a fine balance between amorphous and crystalline phases, which can be tailored by adjusting the heat treatment parameters. The cooling rate during quenching affects the glass transition temperature and the degree of crystallinity. Higher quenching rates typically result in more amorphous structures, while slower rates allow for some degree of crystallization [10].

4.3.1.2 Biomedical Relevance

This method is particularly suitable for producing bioactive glass-ceramics with tailored degradation rates and mechanical properties. The ability to control the crystallization process is essential for applications such as bone grafts, where a balance between mechanical strength and bioactivity is required [12].

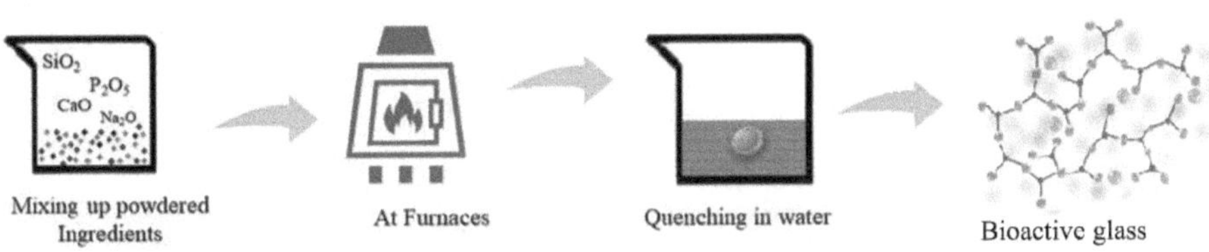

FIGURE 4.2 Melting-quenching process [11]

4.3.2 Sol-Gel Process

The sol-gel process is a versatile and low-temperature technique that allows for the precise control of the composition and microstructure of glass-ceramics [13]. This method involves the transition of a sol (a colloidal suspension of particles) into a gel (a network of interconnected particles) through hydrolysis and polycondensation reactions, followed by drying and heat treatment as illustrated in Figure 4.3.

Process Details:

1. Solution Preparation: Precursors, such as tetraethyl orthosilicate (TEOS) for silica and calcium nitrate for calcium oxide, are dissolved in solvents like ethanol or water. Catalysts such as hydrochloric acid or ammonia are added to control the hydrolysis and condensation rates.
2. Sol Formation: The precursors undergo hydrolysis and condensation reactions to form a sol. The sol is a stable suspension of nanoparticles that can be manipulated to achieve the desired composition.
3. Gelation: The sol gradually transforms into a gel through continued condensation reactions, forming a three-dimensional network.
4. Aging and Drying: The gel is aged to strengthen the network, followed by drying to remove solvents, resulting in a porous xerogel.
5. Heat Treatment: The xerogel is subjected to heat treatment at temperatures typically below 1000°C to densify the material and induce crystallization.

4.3.2.1 Impact on Microstructure and Properties

The sol-gel process allows for the production of glass-ceramics with highly controlled pore sizes and distributions, which are critical for applications requiring specific surface areas and bioactivity. The low processing temperatures reduce the risk of undesirable crystallization and allow for the incorporation of organic or bioactive molecules [15].

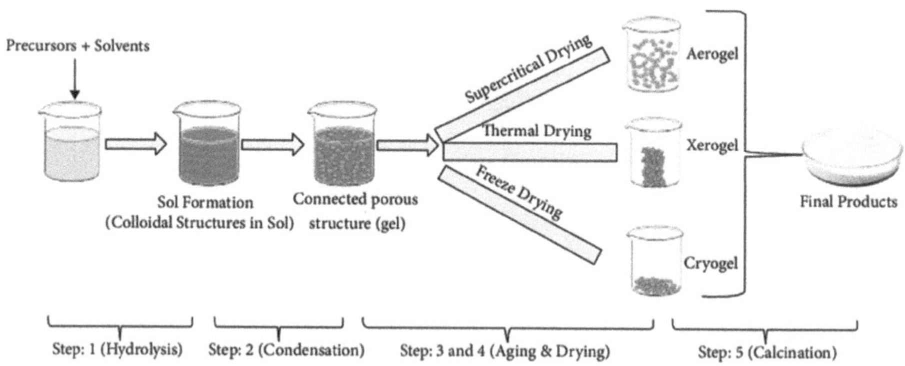

FIGURE 4.3 Sol-gel process [14]

4.3.2.2 Biomedical Relevance

The sol-gel method is particularly advantageous for fabricating bioactive coatings on implants, drug delivery systems, and scaffolds for tissue engineering. The ability to control the porosity and surface area enhances the bioactivity and drug-loading capacity of the glass-ceramics [15].

4.3.3 Sintering Methods

Sintering is a key technique for producing dense and mechanically robust glass-ceramics from powdered raw materials. The process involves compacting the powder into a desired shape and then heating it to a temperature where particle bonding occurs through diffusion without melting [16] (Figure 4.4).

Process Details:

1. Powder Preparation: High-purity powders are synthesized through methods like spray drying or mechanical milling. The particle size and distribution are carefully controlled to ensure uniform compaction and sintering.
2. Compaction: The powder is compacted into a green body using uniaxial pressing, isostatic pressing, or slip casting. The pressure applied during compaction affects the density and mechanical properties of the final product.
3. Sintering: The green body is heated in a controlled atmosphere furnace at temperatures typically between 800–1200°C. During sintering, particle bonding occurs through solid-state diffusion, leading to densification and grain growth.
4. Post-Sintering Treatments: Additional treatments, such as hot pressing or spark plasma sintering, can be employed to enhance densification and mechanical properties.

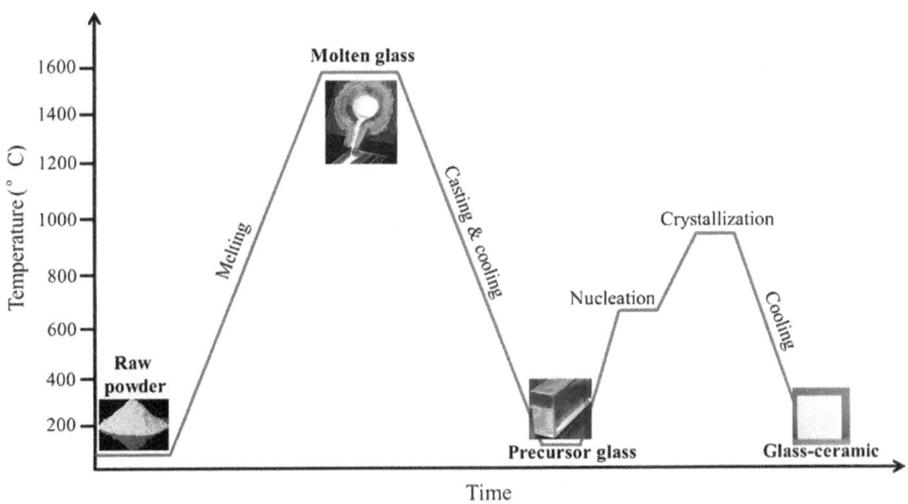

FIGURE 4.4 Sintering process [17]

4.3.3.1 Impact on Microstructure and Properties

Sintering allows for the production of glass-ceramics with high density and mechanical strength. The process parameters, such as temperature, time, and atmosphere, are critical in determining the final microstructure, including grain size and phase composition.

4.3.3.2 Biomedical Relevance

Sintering methods are widely used for manufacturing load-bearing implants and dental restoratives. The high mechanical strength and durability of sintered glass-ceramics make them suitable for applications requiring long-term structural integrity and wear resistance [18].

By understanding and optimizing these processing methods, researchers can tailor the properties of glass-ceramics to meet the specific requirements of various biomedical applications, ensuring their effectiveness and longevity in clinical use.

4.4 TAILORING PROPERTIES FOR BIOLOGICAL APPLICATIONS

Glass-ceramics have proven to be versatile materials with significant potential in various biological applications due to their customizable properties. Tailoring these properties to meet the specific requirements of different biomedical applications is essential for their successful implementation [19]. This section delves into the strategies and methodologies for optimizing glass-ceramics for tissue engineering, drug delivery, and biosensing applications.

4.4.1 Tissue Engineering

Tissue engineering aims to develop functional constructs that restore, maintain, or improve damaged tissues or organs. Glass-ceramics play a critical role as scaffolds in this field due to their biocompatibility, bioactivity, and mechanical properties [20, 21].

4.4.1.1 Scaffold Design

The design of scaffolds involves creating a three-dimensional structure that mimics the extracellular matrix (ECM) of natural tissues. Key factors in scaffold design include porosity, pore size, interconnectivity, and surface chemistry. These parameters influence cell attachment, proliferation, and differentiation, as well as nutrient and waste transport.

- Porosity and Pore Size: High porosity and appropriate pore size (typically 100–500 μm) are crucial for facilitating cell ingrowth and vascularization. Techniques such as freeze casting, 3D printing, and gas foaming are employed to create porous glass-ceramic scaffolds with controlled pore architecture.
- Interconnectivity: Ensuring interconnected pores is vital for tissue integration and vascularization. Methods like salt leaching and phase separation are used to achieve a well-connected porous network.

- Surface Chemistry: Modifying the surface chemistry of glass-ceramics, for example, by incorporating bioactive molecules like peptides or growth factors, can enhance cell adhesion and proliferation. Surface functionalization techniques include silanization and the use of bioactive coatings [21].

4.4.1.2 Bioactivity and Degradation

Bioactivity, the ability of a material to form a bond with biological tissues, is a critical property of glass-ceramic scaffolds. This is often achieved by forming a HA layer on the scaffold surface in physiological environments.

- Hydroxyapatite Formation: The incorporation of calcium and phosphate in the glass-ceramic composition facilitates HA formation. In vitro bioactivity tests, such as immersion in simulated body fluid (SBF), are conducted to evaluate the HA-forming ability of the material.
- Controlled Degradation: The degradation rate of glass-ceramics must be balanced with the rate of new tissue formation. By adjusting the composition and crystallinity of the material, the degradation rate can be tailored to match specific tissue regeneration needs [22].

4.4.2 Drug Delivery

Glass-ceramics are increasingly explored as drug delivery vehicles due to their ability to encapsulate and release therapeutic agents in a controlled manner.

4.4.2.1 Encapsulation Methods

Various techniques are used to encapsulate drugs within glass-ceramics, including sol-gel processing, melt-quenching, and ion exchange. These methods ensure the homogeneous distribution of the drug within the material matrix.

- Sol-Gel Processing: This method allows for the incorporation of drugs at relatively low temperatures, preserving the activity of temperature-sensitive therapeutic agents.
- Melt-Quenching: Involves melting the glass constituents with the drug, followed by rapid cooling to form a glass matrix containing the drug.
- Ion Exchange: Drugs can be loaded into the glass-ceramic through ion exchange processes, which substitute ions in the glass matrix with therapeutic ions [23].

4.4.2.2 Controlled Release

The controlled release of drugs from glass-ceramics is achieved through their degradation and dissolution in physiological conditions.

- Degradation-Controlled Release: The drug release profile can be tailored by adjusting the degradation rate of the glass-ceramic. This can be achieved by modifying the composition and microstructure of the material.

- Diffusion-Controlled Release: In some cases, the release mechanism is dominated by diffusion. The porosity and pore size of the glass-ceramic influence the diffusion rate of the drug molecules.

4.4.2.3 Therapeutic Applications

Glass-ceramics have been explored for delivering a variety of therapeutic agents, including antibiotics, anti-inflammatory drugs, and growth factors. These materials offer localized and sustained release, enhancing the efficacy and reducing systemic side effects.

- Antibiotics: Incorporating antibiotics into glass-ceramics can prevent infections in bone implants and tissue engineering scaffolds.
- Growth Factors: Delivery of growth factors such as bone morphogenetic proteins (BMPs) can promote osteogenesis and enhance bone healing [19].

4.4.3 Biosensing

Glass-ceramics are also used in biosensing applications due to their stability, biocompatibility, and functionalized surfaces [24].

4.4.3.1 Sensor Design

The design of glass-ceramic-based biosensors involves creating materials that can interact specifically with target biomolecules, producing measurable signals [25].

- Surface Functionalization: The surface of glass-ceramics can be functionalized with specific recognition elements, such as antibodies, enzymes, or nucleic acids, to detect target analytes.
- Signal Transduction: Various transduction mechanisms are employed in biosensors, including optical, electrochemical, and piezoelectric methods. The choice of transduction mechanism depends on the specific application and the desired sensitivity.

4.4.3.2 Detection Mechanisms

- Optical Detection: Glass-ceramics can be used in optical biosensors, where changes in light absorption or fluorescence upon binding of the target molecule are measured.
- Electrochemical Detection: Electrochemical biosensors measure changes in current or voltage resulting from the interaction of the target molecule with the functionalized glass-ceramic surface.
- Piezoelectric Detection: Piezoelectric biosensors detect mass changes on the sensor surface due to the binding of target molecules, producing measurable electrical signals [24].

4.4.3.3 Applications in Diagnostics

Glass-ceramic-based biosensors have applications in various diagnostic fields, including medical diagnostics, environmental monitoring, and food safety [26].

- Medical Diagnostics: These sensors can detect biomarkers for diseases, providing rapid and sensitive diagnostic tools.
- Environmental Monitoring: Glass-ceramic biosensors can detect pollutants and pathogens in water and air, contributing to environmental safety.
- Food Safety: They are used to detect contaminants and pathogens in food products, ensuring food quality and safety.

Therefore, the ability to tailor the properties of glass-ceramics through composition, processing, and surface modifications makes them highly suitable for diverse biological applications. By optimizing these materials for specific uses in tissue engineering, drug delivery, and biosensing, one can develop advanced solutions that enhance patient outcomes and contribute to the advancement of biomedical technology.

4.5 CHARACTERIZATION TECHNIQUES

Characterization of glass-ceramics is crucial to understand their structure-property relationships and to tailor them for specific biological applications. Advanced characterization techniques provide detailed insights into the phase composition, crystallinity, microstructure, surface morphology, and mechanical properties of glass-ceramics [27]. This section discusses various characterization methods, including XRD, SEM, TEM, and AFM, highlighting their roles and applications in the analysis of glass-ceramic biomaterials.

4.5.1 X-Ray Diffraction

XRD is a powerful technique used to determine the crystalline structure and phase composition of glass-ceramics [28].

4.5.1.1 Phase Identification

Qualitative Analysis: XRD patterns provide information about the different crystalline phases within the glass-ceramic. By comparing the diffraction peaks to standard reference patterns, the phases can be identified, and their relative proportions estimated.

Quantitative Analysis: The Rietveld refinement method can be used for quantitative phase analysis, providing detailed information about the crystallographic parameters and the phase composition of the material.

4.5.1.2 Crystallinity

Crystallinity Index: The degree of crystallinity can be assessed by analyzing the peak intensities and the background signal in the XRD pattern. A higher degree of crystallinity is indicated by sharper and more intense diffraction peaks.

Crystallite Size: The Scherrer equation can be used to estimate the average crystallite size from the broadening of the diffraction peaks, providing insights into the nanostructure of the glass-ceramic.

4.5.2 Scanning Electron Microscopy

SEM is an essential tool for examining the surface morphology and microstructure of glass-ceramics at high magnifications. SEM uses a focused beam of electrons to generate detailed images of the sample surface.

4.5.2.1 Surface Morphology

Topography: SEM images reveal the surface topography of glass-ceramics, showing features such as grain boundaries, pores, and cracks. This information is crucial for understanding cell-material interactions and optimizing surface properties for biological applications.

Elemental Analysis: Equipped with energy-dispersive X-ray spectroscopy (EDS), SEM can provide elemental composition maps, highlighting the distribution of different elements within the material [29].

4.5.2.2 Microstructure

Microstructural Features: SEM can be used to examine the microstructural features of glass-ceramics, such as the size and shape of crystalline phases, the distribution of different phases, and the presence of any defects or impurities.

Fracture Surface Analysis: SEM analysis of fracture surfaces can provide insights into the fracture mechanisms and the material's mechanical properties, such as toughness and strength [29].

4.5.3 Transmission Electron Microscopy

TEM offers high-resolution imaging and detailed structural analysis of glass-ceramics at the nanometer scale. This technique uses transmitted electrons to form images and diffraction patterns, providing information about the internal structure of the material.

4.5.3.1 High-Resolution Imaging

Nanostructure Analysis: TEM can reveal the fine nanostructure of glass-ceramics, including the size and distribution of nanocrystals, amorphous regions, and interfaces between different phases.

Atomic-Scale Imaging: High-resolution TEM (HRTEM) can achieve atomic-scale resolution, allowing for the direct observation of atomic arrangements and defects within the crystalline lattice.

4.5.3.2 Diffraction Studies

Selected Area Electron Diffraction (SAED): SAED patterns provide information about the crystallographic structure and orientation of different phases within the material. This technique can be used to identify crystalline phases and assess their orientation relationships.

Phase Contrast: TEM phase contrast imaging can be used to visualize the contrast between different phases, providing insights into the phase distribution and interfacial characteristics [30].

4.5.4 Atomic Force Microscopy

AFM is a versatile technique for characterizing the surface topography and mechanical properties of glass-ceramics at the nanometer scale. AFM uses a sharp probe to scan the surface of the material, providing high-resolution topographical maps and quantitative mechanical measurements [31].

4.5.4.1 Surface Topography

3D Imaging: AFM generates three-dimensional images of the surface topography, revealing details such as roughness, texture, and feature sizes. This information is critical for understanding how the surface morphology influences biological interactions, such as cell adhesion and proliferation.

Surface Roughness: Quantitative measurements of surface roughness can be obtained from AFM images, providing data on the smoothness or roughness of the material's surface.

4.5.4.2 Mechanical Properties

Nanoindentation: AFM-based nanoindentation can be used to measure the mechanical properties of glass-ceramics, such as hardness and elastic modulus. These measurements are important for evaluating the material's suitability for load-bearing applications.

Force Spectroscopy: AFM force spectroscopy provides information about the interaction forces between the probe and the material surface, offering insights into the material's stiffness and adhesive properties.

4.5.5 Integration of Characterization Techniques

A comprehensive understanding of glass-ceramics requires the integration of data from multiple characterization techniques. Each method provides unique insights into different aspects of the material's structure and properties, enabling a holistic assessment of their suitability for biological applications.

4.5.5.1 Correlation of Data

Structure-Property Relationships: By correlating data from XRD, SEM, TEM, and AFM, researchers can establish relationships between the microstructure, phase composition, surface morphology, and mechanical properties of glass-ceramics.

Optimization for Applications: The integrated characterization approach allows for the optimization of glass-ceramic materials for specific biological applications, ensuring that they meet the required performance criteria.

4.5.5.2 Advanced Analytical Technique

Synchrotron X-Ray Techniques: Advanced synchrotron-based X-ray techniques, such as X-ray absorption spectroscopy (XAS) and X-ray photoelectron spectroscopy (XPS), can provide additional information about the chemical state and local environment of elements within glass-ceramics.

Combined Microscopy Approaches: Combining different microscopy techniques, such as SEM and TEM, can provide complementary information about the material's microstructure and phase distribution [30].

4.6 CONCLUSION

Glass-ceramics have established themselves as a pivotal material in the realm of biomedical applications, offering a unique combination of biocompatibility, bioactivity, and mechanical robustness. Through a detailed exploration of their nature, processing methods, and characterization techniques, this chapter underscores the multifaceted potential of glass-ceramics in enhancing the efficacy and functionality of biomedical devices and treatments.

4.6.1 Integration of Bioactive Components

The fundamental principles governing the composition and structure of bioactive glasses and glass-ceramics highlight the critical role of specific oxides such as silica, calcium oxide, sodium oxide, and phosphorous pentoxide. These components collectively contribute to the desirable properties of glass-ceramics, including their ability to form HA and support tissue integration. Understanding the interplay between these oxides allows for the precise tailoring of glass-ceramics to meet specific biological requirements, ensuring optimal performance in various biomedical applications.

4.6.2 Versatility in Processing Techniques

The processing techniques discussed—conventional melting-quenching, sol-gel, and sintering—each offer distinct advantages and allow for customization of the microstructure and properties of glass-ceramics. The conventional melting-quenching method provides a straightforward approach to creating glass-ceramics with controlled crystallinity, while the sol-gel process offers superior compositional control and purity. Sintering, on the other hand, is instrumental in producing porous structures conducive to tissue ingrowth. These versatile processing methods enable the production of glass-ceramics that can be precisely engineered to fulfill specific biomedical functions, such as scaffolding for tissue engineering or matrices for drug delivery.

4.6.3 Tailoring for Specific Applications

The adaptability of glass-ceramics makes them suitable for a wide range of biological applications. In tissue engineering, they serve as scaffolds that promote cell attachment and growth, with tailored porosity and degradation rates that match the needs of different tissues. For drug delivery, glass-ceramics can be designed to release therapeutic agents in a controlled manner, enhancing treatment efficacy and reducing side effects. In biosensing, their surface characteristics can be modified to detect specific biological molecules, providing sensitive and specific diagnostic tools.

4.6.4 Advanced Characterization Techniques

The characterizations techniques as discussed earlier provides critical insight on the various characteristics of the materials. Such comprehensive characterization is essential for understanding how processing methods affect the final properties of glass-ceramics and for optimizing their performance in biological settings.

4.6.5 Future Directions

The integration of insights from diverse research areas has established a solid foundation for the continued advancement of glass-ceramics in biomedical applications. Future research should focus on further refining the composition and processing techniques to enhance the bioactivity, mechanical strength, and degradation control of these materials. Additionally, exploring new applications and improving the integration of glass-ceramics with other biomaterials could lead to innovative solutions for complex medical challenges.

In conclusion, glass-ceramics offer a versatile and highly customizable platform for developing advanced biomaterials. By leveraging their unique properties and refining their processing and characterization, researchers can create next-generation materials that significantly improve the outcomes of biomedical applications. This comprehensive understanding and continuous innovation in the field of glass-ceramics promise to drive future developments and breakthroughs, ultimately contributing to better healthcare solutions and enhanced quality of life.

REFERENCES

1. T. Kokubo, "Bioactive glass ceramics: properties and applications," *Biomaterials*, 12, Elsevier, Accessed: May 21, 2024. Online]. Available: https://www.sciencedirect.com/science/article/pii/014296129190194F
2. M. Catauro, and F. Bollino, 2017, "Advanced glass-ceramic materials for biomedical applications," *Journal of Bone Reports & Recommendations*, 3, academia.edu, Accessed: May 21, 2024. [Online]. Available: https://d1wqtxts1xzle7.cloudfront.net/106017115/advanced-glassceramic-materials-forbiomedical-applications-libre.pdf?1695838284=&response-content-disposition=inline%3B+filename%3DAdvanced_Glass_Ceramic_Materials_for_Bio.pdf&Expires=1748247705&Signature=EjFVfdxec373pj6AsD9lIpzalIh-Pa92lBRf1g6~yFPJYvHRFVMXX4AkvxwKT5NFQ3bR7zgQ4OADJvkqhqCZS9RY8v2tuz9nPN0guO4cewm610VzAmnjP6b0sj8QldXqge9TXzgDzxV~nQtIkVeliyeFxpgSMWjJZz8Nx6q6xoHsa4Trjb4-3duVGbwtOibnAFxRqP9f-FbdTLKMP8ObhLfxOfcYg6BSstq6GjJW3UWSnr2l6BQeILtZ507v0LlgG1Qudj3VYBhfRU~UHQsjxLaB-xZyyuWaZMyXcBmDPKYxpO4aGp8zpR-IueM-Xci8S7TFd9CzE1JYvUlsnyIJYg__&Key-Pair-Id=APKAJLOHF5GGSLRBV4ZA
3. M. Montazerian, and E. D. Zanotto, 2016, "History and trends of bioactive glass-ceramics," *Wiley Online Library*, vol. 104, no. 5, pp. 1231–1249, doi: 10.1002/jbm.a.35639.
4. S. Balu, S. Andra, J. Jeevanandam, and M. K. Danquah, 2021, "Bioactive glass composites: from synthesis to application," In Md Enamul Hoque, Ahmed Sharif and Mohammad Jawaid (eds), *Green Biocomposites for Biomedical Engineering: Design, Properties, and Applications*, pp. 65–96, doi: 10.1016/B978-0-12-821553-1.00009-0.

5. P. F. James, 1995, "Glass ceramics: new compositions and uses," *Journal of Non-Crystalline Solids*, Elsevier, Accessed: May 21, 2024. [Online]. Bangladesh: Woodhead Publishing Series in Biomaterial. Available: https://www.sciencedirect.com/science/article/pii/002230939400515X
6. G. H. Beall, 1992, "Design and properties of glass-ceramics," *Annual Review of Materials Science*, vol. 22, no. 1, pp. 91–119, doi: 10.1146/ANNUREV.MS.22.080192.000515.
7. F. Baino, C. Migneco, E. Fiume, M. Miola, S. Ferraris, S. Spriano, M. Ferraris, and E. Verné, 2021, "Glasses and glass–ceramics for biomedical applications," In Francesco Baino, Massimo Tomalino, and Dilshat Tulyaganov (eds), *Ceramics, Glass and Glass-Ceramics*, 153–201, Springer, Accessed: May 21, 2024. [Online]. Available: https://link.springer.com/chapter/10.1007/978-3-030-85776-9_5
8. B. Karmakar, 2017, *Functional glasses and glass-ceramics: processing, properties and applications.* Accessed: May 21, 2024. [Online]. Elsevier. Available: https://books.google.com/books?hl=en&lr=&id=T838DAAAQBAJ&oi=fnd&pg=PP1&dq=role+of+specific+oxides+in+glass+ceramic&ots=60dMfKXQVa&sig=UyuHOpj16KCqx3Lxi1jIoIk3hCU
9. H. Bach, and D. Krause, 2013, *Analysis of the composition and structure of glass and glass ceramics.* Accessed: May 21, 2024. [Online]. Springer Berlin Heidelberg. Available: https://books.google.com/books?hl=en&lr=&id=GgbtCAAAQBAJ&oi=fnd&pg=PA1&dq=role+of+specific+oxides+in+glass-ceramics+&ots=Ek11L1mF1Y&sig=_bx89s-c1vBNxTZ1b7eWccmZ2Nk
10. Z. Khurshid et al., 2018, "Novel techniques of scaffold fabrication for bioactive glasses," *Biomedical, Therapeutic and Clinical Applications of Bioactive Glasses*, Woodhead Publishing. pp. 497–519, doi: 10.1016/B978-0-08-102196-5.00018-5.
11. Y. Gao, M. A. Seles, and M. Rajan, 2023, "Role of bioglass derivatives in tissue regeneration and repair: a review," *Reviews on Advanced Materials Science*, vol. 62, no. 1, 20220318, https://doi.org/10.1515/rams-2022-0318.
12. T. Honma, K. Maeda, S. Nakane, and K. Shinozaki, 2022, "Unique properties and potential of glass-ceramics," *Journal of the Ceramic Society of Japan*, 62, 20220318. https://doi.org/10.2109/jcersj2.22037.
13. D. Arcos, and M. Vallet-Regí, 2010, "Sol-gel silica-based biomaterials and bone tissue regeneration," *Acta Biomater*, vol. 6, no. 8, pp. 2874–2888, doi: 10.1016/j.actbio.2010.02.012.
14. D. Bokov et al., 2021, "Nanomaterial by sol-gel method: synthesis and application," *Advances in Materials Science and Engineering*, vol. 2021, 5102014 doi: 10.1155/2021/5102014.
15. M. S. Shoushtari, D. Hoey, D. R. A. Biak, N. Abdullah, S. Kamarudin, and H. S. Zainuddin, 2024, "Sol–gel-templated bioactive glass scaffold: a review," *Research on Biomedical Engineering*, vol. 40, no. 1, pp. 281–296, https://doi.org/10.1007/s42600-024-00342-x.
16. S. Cetin, 2023, "Production of sintered glass-ceramic composites from low-cost materials," *Ceramics International*, vol. 49, no. 13, pp. 22386–22392, doi: 10.1016/J.CERAMINT.2023.04.068.
17. L. Fu, H. Engqvist, and W. Xia, 2020, "Glass-ceramics in dentistry: a review," *Materials*, vol. 13, no. 5, 1049doi: 10.3390/MA13051049.
18. N. B. Jordanov, I. Georgiev, and A. Karamanov, 2021, "Sintered glass-ceramics, self-glazed materials and foams from metallurgical waste slag," *Materials*, vol. 14, no. 9, doi: 10.3390/MA14092263.
19. L. L. Hench, 2011, "Glass and glass-ceramic technologies to transform the world," *International Journal of Applied Glass Science*, vol. 2, no. 3, pp. 162–176, doi: 10.1111/J.2041-1294.2011.00056.X.

20. M. Arango-Ospina, and A. R. Boccaccini, 2022, "Bioactive glasses and ceramics for tissue engineering," In Aldo R. Boccaccini, Peter X. Ma and Liliana Liverani (eds), *Tissue Engineering Using Ceramics and Polymers, Third Edition,* pp. 111–178, Woodhead Publishing Series in Biomaterials doi: 10.1016/B978-0-12-820508-2.00019-2.
21. M. Vallet-Regí, A. J. Salinas, and D. Arcos, 2016, "Tailoring the structure of bioactive glasses: from the nanoscale to macroporous scaffolds," *International Journal of Applied Glass Science*, vol. 7, no. 2, pp. 195–205, doi: 10.1111/IJAG.12205.
22. R. Kumar, I. Pattanayak, P. A. Dash, and S. Mohanty, 2023, "Bioceramics: a review on design concepts toward tailor-made (multi)-functional materials for tissue engineering applications," *Journal of Materials Science*, Springer, vol. 58, no. 8, pp. 3460–3484, doi: 10.1007/s10853-023-08226-8.
23. L. Hupa, and K. Karlsson, 2016, "Tailoring of bioactive glasses," In Aldo R Boccaccini; Delia S Brauer; Leena Hupa (eds), Accessed: May 21, 2024. [Online]. Royal Society of Chemistry. Available: https://books.rsc.org/books/edited-volume/710/chapter/417257
24. S. Punj, J. Singh, and K. Singh, 2021, "Ceramic biomaterials: properties, state of the art and future prospectives," *Ceramics International*, Elsevier, vol. 47, no. 20, pp. 28059–28074. Accessed: May 21, 2024. [Online]. Available: https://www.sciencedirect.com/science/article/pii/S0272884221019830
25. M. Giardino, D. Pugliese, and D. Janner, 2021, "Glass and glass–ceramic photonic materials for sensors," In Francesco Baino, Massimo Tomalino, Dilshat Tulyaganov (eds.), *Ceramics, Glass and Glass-Ceramics*, Springer, pp. 253–280, doi: 10.1007/978-3-030-85776-9_8.
26. J. Luo, and R. E.-Eitel, 2013, "A biocompatible low temperature co-fired ceramic substrate for biosensors," *Wiley Online Library*, vol. 11, no. 3, pp. 436–442, doi: 10.1111/ijac.12206.
27. T. H. Dang et al., 2020, "Characterization of bioactive glass synthesized by sol-gel process in hot water," *Crystals*, vol. 10, no. 6, p. 529, doi: 10.3390/CRYST10060529.
28. S. Ghosh, N. Dandapat, and V. K. Balla, 2015, "Preparation and in vitro characterization of fluroapatite based bioactive glass-ceramics for biomedical applications," *Materials Today: Proceedings*, vol. 2, no. 4–5, pp. 1326–1331, doi: 10.1016/J.MATPR.2015.07.050.
29. A. Boyde, E. Maconnachie, C. Muller-Mai, and U. Gross, 1990, "SEM study of surface alterations of bioactive glasses and glass-ceramics in a bony implantation bed," *Clinical Materials*, vol. 5, no. 1, pp. 73–88, doi: 10.1016/0267-6605(90)90073-5.
30. R. Ravarian, F. Moztarzadeh, M. S. Hashjin, S. M. Rabiee, P. Khoshakhlagh, and M. Tahriri, 2010, "Synthesis, characterization and bioactivity investigation of bioglass/hydroxyapatite composite," *Ceramics International*, vol. 36, no. 1, pp. 291–297, doi: 10.1016/J.CERAMINT.2009.09.016.
31. I. B. Leonor et al., 2002, "In situ study of partially crystallized bioglass and hydroxylapatite in vitro bioactivity using atomic force microscopy," *Journal of Biomedical Materials Research*, vol. 62, no. 1, pp. 82–88, doi: 10.1002/JBM.10289.

5 In Vivo and In Vitro Behaviours of Bioactive Glass Materials

Che Azurahanim Binti Che Abdullah, H. Jeevan Rao, Krina Goda, Kondaiah Gudimetla, Shakuntala Ojha and Teegala Divya

5.1 INTRODUCTION

Bioactive glasses have attracted considerable attention in the field of biomedical science due to their distinctive properties, including high biocompatibility and bioactivity [1]. These materials are capable of forming a bond with bone and other tissues, which makes them ideal for various medical applications [2]. The ability of bioactive glasses to interact positively with biological systems is largely attributed to their surface chemistry and ion release characteristics, which promote beneficial biological responses.

The primary objective of this chapter is to investigate the in vitro and in vivo behaviours of bioactive glass materials. By examining these behaviours, we aim to understand how these materials perform within different biological environments and how they can be optimized for specific medical applications. In vitro experiments provide initial insights into the material's bioactivity through simulated body fluid (SBF) immersion tests, focusing on surface reactions and ion release kinetics. These tests are critical for assessing the potential of bioactive glasses to form a hydroxyapatite (HA) layer, which is indicative of osteoconductivity.

In vivo studies, on the other hand, provide a more comprehensive understanding of how bioactive glasses interact with living tissues. These studies are conducted using animal models or clinical trials to evaluate biocompatibility, tissue integration, and HA layer formation under real physiological conditions. By comparing in vitro and in vivo data, we can better predict the clinical performance of bioactive glass materials as depicted in Figure 5.1.

This chapter also explores the implications of these findings for the design and optimization of bioactive glass compositions. Understanding the correlation between in vitro behaviour and in vivo performance is crucial for developing materials that can effectively support bone regeneration, dental restoration, and drug delivery

DOI: 10.1201/9781003660781-5

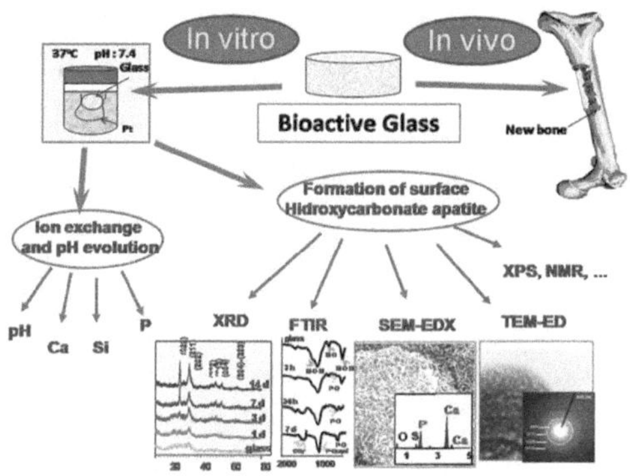

FIGURE 5.1 Different experimental techniques [3]

systems. Through this comprehensive analysis, we aim to highlight the potential of bioactive glasses as versatile biomaterials in the realms of regenerative medicine and tissue engineering.

5.2 IN VITRO BEHAVIOURS OF BIOACTIVE GLASSES

Bioactive glasses are a group of surface-reactive glass-ceramic biomaterials that are used in various medical applications due to their ability to bond with bone and soft tissues. There in vitro behaviours are crucial for understanding their potential effectiveness and safety in clinical applications.

5.2.1 Simulated Body Fluid Immersion Tests

Simulated body fluid (SBF) immersion tests are a fundamental method for evaluating the bioactivity of bioactive glasses. SBF is an aqueous solution with ionic concentrations nearly equal to those of human blood plasma. It serves as an artificial medium to replicate the biological environment in vitro. When bioactive glass materials are immersed in SBF, they undergo a series of surface reactions that are crucial for assessing their potential to form a bond with bone tissue [4].

The primary objective of SBF immersion tests is to observe the formation of a HA layer on the surface of the bioactive glass. HA is a calcium phosphate (Ca-P) mineral that is naturally present in bone, and its formation on the glass surface indicates the material's osteoconductivity. The process begins with the exchange of ions between the glass and the surrounding fluid, leading to the precipitation of HA.

To perform an SBF immersion test, bioactive glass samples are prepared and submerged in the SBF solution, which is maintained at a constant temperature, typically around 37°C, to mimic physiological conditions. The samples are periodically removed, rinsed, and analysed using various techniques such as X-ray diffraction (XRD), Fourier-transform infrared spectroscopy (FTIR), and scanning electron microscopy (SEM) to detect and characterize the formation of HA.

5.2.2 Surface Reactions and Ion Release Kinetics

The primary focus during SBF immersion tests is to monitor the surface reactions and ion release kinetics of the bioactive glasses. The dissolution process involves the release of ions such as calcium, phosphorus, and silicon, which are critical for subsequent biological interactions. The formation of a HA layer on the material's surface is a key indicator of bioactivity and is essential for bone-bonding ability [5].

5.2.2.1 Surface Reactions and Ion Release

1. **Dissolution Mechanisms**
   - **Ion Exchange and Surface Hydrolysis**: Upon immersion in SBF, bioactive glasses undergo ion exchange with the surrounding fluid, leading to the release of calcium, phosphorus, silicon, and other ions from the glass matrix.
   - **Surface Hydrolysis**: Water molecules penetrate the glass network, causing the cleavage of silicate bonds and the generation of silanol (Si-OH) groups on the glass surface.
2. **Ion Release Kinetics**

Monitoring the concentration of released ions over time allows for the characterization of ion release kinetics from bioactive glasses. The composition, structure, and surface area of the glass, as well as the pH and temperature of the immersion medium, influence the kinetics of ion release. Released calcium and phosphorus ions contribute to the formation of Ca-P phases, including HA, which is a major component of bone tissue. Silicon ions stimulate osteogenic differentiation of mesenchymal stem cells and enhance bone matrix mineralization, promoting bone regeneration and integration. The presence of released ions in the surrounding tissue microenvironment facilitates the nucleation and growth of HA crystals, promoting the mineralization of newly formed bone tissue. Osteoblasts and other bone-forming cells exhibit enhanced adhesion, proliferation, and differentiation in the presence of bioactive glass-derived ions. The presence of silanol groups on the bioactive glass surface facilitates the nucleation of HA crystals upon exposure to SBF. Calcium and phosphate ions released from the glass matrix participate in the precipitation and growth of HA crystals on the material's surface. The formation of a HA layer promotes osteoconduction, facilitating the direct bonding of the bioactive glass implant with surrounding bone tissue. The presence of a HA layer enhances the bio integration and stability of bioactive glass implants in vivo, promoting favourable tissue responses and long-term implant success. Measurement of calcium ion concentration in SBF solutions using atomic absorption spectroscopy (AAS) or inductively coupled plasma mass spectrometry (ICP-MS) quantifies the extent of ion release and bioactivity. Brunauer–Emmett–Teller (BET) analysis determines the surface area of bioactive glasses, influencing their reactivity and ion release kinetics.

5.2.3 Assessment of Bioactivity

The bioactivity of bioactive glasses is primarily governed by the surface reactions that occur when they are exposed to physiological fluids. These reactions include the rapid exchange of ions, such as calcium (Ca^{2+}), phosphate (PO_4^{3-}), and silicon (SiO_4^{4-}), between the glass and the surrounding environment [4]. The kinetics of ion release are crucial for understanding the material's behaviour and its ability to support tissue regeneration. Initially, rapid exchange of alkali ions (such as Na^+) from the glass with hydrogen ions (H^+) or hydronium ions (H_3O^+) from the solution, leading to the formation of a silica-rich layer. Hydrolysis of the silica network forms silanols (Si-OH), which then re-polymerize to form a gel-like silica layer on the glass surface. The silica layer serves as a template for the nucleation and growth of Ca-P clusters, eventually leading to the formation of an amorphous Ca-P layer. The amorphous Ca-P layer gradually transforms into a crystalline HA layer, mimicking the mineral phase of bone.

The rate of these reactions and the kinetics of ion release depend on the composition of the bioactive glass. For instance, glasses with higher silica content tend to form a more robust silica gel layer, while those with higher calcium content facilitate quicker HA formation. Monitoring the release of ions such as calcium and silicon using techniques like inductively coupled plasma optical emission spectrometry (ICP-OES) provides insights into the dissolution behaviour and bioactivity of the glass [5]. These in vitro assessments are crucial as they provide preliminary data on the bioactive potential of the glass, which is essential for predicting its performance in vivo. Understanding the surface reactions and ion release kinetics helps in designing bioactive glasses with optimized compositions for specific biomedical applications, such as bone regeneration and tissue engineering.

5.3 IN VIVO BEHAVIOURS OF BIOACTIVE GLASSES

Bioactive glasses exhibit several important behaviours in vivo that make them suitable for medical applications, particularly in bone repair and regeneration. These behaviours include bio integration, osteoconductive, osteoinductivity, and their impact on surrounding tissues and systemic responses. Understanding these in vivo behaviours is crucial for developing effective bioactive glass-based therapies.

5.3.1 Animal Models

In vivo studies using animal models are essential for understanding the biological performance of bioactive glasses. These studies provide insights into how these materials interact with living tissues, which cannot be fully replicated by in vitro experiments. Animal models are chosen based on the specific application being studied, with common choices including rats, rabbits, and larger animals like sheep or dogs for more complex assessments as illustrated in Figure 5.2.

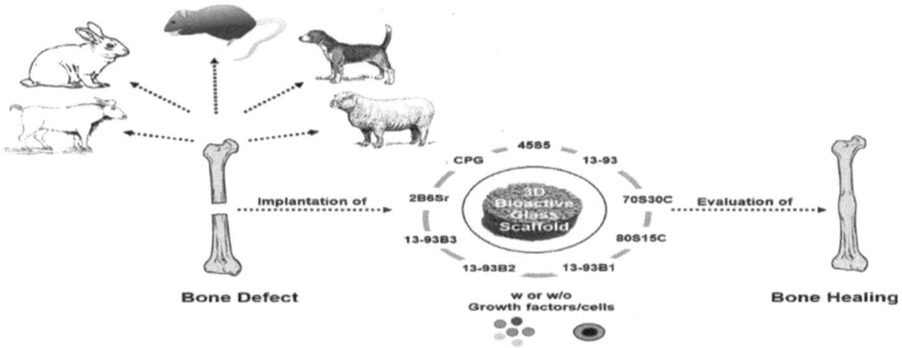

FIGURE 5.2 In vivo study [6]

5.3.1.1 Biocompatibility

Biocompatibility is a fundamental requirement for any biomaterial intended for medical use. In vivo biocompatibility tests assess the local and systemic reactions of the host organism to the bioactive glass. This includes evaluating any inflammatory responses, toxicity, or adverse effects that might arise from the material. Histological analyses are performed to examine the tissue surrounding the implanted bioactive glass, looking for signs of inflammation, fibrosis, or necrosis [7].

The initial immune response to the implanted bioactive glass involves the recruitment of neutrophils and macrophages to the site of implantation. These cells attempt to phagocytize the material, and their presence is a critical indicator of the body's immediate reaction. If the bioactive glass induces prolonged inflammation, it can lead to chronic inflammatory states characterized by the presence of macrophages, lymphocytes, and plasma cells. Chronic inflammation can impede healing and may lead to the development of granulomas. Histological analysis of the tissue surrounding the bioactive glass implant provides insight into how well the material integrates with the host tissue. This includes examining the formation of new tissue, the presence of any fibrous capsule, and the degree of vascularization. The tissue is also evaluated for pathological signs such as fibrosis (excessive formation of fibrous connective tissue), necrosis (death of tissue), and foreign body reactions. These adverse responses can indicate that the material is not well-tolerated.

Systemic toxicity is assessed by monitoring the function of vital organs, such as the liver, kidneys, and heart. Blood tests can reveal changes in biomarkers that indicate organ stress or damage. Evaluating the metabolic effects of the bioactive glass involves analysing blood chemistry and urine samples for any alterations that might suggest systemic toxicity. The production of antibodies against the bioactive glass is measured to determine if the material elicits an adaptive immune response. Elevated antibody levels can indicate that the material is recognized as foreign and potentially harmful. The activity of immune cells such as T-lymphocytes is also assessed, as these cells play a crucial role in mediating immune responses and maintaining immunological memory. Animal models, such as rodents or larger mammals, are commonly used for in vivo biocompatibility testing. The choice of model depends on the anatomical and physiological relevance to human biology.

Tissue samples are typically stained using hematoxylin and eosin (H&E) for general morphology, Masson's trichrome for collagen deposition, and specific immunohistochemical markers for identifying inflammatory cells and other relevant proteins. Blood and urine samples are analysed using biochemical assays to detect changes in levels of enzymes, electrolytes, and other markers indicative of organ function and systemic health. In vivo biocompatibility testing of bioactive glass involves a multifaceted approach to thoroughly evaluate the material's performance within a living organism. By assessing local tissue responses, systemic effects, and immune reactions, researchers can ensure that the bioactive glass is safe and effective for medical applications. This rigorous evaluation helps in identifying any potential risks and mitigating them before clinical use.

5.3.1.2 Tissue Integration

The ability of bioactive glass to integrate with host tissues is crucial for its effectiveness in applications such as bone regeneration. In vivo studies focus on the degree of integration between the bioactive glass and the surrounding tissue. This involves examining the formation of new tissue, such as bone or connective tissue, around the implant. Techniques such as micro-computed tomography (micro-CT) and histological staining are used to visualize and quantify tissue integration [8]. Micro-CT is a non-invasive imaging technique that offers a high-resolution, three-dimensional view of the implant and surrounding tissue. It allows researchers to visualize the extent of new bone growth and the density of the tissue interface. Here, tissue samples are extracted and meticulously treated with specialized dyes. These dyes highlight specific cell types and tissue structures. By examining these stained samples under a microscope, researchers can gain a deeper understanding of the quality and composition of the newly formed tissue at the implant site. This technique is referred to as histological staining. Successful integration of bioactive glass with host tissues is paramount for several reasons. A robust bond between the implant and surrounding tissue ensures the long-term stability and functionality of the implant. Bioactive glass can actively stimulate tissue growth, accelerating the healing process and promoting tissue regeneration. Seamless integration minimizes the risk of the body rejecting the implant, leading to fewer complications. The exceptional ability of bioactive glass to integrate with host tissues paves the way for significant advancements in regenerative medicine. By closely examining this integration process through in vivo studies and utilizing powerful techniques like micro-CT and histological staining, researchers can optimize the design and functionality of bioactive glass for promoting tissue repair and regeneration.

5.3.1.3 Osteoconductivity

Osteoconductivity refers to the ability of a material to support the growth of new bone along its surface. The formation of a HA layer on the bioactive glass is a key indicator of osteoconductivity. In vivo studies measure the extent and quality of new bone formation around the bioactive glass implants. This is typically assessed through histological examination and imaging techniques, which reveal the direct bonding of new bone to the HA layer formed on the glass surface [8, 9]. A crucial factor influencing osteoconductivity is the formation of a HA layer on the bioactive glass. HA, the main mineral component of natural bone, acts as a chemical bridge. It creates a surface that mimics natural bone, attracting bone-forming cells (osteoblasts) and facilitating their adhesion. This sets the stage for the magic of bone regeneration to unfold. To truly understand how effectively bioactive glass promotes bone growth, scientists conduct in vivo studies. These studies involve implanting the material within a living organism, allowing researchers to directly observe its interaction with bone tissue. Tiny tissue samples are extracted and meticulously stained with specialized dyes. When viewed under a microscope, these stained samples reveal the intricate details of the newly formed bone at the implant site. Researchers can assess the density, organization, and maturity of the new bone, providing valuable insights into the osteoconductive potential of the bioactive glass. Micro-CT scans offer a high-resolution, three-dimensional view of the implant and surrounding tissue. This allows researchers to quantify the amount of new bone growth and analyse the interface between the implant and the newly formed bone.

The ability of new bone to directly bond to the HA layer formed on the bioactive glass surface is a critical indicator of successful osteoconduction. This strong connection ensures the long-term stability and functionality of the implant, promoting a seamless integration between the artificial and natural bone. By understanding the intricate link between osteoconductivity, HA formation, and in vivo studies, researchers can refine bioactive glass to create even more effective bone regeneration solutions. This paves the way for faster healing, improved bone repair outcomes, and ultimately, a brighter future for patients suffering from bone defects and injuries.

5.3.2 Clinical Trials

Clinical trials are the final step in evaluating the performance of bioactive glasses in human applications. These trials are designed to assess the safety and efficacy of the material in real-world medical settings, building on the data obtained from in vitro and animal studies. Clinical trials don't exist in isolation. They rely heavily on the insights gleaned from previous stages of research. In vitro studies, conducted in a controlled laboratory environment, provide a fundamental understanding of how bioactive glass interacts with cells and tissues. Animal studies, where the material is implanted in living organisms, offer valuable data on its biocompatibility and preliminary effectiveness in promoting bone growth or tissue regeneration. The primary objective of clinical trials involving bioactive glass is to ensure patient safety. Researchers meticulously monitor participants for any adverse reactions or complications that might arise from the material. This data is crucial for determining the safe dosage, application method, and potential side effects of bioactive glass. Beyond safety, clinical trials also rigorously assess the effectiveness of bioactive glass in achieving its intended purpose. This could involve evaluating its ability to:

- Promote bone growth in patients with fractures or bone defects.
- Facilitate tissue repair in cases of chronic wounds or surgical procedures.
- Provide structural support and stability in orthopaedic applications.

Clinical trials are not merely a final hurdle; they are a vital stepping stone for bioactive glass to reach its full potential. The data obtained from these trials paves the way for regulatory approval, allowing this innovative material to be used in real-world medical settings and potentially improve the lives of countless patients.

5.3.2.1 Safety and Biocompatibility

Clinical trials begin with assessing the safety and biocompatibility of bioactive glasses in human subjects. This involves monitoring patients for any adverse reactions or complications associated with the use of the material. Blood tests, imaging, and other diagnostic tools are used to detect any systemic effects or local reactions at the implantation site.

5.3.2.1.1 Multifaceted Safety Net: Monitoring for Adverse Events

The cornerstone of safety evaluation lies in comprehensive monitoring of human subjects for any adverse reactions or complications associated with the bioactive glass implant. Researchers employ a multi-pronged approach: Throughout the trial, participants undergo regular physical examinations to detect any potential signs or symptoms of adverse events, such as inflammation, pain, or infection at the implantation site. Blood tests are routinely conducted to assess for systemic effects, monitoring for changes in complete blood count, inflammatory markers, or organ function that might indicate a negative response to the bioactive glass. Depending on the application, advanced imaging modalities like X-rays, CT scans, or MRIs can be used to visualize the implant site and surrounding tissues. This allows for the detection of any local reactions like unexpected bone resorption, implant loosening, or soft tissue abnormalities. Particular attention is paid to the area surrounding the implant. Researchers closely monitor for signs of infection, inflammation, or tissue necrosis at the implantation site. Biopsies may be performed in specific cases to obtain a deeper understanding of the tissue response to the bioactive glass. Blood tests and other diagnostic tools are used to detect any potential widespread effects of the bioactive glass on the body. This includes monitoring for immune responses, changes in organ function, or the presence of any bioactive glass particles in the bloodstream.

5.3.2.1.2 A Data-Driven Approach to Safety

By meticulously collecting and analysing data from clinical observations, laboratory testing, and imaging techniques, researchers can establish a comprehensive safety profile for bioactive glass in humans. This data is instrumental in determining the safe dosage, application method, and potential side effects associated with the material. Furthermore, it allows for the identification of any at-risk patient populations who might require specific precautions when using bioactive glass implants. The safety assessment within clinical trials plays a critical role in ensuring the responsible translation of innovative bioactive glass technologies into mainstream medical practice. By prioritizing patient safety, researchers pave the way for the safe and effective utilization of bioactive glass in improving human health.

5.3.2.2 Efficacy in Medical Applications

The primary focus of clinical trials is to evaluate the efficacy of bioactive glasses in their intended medical applications, such as bone regeneration, dental restoration, or drug delivery. For bone regeneration, this might include measuring the rate of bone healing and the quality of the new bone formed. In dental applications, trials assess the durability and performance of bioactive glass-based restorations.

5.3.2.2.1 Bone Regeneration

Clinical trials aim to determine the rate and extent of bone healing when bioactive glass is used as a scaffold or filler in bone defects. This involves assessing the integration of the material with host bone and the quality of the new bone formed. The trials focus on the microarchitecture, density, and mechanical properties of the newly formed bone to ensure it is comparable to native bone. Imaging techniques such as X-rays, CT scans, and MRI are used to monitor the progression of bone healing. These modalities provide detailed insights into the morphology and volume of new bone formation. Histomorphometry involves the microscopic examination of bone tissue samples to quantify parameters such as bone volume fraction, trabecular thickness, and osteoid formation. Biomechanical Testing of bone samples assesses the strength and resilience of the regenerated bone, ensuring it can withstand physiological loads.

5.3.2.2.2 Dental Restoration

Clinical trials evaluate the performance of bioactive glass-based dental restorations, focusing on their ability to withstand masticatory forces over time. The trials also assess the material's compatibility with oral tissues and its aesthetic properties, ensuring it blends well with natural teeth. Dental restorations are examined at regular intervals for signs of wear, fracture, or failure. Standardized indices such as the United States Public Health Service (USPHS) criteria are often used. Surveys and questionnaires are administered to gather patient feedback on comfort, satisfaction, and any adverse symptoms. Microleakage studies involving dye penetration tests to assess the sealing ability of restorations, preventing the ingress of bacteria and fluids that could lead to secondary caries.

5.3.2.2.3 Drug Delivery

Trials aim to demonstrate the ability of bioactive glass to deliver drugs at a controlled and sustained rate, maintaining therapeutic levels over a desired period. The effectiveness of the drug delivery system is evaluated in terms of achieving the desired pharmacological response while minimizing side effects. Blood samples are analysed to determine the concentration of the drug over time, providing data on absorption, distribution, metabolism, and excretion. The clinical effects of the drug, such as reduction in symptoms or biomarkers, are measured to correlate with the drug release profiles. Tissue samples are examined to assess the local effects of the drug-loaded bioactive glass, ensuring there is no adverse tissue reaction.

5.3.2.3 Long-Term Performance

The long-term performance of bioactive glasses is critical for their success in clinical applications. Clinical trials monitor the durability and stability of the material over extended periods. This includes assessing the long-term integration with host tissues and the maintenance of the material's bioactive properties. Follow-up studies and patient monitoring provide valuable data on the longevity and reliability of bioactive glass implants [10].

Clinical trials involve longitudinal studies to evaluate how bioactive glasses withstand physiological conditions over the years. This includes measuring degradation rates, resistance to mechanical wear, and structural integrity under cyclic loading conditions that mimic normal bodily movements. A key indicator of bioactive glass performance is its ability to form stable bonds with surrounding tissues. This is assessed through examining tissue samples at various intervals to observe the interface between the bioactive glass and host tissues, looking for signs of successful osteointegration or integration with dental tissues and utilizing advanced imaging methods such as micro-CT, MRI, and electron microscopy to visualize and quantify the extent of integration and detect any signs of detachment or degradation. It is crucial that bioactive glasses maintain their ability to stimulate cellular responses and promote tissue regeneration. Long-term studies on the ability of the glass to form a hydroxycarbonate apatite (HCA) layer on the surface is indicative of bioactivity, in physiological conditions. Whereas, in vitro and in vivo assays evaluate sustained cellular proliferation, differentiation, and extracellular matrix production in the presence of bioactive glass. Participants with bioactive glass implants are monitored over the years to gather comprehensive data on the performance and safety of the material. This includes regular clinical evaluations, imaging studies, and patient-reported outcomes to assess pain, functionality, and overall satisfaction. Monitoring for any long-term complications, such as chronic inflammation, infection, or adverse immune responses. Assessing the functional improvements in terms of mobility, strength, and quality of life for orthopaedic applications, or restoration longevity and comfort in dental applications.

5.3.3 Hydroxyapatite Layer Formation

The formation of a HA layer on the surface of bioactive glasses is a crucial factor in evaluating in vivo performance. This layer facilitates the bonding between the material and bone tissue, enhancing the healing process and ensuring the stability of the implant. In vivo studies focus on the kinetics and quality of HA formation, which are influenced by the composition and surface properties of the bioactive glass.

5.3.3.1 Hydroxyapatite Formation kinetics

When bioactive glasses are exposed to physiological fluids, a series of ion exchange reactions occur at the material's surface. This leads to the release of soluble silica and other ions such as calcium and phosphate, which subsequently precipitate to form a Ca-P-rich layer. This layer then crystallizes into HA, mimicking the mineral phase of natural bone. The rate at which HA forms on the surface of bioactive glasses is a key focus in in vivo studies. This involves measuring. Assessing the early stages of ion release and layer formation using techniques like inductively coupled plasma (ICP) spectroscopy and surface analytical methods such as X-ray photoelectron spectroscopy (XPS) and secondary ion mass spectrometry (SIMS). Determining the time required for the amorphous Ca-P layer to crystallize into HA, using XRD and Fourier-transform infrared spectroscopy (FTIR).

The quality of the HA layer is assessed by employing SEM and transmission electron microscopy (TEM) to observe the surface topography and crystalline structure of the formed HA layer. And use of energy-dispersive X-ray spectroscopy (EDS) and Raman spectroscopy analyse the elemental composition and confirm the presence of HA. Evaluating the bond strength between the HA layer and the underlying bioactive glass substrate is crucial. This is typically measured using mechanical testing methods such as tensile and shear tests to ensure the HA layer can withstand physiological loads.

5.3.3.2 Quality of the Hydroxyapatite Layer

The quality of the HA layer is assessed through various characterization techniques, such as XRD and SEM. A high-quality HA layer is characterized by its crystallinity, thickness, and uniformity. These properties are crucial for ensuring strong and stable bonding between the bioactive glass and the surrounding bone tissue (Figure 5.3).

5.3.3.2.1 Translating In Vitro to In Vivo Success

The translation of promising in vitro results into successful clinical outcomes requires thorough in vivo validation. In vitro experiments provide initial insights into the bioactivity and compatibility of bioactive glasses, but in vivo studies are essential to confirm these findings under complex physiological conditions. By systematically evaluating biocompatibility, tissue integration, and HA layer formation in vivo, researchers can refine the composition and design of bioactive glasses to maximize their clinical efficacy.

5.4 CORRELATION BETWEEN IN VITRO AND IN VIVO BEHAVIOURS

Understanding the correlation between in vitro and in vivo performance of bioactive glass materials is essential for optimizing their design and application in biomedical fields. By linking the results obtained from in vitro experiments with the observations from in vivo studies, researchers can better predict the clinical outcomes and effectiveness of these materials.

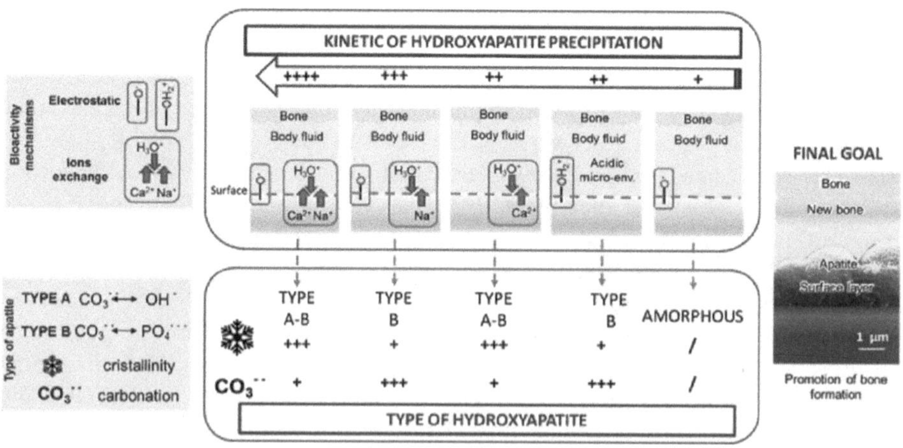

FIGURE 5.3 Hydroxyapatite formation [11]

5.4.1 Biocompatibility and Tissue Integration

5.4.1.1 In Vitro Biocompatibility

In vitro biocompatibility tests represent a critical initial phase in evaluating the potential of bioactive glasses for medical applications. These tests are designed to assess how cells interact with bioactive glass materials, providing essential insights into their cytocompatibility. The primary parameters measured include cell viability, proliferation, and differentiation. Several well-established techniques are employed to obtain these measurements.

The MTT assay is a colorimetric assay that measures cellular metabolic activity as an indicator of cell viability. In this test, cells cultured with bioactive glass extracts or directly on bioactive glass surfaces are exposed to MTT reagent, which is metabolized by mitochondrial enzymes in living cells to form a purple formazan product. Cells are incubated with MTT reagent for a specified period, after which the formazan product is solubilized and quantified using a spectrophotometer. The absorbance correlates with the number of viable cells. This technique uses fluorescent dyes to distinguish between live and dead cells. Live cells are stained with calcein-AM, which produces green fluorescence, while dead cells are stained with ethidium homodimer-1, resulting in red fluorescence. Fluorescence microscopy is used to capture images of the stained cells. Quantitative analysis is performed by counting the green (live) and red (dead) cells to calculate cell viability.

Direct counting of cells using a hemocytometer or automated cell counter after detaching cells from the bioactive glass surface or collecting cells from culture media. This method provides a straightforward measure of cell proliferation over time. Techniques such as BrdU (bromodeoxyuridine) incorporation or EdU (5-ethynyl-2′-deoxyuridine) assays, which measure DNA synthesis in proliferating cells. Cells incorporating BrdU or EdU are detected using specific antibodies or fluorescent tags, respectively. For applications in bone regeneration, the ability of bioactive glasses to promote osteogenic differentiation is crucial. This is typically assessed by measuring markers such as alkaline phosphatase (ALP) activity, calcium deposition, and the expression of osteogenic genes. Cells cultured with bioactive glasses are lysed, and the ALP activity is quantified using a colorimetric substrate that produces a measurable product. Staining techniques like Alizarin Red S staining are used to detect and quantify mineralized calcium deposits produced by differentiating osteoblasts.

This technique is used to analyse cell populations for specific markers of viability, proliferation, and differentiation. Cells are labelled with fluorescent antibodies or dyes and passed through a flow cytometer, which measures the fluorescence intensity and provides data on the expression of specific proteins or cellular states. Flow cytometry allows for the simultaneous measurement of multiple parameters, providing a comprehensive profile of cell behaviour in response to bioactive glass materials. Quantitative PCR (qPCR) and RNA sequencing are employed to measure the expression levels of genes associated with cell viability, proliferation, and differentiation. These molecular techniques provide insights into the underlying biological processes influenced by bioactive glass materials. RNA sequencing offers a global view of the cellular response, identifying key regulatory pathways activated or suppressed by the bioactive glass. By employing these in vitro biocompatibility tests, researchers can obtain a detailed understanding of how bioactive glass materials interact with cells. This information is critical for predicting in vivo performance and optimizing the design of bioactive glasses for specific medical applications. Successful in vitro results are a prerequisite for advancing bioactive glass materials to in vivo studies and subsequent clinical trials.

5.4.1.2 In Vivo Biocompatibility

In vivo biocompatibility testing extends the evaluation of bioactive glass implants to a complex biological environment, offering a comprehensive understanding of the material's interactions within a living organism. These tests are pivotal for validating in vitro findings and ensuring the material's safety and compatibility with living tissues. Animal models are commonly employed to observe the host response to bioactive glass implants, providing critical insights into various biological reactions and integration processes. Animal models, such as rodents, rabbits, or larger mammals, are chosen based on their anatomical and physiological similarities to humans. The selection is crucial for ensuring the relevance and translatability of the findings to clinical applications. Different models may be selected depending on the specific medical application of the bioactive glass, such as bone regeneration, dental restoration, or soft tissue integration. The initial host response to bioactive glass implantation involves the recruitment of immune cells, such as neutrophils and macrophages, to the site. This acute inflammatory phase is monitored to assess the immediate reaction and the material's immunogenicity. Prolonged inflammation is a critical parameter, as it can lead to chronic inflammatory states characterized by the continuous presence of macrophages, lymphocytes, and foreign body giant cells. Persistent inflammation can impede healing and lead to adverse outcomes.

The formation of a fibrous capsule around the implant is evaluated. Excessive fibrosis can indicate a negative reaction, as it can isolate the implant from surrounding tissues, impairing its integration and function. Histological staining techniques, such as Masson's trichrome, are used to quantify collagen deposition and assess the extent of fibrotic tissue formation.

5.4.1.3 Correlating In Vitro and In Vivo Data

Correlating in vitro and in vivo biocompatibility data involves comparing cell responses observed in laboratory settings with tissue responses in animal models. Consistencies in cell viability, minimal inflammatory reactions, and healthy tissue integration across both settings strengthen the confidence in the material's suitability for clinical applications. Discrepancies highlight areas needing further investigation and optimization. Correlating in vitro and in vivo biocompatibility data is crucial for validating the performance and safety of bioactive glass materials and for predicting their clinical outcomes. This process involves a detailed comparison of cellular responses observed in controlled laboratory settings with tissue responses in animal models. Establishing consistencies between these two types of studies reinforces the material's suitability for clinical applications, while discrepancies can identify areas requiring further investigation and optimization.

5.4.1.3.1 Comparative Analysis

1. **Cell Viability and Proliferation**: In vitro assays such as MTT, live/dead staining, and cell counting provide initial data on cell viability and proliferation when exposed to bioactive glass extracts or surfaces.
    - **In Vivo Correlation**: These in vitro results are compared with histological and immunohistochemical analyses of tissue samples from animal models. Metrics such as cell density, tissue morphology, and presence of viable, proliferating cells in the tissue surrounding the implant site are examined.
    - **Consistency**: Consistent findings of high cell viability and proliferation in both in vitro and in vivo studies indicate the bioactive glass's favourable biocompatibility.
2. **Inflammatory Response**: In vitro studies measure the expression of inflammatory markers and cytokines released by cells in response to bioactive glass.
    - **In Vivo Correlation**: These markers are compared with in vivo data, including histopathological assessments of inflammatory cell infiltration and cytokine profiling in tissues around the implant. Reduced inflammation in both settings suggests a low immunogenicity of the material.
    - **Consistency**: Minimal inflammatory responses observed in vitro and in vivo confirm the material's compatibility with biological systems.
3. **Tissue Integration and Differentiation**: In vitro differentiation assays (e.g., osteogenic differentiation of stem cells) provide insights into the material's potential to support tissue-specific cell differentiation.
    - **In Vivo Correlation**: These findings are correlated with in vivo evidence of new tissue formation, integration, and functional outcomes, such as bone-implant contact (BIC) and mechanical stability.
    - **Consistency**: Successful differentiation and integration observed in both settings suggest the material's effectiveness in promoting tissue regeneration and integration.

5.4.1.3.2 Identifying Discrepancies

Any inconsistencies between in vitro and in vivo data highlight areas needing further investigation. For instance, if in vitro studies show high cell viability but in vivo studies indicate significant inflammation or poor integration, additional factors influencing the in vivo environment must be considered. Discrepancies may arise from differences in surface properties of bioactive glass when transitioning from in vitro to in vivo environments. Surface modifications or coatings might be necessary to enhance in vivo performance. Variations in ion release kinetics between in vitro and in vivo conditions can affect cellular responses. In vivo conditions often involve dynamic fluid flow and complex interactions with body fluids that are not fully replicated in vitro.

Addressing discrepancies involves refining the bioactive glass composition, surface treatments, and fabrication techniques to enhance compatibility and performance in vivo. Modifying the ratios of silicon, calcium, and other constituents in the bioactive glass can improve its biological interactions and degradation behaviour. Techniques such as surface roughening, coating with bioactive molecules, or creating specific topographies can enhance cell adhesion, proliferation, and integration in vivo.

5.4.2 Hydroxyapatite Layer Formation

5.4.2.1 In Vitro Hydroxyapatite Formation

In vitro studies using SBF immersion tests provide insights into the bioactivity of bioactive glasses by examining the formation of a HA layer on their surfaces. Techniques such as XRD, FTIR, and SEM are used to detect and characterize the HA. The rate of formation, as well as the quality and thickness of the HA layer, are key indicators of the material's osteoconductivity.

5.4.2.1.1 Simulated Body Fluid Immersion Tests

Preparation and Procedure

- **Simulated Body Fluid**: SBF is an aqueous solution with ion concentrations similar to those of human blood plasma. It is prepared following established protocols to ensure consistency and reproducibility in testing.
- **Immersion Process**: Bioactive glass samples are immersed in SBF at 37°C, typically for varying periods ranging from a few hours to several weeks. The solution is periodically refreshed to maintain constant ion concentrations.
- **Monitoring**: The immersion process is monitored to observe the formation and growth of the HA layer on the bioactive glass surface.

Characterization Techniques

1. **X-ray Diffraction**
    - **Phase Identification**: XRD is used to identify crystalline phases present on the surface of bioactive glass after immersion in SBF. The appearance of characteristic peaks corresponding to HA confirms its formation.
    - **Crystallinity**: The degree of crystallinity of the HA layer is assessed, as higher crystallinity often correlates with better biological performance and mechanical properties.
2. **Fourier-Transform Infrared Spectroscopy**
    - **Chemical Composition**: FTIR provides information on the chemical bonds and functional groups present in the HA layer. The presence of phosphate (PO_4^{3-}) and hydroxyl (OH^-) groups is indicative of HA formation.
    - **Structural Analysis**: FTIR spectra can reveal the structural similarities between the formed HA layer and natural bone mineral, providing insights into the quality of the HA.
3. **Scanning Electron Microscopy**
    - **Morphological Analysis**: SEM is employed to visualize the surface morphology of the bioactive glass after SBF immersion. High-resolution images reveal the topographical features and uniformity of the HA layer.

- **Thickness Measurement**: Cross-sectional SEM analysis can be used to measure the thickness of the HA layer, which is critical for evaluating the extent of bioactivity.
- **Elemental Analysis**: EDS, often coupled with SEM, provides elemental composition data, confirming the presence of calcium (Ca) and phosphorus (P) in the correct ratios for HA.

5.4.2.1.2 Key Indicators of Osteoconductivity

1. **Rate of Formation**
   - **Kinetics**: The rate at which the HA layer forms on the bioactive glass surface is a crucial indicator of bioactivity. Faster formation rates suggest higher bioactivity and better potential for promoting bone regeneration.
2. **Quality of the Hydroxyapatite Layer**
   - **Crystallinity and Purity**: High-quality HA layers are characterized by high crystallinity and purity, which are essential for optimal biological performance.
   - **Structural Integrity**: The structural integrity of the HA layer, including its ability to withstand mechanical stresses without degradation, is important for its functionality in vivo.
3. **Thickness of the Hydroxyapatite Layer**
   - **Uniformity and Coverage**: A uniform and adequately thick HA layer covering the entire bioactive glass surface ensures consistent bioactivity and effective bonding with bone tissue.
   - **Functional Thickness**: The thickness of the HA layer should be sufficient to provide a conducive environment for cell attachment and proliferation, but not so thick as to impede the material's mechanical properties.

In vitro HA formation studies using SBF immersion tests are fundamental for evaluating the bioactivity of bioactive glasses. Techniques such as XRD, FTIR, and SEM are employed to detect and characterize the HA layer formed on the material's surface. Key indicators of osteoconductivity include the rate of HA formation, and the quality and thickness of the HA layer. These studies provide essential data that help optimize the composition and design of bioactive glasses for effective bone regeneration and other medical applications.

5.4.2.2 In Vivo Hydroxyapatite Formation

In vivo, the formation of a HA layer on bioactive glass implants is assessed through histological and imaging techniques. The presence of HA on the material surface, along with new bone growth around the implant, signifies successful integration and osteoconductivity. The quality and uniformity of the HA layer are critical for ensuring strong bonding between the implant and bone tissue.

5.4.2.2.1 Assessment Techniques

1. **Histological Analysis**
   - **Tissue Sampling**: Tissue samples from around the implant site are collected at various time points post-implantation. These samples are processed and stained to visualize the bone-implant interface.

- **Staining Methods:** Common staining methods include H&E for general tissue structure, Masson's Trichrome for collagen and bone matrix, and Von Kossa or Alizarin Red for mineralized tissue.
- **Histomorphometry:** Quantitative histological techniques measure parameters such as new bone area, BIC, and HA layer thickness. These metrics are critical for assessing the extent and quality of HA formation and bone integration.

2. **Imaging Techniques**
   - **X-ray Microtomography (Micro-CT)**
     - **3D Visualization**: Micro-CT provides high-resolution, three-dimensional images of the implant and surrounding bone, allowing for detailed analysis of bone architecture and density.
     - **Quantitative Analysis**: Micro-CT scan quantify bone volume, trabecular thickness, and other parameters that indicate the degree of bone regeneration and integration with the bioactive glass.
   - **Scanning Electron Microscopy**
     - **Surface Morphology**: SEM is used to examine the surface morphology of explanted bioactive glass. It reveals the presence and uniformity of the HA layer, as well as the microstructural details of the bone-implant interface.
     - **Elemental Composition**: EDS coupled with SEM provides elemental analysis, confirming the presence of calcium and phosphorus indicative of HA.
   - **Transmission Electron Microscopy**
     - **Nanoscale Analysis**: TEM offers insights into the ultrastructural organization of the HA layer and the bone-implant interface at the nanoscale level, providing detailed information on crystallinity and bonding characteristics.

5.4.2.2.2 Indicators of Successful HA Formation

1. **Presence of Hydroxyapatite**
   - **Detection**: The formation of HA on the surface of the bioactive glass implant is confirmed through imaging and histological staining. The presence of characteristic mineral deposits around the implant site indicates bioactivity.
   - **Integration**: Successful integration is marked by the seamless transition between the HA layer and newly formed bone, with no significant gaps or fibrotic tissue intervening.

2. **New Bone Growth**
   - **Osteoconductivity**: The ability of the bioactive glass to support new bone growth is a direct measure of its osteoconductivity. Histological and imaging studies assess the extent and quality of new bone formation around the implant.
   - **Bone-Implant Contact**: High levels of direct BIC are indicative of strong bonding and effective integration. This contact is essential for the mechanical stability of the implant.

3. **Quality and Uniformity of Hydroxyapatite Layer**
   - **Crystallinity**: High crystallinity of the HA layer is crucial for mimicking the mineral phase of natural bone and ensuring optimal mechanical properties.
   - **Uniformity and Coverage**: A uniform HA layer with consistent thickness across the implant surface ensures comprehensive bioactivity and effective bonding with the host bone tissue.

In vivo assessment of HA formation on bioactive glass implants is a critical step in validating their efficacy and biocompatibility. Advanced histological and imaging techniques, such as histomorphometry, micro-CT, SEM, and TEM, provide comprehensive insights into the presence, quality, and uniformity of the HA layer. The successful formation of HA and new bone growth around the implant signify effective osteoconductivity and integration, ensuring strong bonding between the bioactive glass and bone tissue. These in vivo evaluations are essential for optimizing bioactive glass materials for clinical applications in bone regeneration and other medical fields.

5.4.3 Ion Release Kinetics

5.4.3.1 In Vitro Ion Release

In vitro ion release studies involve immersing bioactive glasses in SBF or other relevant solutions and measuring the concentrations of released ions over time. Techniques like ICP-OES are used to quantify the release of key ions such as calcium, phosphate, and silicon. The kinetics of ion release are important for understanding the material's dissolution behaviour and subsequent bioactivity.

5.4.3.1.1 Experimental Procedure

1. **Preparation of Bioactive Glass Samples**
   - **Sample Selection**: Bioactive glass samples are prepared in various forms, such as powders, pellets, or thin films, depending on the specific study requirements.
   - **Surface Area Considerations**: The surface area of the samples is carefully measured as it influences the rate of ion release.
2. **Immersion in Simulated Body Fluid**
   - **Solution Composition**: SBF is prepared to mimic the ionic composition of human blood plasma, ensuring that the experimental conditions closely replicate physiological environments.
   - **Immersion Conditions**: Bioactive glass samples are immersed in SBF at 37°C, with the solution typically refreshed periodically to maintain constant ionic concentrations.
3. **Measurement of Ion Release**
   - **Time Points**: Samples of the immersion solution are collected at various time points, ranging from a few hours to several days or weeks, to monitor the kinetics of ion release.
   - **Quantification Techniques**: Inductively ICP-OES is commonly used to quantify the concentrations of released ions such as calcium (Ca^{2+}), phosphate (PO_4^{3-}), and silicon (Si^{4+}).

5.4.3.1.2 *Analytical Techniques*

1. **Inductively Coupled Plasma Optical Emission Spectrometry**
   - **Principle**: ICP-OES involves ionizing the sample solution with an inductively coupled plasma and measuring the emitted light at specific wavelengths corresponding to the ions of interest.
   - **Quantification**: This technique provides precise and accurate measurements of ion concentrations, allowing for detailed analysis of the dissolution behaviour of bioactive glasses.
2. **Complementary Techniques**
   - **Atomic Absorption Spectroscopy**: Sometimes used alongside ICP-OES for cross-validation of ion concentration data.
   - **Ion Chromatography (IC)**: Can be employed for the separation and quantification of specific ions in the solution.

5.4.3.1.3 *Kinetics of Ion Release*

1. **Initial Burst Release**
   - **Surface Dissolution**: The initial stage of ion release often involves a burst release of ions from the bioactive glass surface. This is attributed to the rapid dissolution of the surface layer when first exposed to SBF.
   - **Bioactivity Indication**: A significant initial release of calcium and phosphate ions is indicative of the glass's bioactivity, as these ions play a critical role in the formation of HA.
2. **Sustained Release**
   - **Controlled Dissolution**: Following the initial burst, the ion release typically transitions to a more controlled, sustained release phase. This phase is influenced by the glass composition and the network connectivity of the material.
   - **Long-term Behaviour**: The sustained release of silicon and other ions supports ongoing biological processes such as angiogenesis and osteogenesis over extended periods.
3. **Factors Influencing Ion Release**
   - **Glass Composition**: The specific composition of the bioactive glass, including the types and proportions of constituent oxides, significantly affects the rate and pattern of ion release.
   - **pH and Ionic Strength of Solution**: The pH and ionic strength of the SBF or other immersion solutions can alter the dissolution kinetics, impacting the overall bioactivity of the material.
   - **Surface Area and Porosity**: The physical characteristics of the bioactive glass, including surface area and porosity, influence the rate at which ions are released into the solution.

In vitro ion release studies provide critical data on the dissolution behaviour and bioactivity of bioactive glasses. By immersing bioactive glass samples in SBF and measuring the concentrations of released ions over time using techniques such as ICP-OES, researchers can gain valuable insights into the kinetics of ion release. This information is essential for understanding how bioactive glasses interact with biological environments, predicting their performance in vivo, and optimizing their compositions for various medical applications.

5.4.3.2 In Vivo Ion Release

In vivo, the release of ions from bioactive glass implants into the surrounding tissues and fluids is monitored to understand their role in promoting tissue regeneration and healing. The ionic composition of local biological fluids and tissues is analysed to detect any changes induced by the bioactive glass. These studies help in assessing the biological impact of ion release and its contribution to the overall performance of the implant.

5.4.3.2.1 Monitoring Ion Release In Vivo

1. **Implantation and Sample Collection**
   - **Animal Models**: Bioactive glass implants are typically evaluated in appropriate animal models, such as rodents, rabbits, or larger mammals, depending on the study's objectives and relevance to human physiology.
   - **Implantation Sites**: The bioactive glass can be implanted in various anatomical locations, such as bone defects, dental sites, or soft tissue, to study its specific application.
   - **Sampling Intervals**: Biological fluids (e.g., blood, serum, interstitial fluid) and tissue samples are collected at predefined time points post-implantation to monitor ion release over time.
2. **Quantification of Released Ions**
   - **Analytical Techniques**: Techniques such as inductively ICP-OES, ICP-MS, and AAS are used to measure the concentrations of key ions, including calcium (Ca^{2+}), phosphate (PO_4^{3-}), and silicon (Si^{4+}).
   - **Localization**: Spatial analysis of ion concentrations within different tissue compartments helps in understanding the diffusion and distribution of released ions.

5.4.3.2.2 Biological Impact of Ion Release

1. **Tissue Regeneration and Healing**
   - **Osteogenesis**: The release of calcium and phosphate ions from bioactive glass implants supports the formation of new bone by providing essential building blocks for HA formation and stimulating osteoblast activity.
   - **Angiogenesis**: Silicon ions have been shown to promote angiogenesis, the formation of new blood vessels, which is critical for supplying nutrients and oxygen to regenerating tissues.
2. **Modulation of Cellular Activity**
   - **Cell Proliferation and Differentiation**: Released ions can influence the behaviour of various cell types, including osteoblasts, fibroblasts, and endothelial cells, enhancing their proliferation and differentiation.
   - **Inflammatory Response**: The ionic environment created by the dissolution of bioactive glass can modulate the inflammatory response, potentially reducing chronic inflammation and promoting a conducive environment for healing.

5.4.3.2.3 Analysis of Biological Fluids and Tissues

1. **Ionic Composition Analysis**
   - **Fluid Analysis**: The ionic composition of local biological fluids, such as blood plasma or interstitial fluid, is analysed to detect changes induced by the bioactive glass implant. This includes measuring the concentrations of calcium, phosphate, silicon, and other relevant ions.
   - **Tissue Analysis**: Tissue samples from the implant site are analysed for ion content and distribution. Techniques such as EDS coupled with SEM provide detailed elemental analysis.
2. **Histological and Histochemical Studies**
   - **Histological Staining**: Techniques such as H&E staining, Masson's Trichrome, and Von Kossa staining are used to visualize tissue structure, collagen deposition, and mineralization, respectively.
   - **Histochemical Analysis**: Immunohistochemical staining for markers of osteogenesis (e.g., osteocalcin, osteopenia) and angiogenesis (e.g., CD31, VEGF) provides insights into the biological processes influenced by ion release.

5.4.3.2.4 Assessing Implant Performance

1. **Integration and Bonding**
   - **Bone-Implant Interface**: The quality of the bond between the bioactive glass implant and the surrounding bone is assessed through histomorphometric analysis and imaging techniques. A strong, continuous bond is indicative of successful integration.
   - **Mechanical Stability**: The mechanical properties of the regenerated tissue and the implant's ability to withstand physiological loads are evaluated through mechanical testing and finite element analysis.
2. **Long-Term Effects**
   - **Sustained Ion Release**: Long-term studies monitor the sustained release of ions and their effects on tissue health and regeneration over extended periods. This is crucial for understanding the durability and effectiveness of the implant.
   - **Biocompatibility and Safety**: The systemic effects of ion release, including potential toxicity and overall biocompatibility, are assessed through blood tests, organ function analysis, and histopathological examination.

5.4.3.3 Correlating In Vitro and In Vivo Ion Release Data

Correlating ion release data from in vitro and in vivo studies involves comparing the kinetics and concentrations of released ions in both environments. Consistent ion release profiles across both settings indicate a predictable dissolution behaviour and bioactivity of the material. Variations in ion release can highlight differences in the biological environment and help in adjusting the glass composition for optimal performance.

5.4.3.3.1 Comparative Analysis of Ion Release Data

1. **Kinetics of Ion Release**
   - **Initial Burst Release**: Both in vitro and in vivo studies often show an initial rapid release of ions, particularly calcium (Ca^{2+}), phosphate

(PO_4^{3-}), and silicon (Si^{4+}), due to the dissolution of the bioactive glass surface. Comparing the rate and extent of this initial release helps to validate the material's bioactivity.
- **Sustained Release Phase**: After the initial burst, a more controlled, sustained release phase follows. Correlating the duration and rate of this phase in vitro and in vivo is crucial for predicting the long-term performance and bioactivity of the implant.

2. **Concentrations of Released Ions**
   - **Quantitative Measurement**: Techniques such as ICP-OES and ICP-MS are used to measure the concentrations of released ions in both in vitro and in vivo samples. Consistent concentration profiles suggest that the in vitro environment successfully mimics the in vivo conditions.
   - **Threshold Levels**: Ensuring that the ion concentrations reach therapeutic levels necessary for promoting osteogenesis, angiogenesis, and other regenerative processes without causing toxicity or adverse reactions.

5.4.3.3.2 Interpretation of Correlation Data

1. **Predictable Dissolution Behaviour**
   - **Consistency in Data**: Consistent ion release profiles in vitro and in vivo indicate that the bioactive glass has a predictable dissolution behaviour, enhancing confidence in its performance for clinical applications.
   - **Validation of In Vitro Models**: When in vitro ion release data accurately predict in vivo behaviour, it validates the use of in vitro models for initial screening and optimization of bioactive glass compositions.
2. **Variations and Their Implications**
   - **Biological Environment Differences**: Variations in ion release profiles between in vitro and in vivo studies can highlight differences in the biological environment, such as pH variations, presence of enzymes, and dynamic fluid flow in vivo.
   - **Adjustment of Composition**: Identifying these differences allows researchers to adjust the composition of the bioactive glass to better suit the in vivo conditions, enhancing its bioactivity and overall performance.

5.4.3.3.3 Applications of Correlated Data

1. **Optimization of Bioactive Glass Compositions**
   - **Tailoring Ion Release**: By understanding the specific ion release kinetics required for different medical applications, bioactive glass compositions can be tailored to optimize their therapeutic effects.
   - **Enhanced Bioactivity**: Adjustments based on correlated data can enhance the material's ability to support bone regeneration, wound healing, and other regenerative processes.
2. **Clinical Translation**
   - **Predictive Modelling**: Reliable in vitro to in vivo correlation allows for the development of predictive models that can expedite the translation of bioactive glass materials from the laboratory to clinical settings.

- **Regulatory Approval**: Consistent and predictable ion release profiles support the case for regulatory approval by demonstrating the material's safety, efficacy, and reliability.

5.4.3.3.4 Methodological Considerations

1. **Standardized Protocols**
   - **Reproducibility**: Using standardized protocols for both in vitro and in vivo studies ensure reproducibility and comparability of ion release data.
   - **Controlled Variables**: Carefully controlling variables such as temperature, pH, and immersion fluid composition in vitro can help achieve more accurate correlations with in vivo data.
2. **Advanced Analytical Techniques**
   - **High-Resolution Imaging**: Techniques such as SEM, TEM, and XRD provide detailed information on the microstructural changes in bioactive glass during dissolution, complementing ion release data.
   - **Elemental Analysis**: Combining ion concentration measurements with elemental analysis of tissues and fluids provides a comprehensive understanding of the material's behaviour in vivo.

5.5 APPLICATIONS OF BIOACTIVE GLASS MATERIALS IN BIOMEDICAL FIELDS

In vitro tests, although simplified, offer valuable predictive data regarding the potential performance of bioactive glasses in vivo. Consistent findings between in vitro and in vivo studies enhance the reliability of preliminary laboratory tests as predictors of clinical outcomes. The unique properties of bioactive glass materials make them highly versatile for a range of biomedical applications. This section explores the specific uses of bioactive glasses in bone regeneration, dental restoration, and drug delivery systems, highlighting their advantages and contributions to advancing medical treatments (Figure 5.4).

5.5.1 Bone Regeneration

Bone regeneration is a complex process that aims to repair or replace damaged or lost bone tissue. Bioactive glasses have emerged as a promising class of biomaterials for this purpose due to their unique ability to, unlike traditional biomaterials, bioactive glasses don't simply sit inertly within the body. They actively participate in the healing process by forming a hydroxyapatite (HA) layer on their surface. HAp is the primary mineral component of bone, and its presence facilitates a strong bond between the implant and surrounding bone tissue, known as osseointegration. This strong bond is crucial for long-term implant stability and functionality. Beyond osseointegration, bioactive glasses actively stimulate new bone formation. As the HAp layer forms, it serves as a scaffold, attracting and guiding bone-forming cells (osteoblasts) to migrate towards the implant. These osteoblasts then deposit new bone matrix on the HAp surface, promoting bone regeneration at the defect site [13].

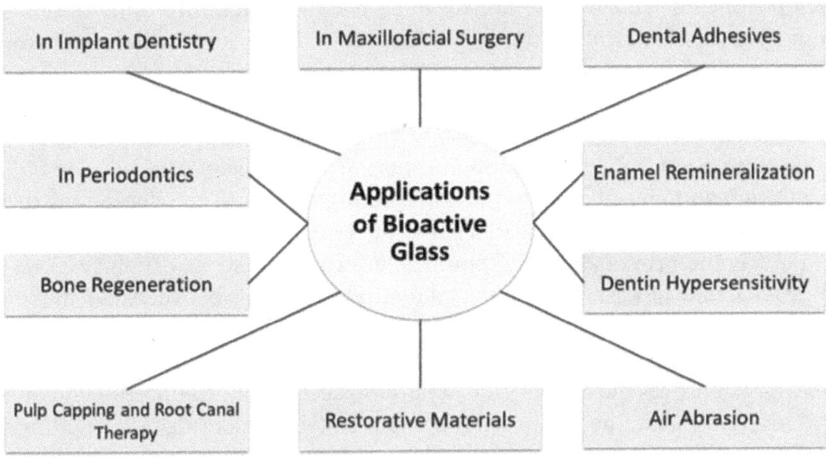

FIGURE 5.4 Application of bioactive glass in dentistry [12]

5.5.2 Applications in Orthopaedics and Dentistry

Bioactive glasses find numerous applications in orthopaedics and dentistry for bone regeneration, including:

- **Bone Defect Repair**: Filling gaps or voids in bone caused by trauma, disease, or surgery.
- **Spinal Fusion**: Promoting bone growth between vertebrae for spinal stabilization.
- **Treatment of Bone Fractures**: Assisting the healing process in complex fractures.
- **Dental Implants**: Providing a strong and biocompatible foundation for dental restorations.
- **Periodontal Regeneration**: Encouraging bone regrowth around teeth with bone loss.

Bioactive glasses represent a significant advancement in bone regeneration strategies. Their ability to mimic the natural bone environment and actively participate in the healing process makes them valuable tools for orthopaedic surgeons and dentists. As research continues to explore their full potential, bioactive glasses hold promise for revolutionizing the treatment of bone-related conditions and improving patient outcomes.

5.5.1.1 Orthopaedic Implants

Bioactive glasses are used in various orthopaedic implants to repair and regenerate bone tissue. Their bioactivity promotes the formation of a HA layer, which facilitates the bonding of the implant to the bone. This property is particularly beneficial in treating bone defects and fractures, enhancing the stability and integration of implants [14, 15]. Unlike traditional implant materials, bioactive glasses possess the remarkable ability to actively interact with bone tissue. This bioactivity stems from their controlled dissolution behaviour, which leads to several key benefits:

- Hydroxyapatite Layer Formation: Upon implantation, bioactive glasses undergo a controlled dissolution process. This releases beneficial ions like calcium and phosphate into the surrounding environment. These ions then participate in the formation of a bone-like HAp layer on the implant surface. HAp is the primary mineral component of bone, and its presence plays a crucial role in osseointegration, the strong bonding between the implant and bone tissue.
- Enhanced Implant Stability: The formation of a strong HAp layer significantly improves the stability and long-term success of orthopaedic implants. This is because the HAp layer acts as a biological bridge, facilitating a tight connection between the implant and surrounding bone. Traditional implants, lacking this bioactivity, may experience loosening or failure over time due to weak integration with bone.

5.5.1.1.1 Applications in Orthopaedic Implants

Bioactive glasses are finding increasing use in various orthopaedic implant applications, including:

- Bone Defect Repair: Filling bone voids or gaps caused by trauma, disease, or surgery. Bioactive glasses promote bone ingrowth into the defect site, aiding in faster and more complete healing.
- Fracture Fixation: Providing internal fixation for complex fractures. Bioactive glasses not only stabilize the fracture but also encourage bone healing at the fracture site.
- Spinal Fusion: Promoting bone growth between vertebrae for spinal stabilization procedures. Bioactive glasses can enhance the success rate of spinal fusion by facilitating a strong connection between the implant and surrounding bone.
- Joint Replacements: Bioactive coatings on joint replacement implants can improve their long-term stability and integration with surrounding bone tissue.

Bioactive glasses represent a paradigm shift in orthopaedic implant design. Their bioactivity fosters a more natural and efficient healing process, offering significant advantages over traditional implant materials. As research delves deeper into their potential, bioactive glasses hold immense promise for improving patient outcomes and revolutionizing the treatment of bone-related disorders in orthopaedics.

5.5.1.2 Bone Grafts

Bioactive glass materials are also employed as bone grafts, either alone or in combination with other materials. They serve as scaffolds that support new bone formation and provide structural integrity to the defect site. The osteoconductive nature of bioactive glasses ensures that new bone grows along the scaffold, eventually replacing it with natural bone tissue [16].

5.5.1.2.1 Scaffolding for Bone Growth

- **Structural Support**: Bioactive glasses can be shaped into various forms (blocks, granules, etc.) to fill bone defects and provide initial structural support. This allows the body time to initiate the healing process and regenerate new bone tissue.
- **Osteoconduction**: Bioactive glasses are inherently osteoconductive. This means they act as a scaffold that attracts and guides bone-forming cells (osteoblasts) to migrate towards the defect site. These osteoblasts then adhere to the bioactive glass surface and start depositing new bone matrix.

5.5.1.2.2 Gradual Degradation and Replacement

Unlike some traditional bone graft materials, bioactive glasses are not permanent implants. They offer a distinct advantage: glasses degrade at a controlled rate over time within the body. This gradual degradation process allows for the gradual replacement of the scaffold with newly formed bone tissue. As the new bone grows and strengthens, the bioactive glass material slowly dissolves, leaving behind a fully functional and natural bone structure.

5.5.1.2.3 Optimizing Bone Regeneration

Bioactive glasses offer additional benefits that enhance the bone grafting process: Their bioactivity promotes the formation of a HAp layer on the surface. This HAp layer mimics the natural composition of bone and further facilitates bone cell adhesion and growth. Bioactive glasses can be engineered to incorporate therapeutic agents within their structure. These agents, such as growth factors, can be released locally over time, stimulating and accelerating bone regeneration at the defect site.

5.5.1.2.4 Applications in Bone Grafting

Bioactive glasses are being utilized in various bone grafting applications, including:

- **Filling Bone Defects**: They can be used to fill voids or gaps in bone caused by trauma, disease, or surgery. Bioactive glasses provide both initial support and promote new bone growth, leading to complete repair of the defect.
- **Spinal Fusion Procedures**: Bioactive glasses can be used as bone graft substitutes or extenders in spinal fusion surgeries. They promote bone growth between vertebrae, facilitating successful spinal stabilization.
- **Dental Applications**: Bioactive glasses are being explored for applications in alveolar ridge augmentation (increasing jawbone height) and sinus lift procedures (increasing bone volume in the upper jaw) in dentistry.

Bioactive glasses offer a revolutionary approach to bone grafting. Their ability to act as scaffolds, promote bone growth, and degrade over time positions them as a valuable tool for surgeons. As research continues to optimize their properties and applications, bioactive glasses hold immense promise for improving the success rate of bone grafting procedures and enhancing patient outcomes in various bone repair scenarios.

5.5.1.3 Spinal Fusion

In spinal fusion procedures, bioactive glass can be used to facilitate the fusion of vertebrae. The material's ability to promote bone growth and integration helps in achieving a solid fusion, reducing the risk of implant failure and improving patient outcomes [17].

Spinal fusion is a surgical procedure that aims to permanently join two or more vertebrae together to provide stability and alleviate pain caused by spinal instability. Traditionally, this procedure relies on bone grafts, which can have drawbacks. Bioactive glasses offer a promising alternative due to their ability to promote bone growth and integration, leading to a more successful and stable fusion.

5.5.1.3.1 Advantages over Traditional Methods

Bioactive glasses offer several advantages over traditional bone grafts in spinal fusion:

Traditional bone grafts often require harvesting bone from another part of the patient's body, leading to additional pain and potential complications. Bioactive glasses eliminate the need for a secondary surgery and its associated risks. The ability of bioactive glasses to actively promote bone growth leads to higher fusion rates compared to traditional methods. This translates to a faster recovery time and improved patient outcomes. The strong bond formed between the bioactive glass and bone tissue leads to a more stable fusion, minimizing the risk of implant failure and the need for revision surgery.

5.5.2 Dental Restoration

Dental restorations aim to repair or replace damaged teeth, restoring functionality and aesthetics. Bioactive glasses are emerging as a revolutionary force in this field due to their unique properties that mimic natural tooth structures and promote a more natural and long-lasting repair process [18].

Bioactive glasses can be formulated to possess properties similar to tooth dentin, the hard layer beneath the enamel. This allows for restorations that more closely resemble the natural tooth structure in terms of strength, elasticity, and wear resistance. Unlike traditional dental materials, bioactive glasses can form a strong chemical bond with dentin. This bond creates a more stable and durable restoration, minimizing the risk of leakage and future complications.

5.6 BENEFITS OF BIOACTIVE GLASSES IN DENTAL RESTORATION

- **Enhanced Aesthetics:** The biomimetic properties of bioactive glasses allow for restorations that are virtually indistinguishable from natural teeth, achieving superior aesthetic results.
- **Long-Term Durability:** The strong bond between the bioactive glass and dentin contributes to the long-term durability of the restoration. This

reduces the need for frequent replacements, saving patients time and money.

- **Reduced Microleakage:** The tight bond formed with dentin minimizes the risk of microleakage, where bacteria can seep into the tooth and cause decay. This promotes better oral health and reduces the risk of future complications.

5.6.1 Beyond Basic Restorations

The versatility of bioactive glasses extends beyond traditional fillings:

- **Pulp Revascularization:** Bioactive glasses can be used in procedures aiming to regenerate damaged tooth pulp, the inner layer containing nerves and blood vessels. This approach could potentially save teeth that would otherwise require extraction.
- **Periodontal Regeneration:** Bioactive glasses show promise in promoting bone regrowth around teeth with periodontal disease. This can help restore lost supporting bone tissue and improve long-term tooth stability.

5.6.2 Optimizing Bioactive Glasses for Dentistry

Researchers are constantly exploring ways to refine bioactive glasses for dental applications:

- **Tailored Compositions:** Bioactive glasses can be formulated with specific compositions to optimize their biocompatibility, bonding strength, and aesthetic properties for different dental restoration needs.
- **Antimicrobial Properties:** Bioactive glasses can be engineered to incorporate antimicrobial agents that can help fight bacteria and reduce the risk of infection around the restoration site.

Bioactive glasses represent a paradigm shift in dental restoration. Their ability to mimic natural tooth structures, bond strongly with dentin, and offer potential for advanced procedures like pulp revascularization positions them as a game-changer in this field. As research progresses and explores their full potential, bioactive glasses hold immense promise for creating more natural, durable, and biocompatible dental restorations, ultimately improving patient outcomes and oral health.

5.6.2.1 Fillings and Crowns

Bioactive glass materials are used in dental fillings and crowns to restore decayed or damaged teeth. Their bioactivity promotes the formation of a hydroxyapatite layer, which bonds with the tooth structure, providing a durable and stable restoration. This bonding reduces the risk of secondary decay and enhances the longevity of the restoration [19].

Unlike traditional materials that simply fill the cavity, bioactive glasses boast a unique property – bioactivity. This translates to:

- **Hydroxyapatite Formation:** Upon placement, bioactive glasses interact with surrounding fluids, leading to the formation of a HAp layer on their surface. HAp is the primary mineral component of dentin, the hard layer beneath tooth enamel.
- **Strong Chemical Bond:** The HAp layer acts as a bridge, forming a strong chemical bond with the remaining tooth structure. This bond is significantly stronger than the mechanical interlocking achieved by traditional materials.

5.6.2.1.1 Benefits of Bioactive Glasses in Fillings and Crowns

- **Reduced Microleakage:** The tight chemical bond minimizes the risk of microleakage, where bacteria and fluids can seep into the tooth through microscopic gaps. This significantly reduces the risk of secondary decay around the restoration.
- **Enhanced Longevity:** The strong bond between the bioactive glass and tooth structure contributes to the long-term durability of the restoration. This translates to fewer replacements and potentially lower costs for patients.
- **Improved Aesthetics:** Bioactive glasses can be formulated to mimic the natural translucency of tooth dentin. This allows for restorations that blend seamlessly with surrounding teeth, achieving superior aesthetics compared to some traditional materials.

5.6.2.1.2 Beyond Basic Fillings

The potential of bioactive glasses extends beyond routine fillings:

- **Large Restorations:** Their bonding strength makes bioactive glasses suitable for larger restorations, potentially reducing the need for crowns in some cases. This can preserve more natural tooth structure.
- **Minimally Invasive Dentistry:** The biocompatibility and bonding properties of bioactive glasses may allow for more minimally invasive procedures, potentially requiring less removal of healthy tooth structure.

5.6.2.1.3 Optimizing Bioactive Glasses for Dentistry

Researchers are constantly working to refine bioactive glasses for optimal performance:

- **Tailored Compositions:** Bioactive glasses can be formulated with specific compositions to adjust their setting time, aesthetics, and bonding strength to meet the specific needs of a filling or crown.
- **Antimicrobial Properties:** Incorporating antimicrobial agents into the bioactive glass composition can further reduce the risk of bacterial growth around the restoration site.

Bioactive glasses represent a significant advancement in dental fillings and crowns. Their ability to form a strong chemical bond with tooth structure, minimize microleakage, and potentially offer aesthetic benefits positions them as a transformative technology in dentistry. As research continues to optimize their properties and applications, bioactive glasses hold immense promise for creating more durable, biocompatible, and long-lasting dental restorations, ultimately improving patient outcomes and oral health.

5.6.2.2 Root Canal Therapy

In root canal therapy, bioactive glass can be used as a filler material to seal the root canal and promote healing. Its bioactivity encourages the regeneration of periapical tissue and the formation of a strong bond between the filler and the tooth, improving the success rate of the treatment [20, 21].

Unlike traditional root canal sealers, bioactive glasses offer more than just a physical barrier. Their bioactivity unlocks a cascade of beneficial processes:

- **Periapical Tissue Regeneration:** The bioactivity of the glass stimulates the regeneration of periapical tissue, the bone and ligament surrounding the tooth root. This promotes healing and reduces the risk of post-treatment complications like inflammation and infection.
- **Enhanced Sealing:** The formation of a hydroxyapatite (HAp) layer on the surface of the bioactive glass further strengthens the seal within the root canal. HAp mimics the natural mineral component of bone, creating a tight and durable bond with surrounding dentin.

5.6.2.2.1 Benefits of Bioactive Glasses in Root Canal Therapy

- **Improved Success Rates:** By promoting periapical tissue regeneration and providing a stronger seal, bioactive glasses potentially contribute to higher success rates for root canal therapy.
- **Reduced Risk of Complications:** The stimulation of healing and the tight seal minimize the risk of post-treatment complications like infections and inflammation.
- **Biocompatibility:** Bioactive glasses are generally well-tolerated by the body, minimizing the risk of adverse reactions.

5.6.2.2.2 Beyond Basic Sealing

The potential of bioactive glasses in root canal therapy extends further:

- **Antimicrobial Properties:** Bioactive glasses can be engineered to incorporate antimicrobial agents, providing an additional layer of defence against bacteria within the root canal.
- **Drug Delivery:** Bioactive glasses can be designed to slowly release therapeutic drugs like antibiotics or anti-inflammatory agents, promoting healing and reducing the risk of future infections.

5.6.2.2.3 Optimizing Bioactive Glasses for Root Canal Therapy

Researchers are actively exploring ways to refine bioactive glasses for optimal performance in root canal fillings:

- **Tailored Compositions:** Bioactive glasses can be formulated with specific compositions to control their setting time, biocompatibility, and potential for drug delivery, catering to the specific needs of each patient.
- **Injectable Formulations:** Developing injectable bioactive glass formulations could facilitate easier placement and filling of complex root canal systems.

Bioactive glasses represent a novel approach to root canal therapy. Their ability to promote periapical tissue regeneration, create a strong seal, and potentially offer additional functionalities like drug delivery positions them as a promising advancement in this field. As research continues to optimize their properties and applications, bioactive glasses hold immense promise for improving the success rate of root canal therapy and enhancing patient outcomes.

5.6.2.3 Bone Augmentation

Bioactive glass materials are also used in bone augmentation procedures to support the placement of dental implants. They help in regenerating the bone tissue around the implant site, ensuring a stable foundation for the implant and reducing the risk of implant failure [22, 23].

Unlike traditional bone augmentation materials that simply fill the void, bioactive glasses possess a unique property – bioactivity. This translates to:

- **Osteoconduction:** Bioactive glasses act as a scaffold, attracting and guiding bone-forming cells (osteoblasts) towards the implant site. These osteoblasts then adhere to the bioactive glass surface and start depositing new bone matrix.
- **Stimulating New Bone Growth:** The bioactivity of the glasses can further stimulate the growth of new bone tissue around the implant site. This process is crucial for creating a strong and durable foundation for the implant.

5.6.2.3.1 Benefits of Bioactive Glasses in Bone Augmentation

- **Enhanced Implant Stability:** By promoting new bone growth, bioactive glasses contribute to a more stable and integrated implant. This reduces the risk of implant failure and ensures long-term functionality.
- **Reduced Risk of Infection:** The biocompatibility of bioactive glasses minimizes the risk of inflammation or infection around the implant site, promoting a healthy healing environment.
- **Faster Integration:** The ability of bioactive glasses to stimulate bone growth can potentially lead to faster integration of the implant with surrounding bone tissue, accelerating the treatment process.

5.6.2.3.2 Optimizing Bioactive Glasses for Bone Augmentation

Researchers are continuously exploring ways to refine bioactive glasses for optimal performance in bone augmentation:

- **Tailored Compositions:** Bioactive glasses can be formulated with specific compositions to optimize their osteoconductive properties, resorption rate, and potential for delivering growth factors. This allows for customization based on the specific needs of each patient's bone defect.
- **Injectable Formulations:** Developing injectable bioactive glass formulations could facilitate easier placement of the material during bone augmentation procedures.
- **Combination Strategies:** Bioactive glasses can be combined with other bone grafting materials to leverage the strengths of each approach and achieve optimal results.

5.6.3 Drug Delivery Systems

The versatility of bioactive glass materials extends to their use in drug delivery systems, which is depicted in Figure 5.5. Their porous structure and ability to degrade in a controlled manner make them suitable carriers for therapeutic agents [24].

5.6.3.1 Controlled Release

Bioactive glasses can be engineered to release drugs in a controlled manner over a specific period. This controlled release is beneficial for delivering medications directly to the site of injury or disease, enhancing the effectiveness of the treatment and reducing side effects [25].

5.6.3.1.1 Mechanism of Controlled Release

The controlled release from bioactive glasses is primarily governed by their degradation behaviour in physiological environments. Upon implantation, bioactive glasses undergo a series of surface reactions, including ion exchange, dissolution, and precipitation of an HCA layer. These processes are influenced by factors such as glass

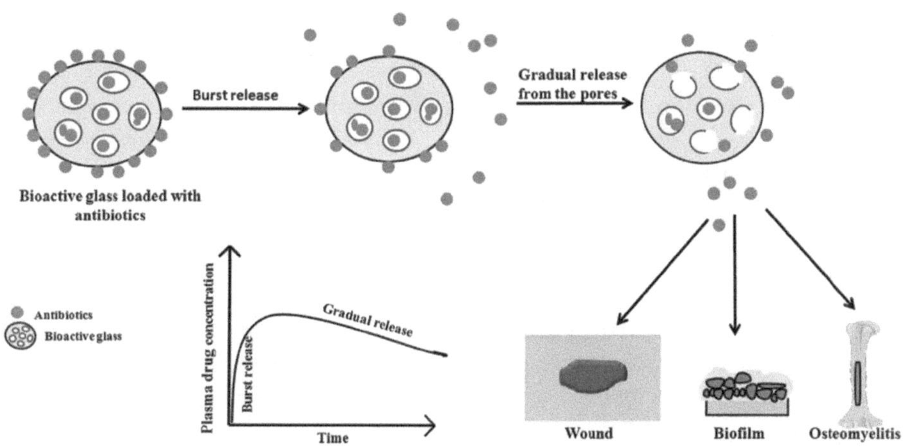

FIGURE 5.5 Drug delivery using bioactive glass [24]

composition, particle size, and the presence of dopants, which can be manipulated to achieve desired release profiles.

1. **Glass Composition**: The SiO_2, CaO, P_2O_5, and other oxide components can be varied to adjust the degradation rate. Higher SiO_2 content generally slows down the degradation, while increasing CaO or P_2O_5 accelerates it.
2. **Particle Size and Porosity**: Smaller particles and higher porosity enhance the surface area available for interaction with body fluids, thus increasing the degradation rate and drug release.
3. **Incorporation of Dopants**: Elements such as silver, strontium, and magnesium can be introduced to modify the glass network and its bioactivity, offering additional control over the release kinetics.

5.6.3.1.2 Advantages of Controlled Drug Release

1. **Targeted Delivery**: By delivering drugs directly to the site of injury or disease, bioactive glasses minimize systemic exposure and potential side effects. This localized delivery is particularly beneficial for treatments requiring high local concentrations of the drug.
2. **Sustained Release**: The controlled degradation of bioactive glasses allows for a sustained release of therapeutic agents over extended periods, reducing the need for frequent administration and enhancing patient compliance.
3. **Enhanced Therapeutic Efficacy**: The continuous release of drugs maintains therapeutic levels at the target site, improving the overall effectiveness of the treatment. This is especially crucial for chronic conditions and infections where prolonged drug presence is necessary.

5.6.3.1.3 Applications

Bioactive glasses with controlled release properties are utilized in various medical applications, including:

- **Bone Regeneration**: Delivery of growth factors or antibiotics to promote bone healing and prevent infections.
- **Wound Healing**: Sustained release of antimicrobial agents to enhance wound healing and prevent bacterial colonization.
- **Cancer Therapy**: Localized delivery of chemotherapeutic agents to tumour sites, minimizing systemic toxicity and improving therapeutic outcomes.

In summary, the ability to engineer bioactive glasses for controlled drug release offers a promising strategy for enhancing the efficacy of medical treatments. By tailoring the glass composition, particle characteristics, and incorporating specific dopants, researchers can develop bioactive glass systems that provide precise, sustained, and localized delivery of therapeutic agents, significantly improving patient outcomes.

5.6.3.2 Localized Delivery

The use of bioactive glasses in localized drug delivery systems allows for high concentrations of drugs to be delivered directly to the target area. This localized delivery is particularly useful in treating infections, inflammation, and cancer, where high doses of medication are required without affecting the entire body [26].

5.6.3.2.1 Mechanism of Localized Drug Delivery

Localized drug delivery using bioactive glasses leverages their unique physicochemical properties. Upon implantation, bioactive glasses interact with physiological fluids, undergoing surface reactions that lead to the formation of a bioactive layer. This interaction facilitates the gradual and controlled release of incorporated drugs directly at the target site. The mechanisms can be outlined as follows:

1. **Surface Reactions and Layer Formation**: Bioactive glasses, upon contact with body fluids, undergo rapid ion exchange, dissolution, and precipitation reactions, resulting in the formation of an HCA layer. This bioactive layer not only promotes tissue bonding but also modulates drug release.
2. **Drug Incorporation and Release Kinetics**: Therapeutic agents can be incorporated into the glass matrix during the synthesis process or loaded onto the surface of preformed glass particles. The release kinetics are controlled by the glass composition, degradation rate, and the physicochemical properties of the incorporated drug.

5.6.3.2.2 Advantages of Localized Drug Delivery

1. **High Local Concentration**: By delivering drugs directly to the target area, bioactive glasses enable high local concentrations of the therapeutic agent. This is particularly beneficial in treating infections, where high doses of antibiotics are required to eradicate pathogens effectively.
2. **Minimized Systemic Exposure**: Localized delivery reduces the systemic distribution of the drug, minimizing potential side effects and toxicity associated with high systemic concentrations. This is critical in treatments such as chemotherapy, where systemic toxicity can be a significant concern.
3. **Improved Therapeutic Efficacy**: Concentrating the drug at the site of action ensures that therapeutic levels are achieved and maintained, enhancing the overall efficacy of the treatment. This is crucial in managing conditions like chronic inflammation and localized cancerous tumours.

5.6.3.2.3 Applications in Treating Infections, Inflammation, and Cancer

1. **Infections**: Bioactive glasses can be loaded with antibiotics or antimicrobial agents to treat localized infections. The sustained release of these agents ensures a prolonged antibacterial effect, preventing bacterial colonization and biofilm formation. This approach is particularly useful in treating bone infections (osteomyelitis) and soft tissue infections.
2. **Inflammation**: Anti-inflammatory drugs can be incorporated into bioactive glasses to manage localized inflammation. This is beneficial in conditions such as arthritis or periodontal disease, where targeted anti-inflammatory therapy can reduce symptoms and improve healing.
3. **Cancer Therapy**: Bioactive glasses can be used to deliver chemotherapeutic agents directly to tumour sites. This localized delivery maximizes

the drug concentration at the tumour, enhancing its cytotoxic effects while minimizing systemic toxicity. Additionally, bioactive glasses can be engineered to release drugs in response to the tumour microenvironment, providing a smart delivery system for cancer therapy.

The use of bioactive glasses for localized drug delivery represents a significant advancement in therapeutic strategies. By enabling high concentrations of drugs at the target site while minimizing systemic exposure, bioactive glasses offer an effective solution for treating infections, inflammation, and cancer. Their ability to be engineered for specific release profiles and tailored to various medical applications makes them a versatile and powerful tool in modern medicine.

5.6.3.3 Multi-Functional Carriers

Bioactive glass materials can be combined with other therapeutic agents, such as growth factors and antibiotics, to create multi-functional drug delivery systems. These systems can simultaneously promote tissue regeneration and combat infections, offering a comprehensive approach to treatment [24].

5.6.3.3.1 Mechanism of Multi-Functional Drug Delivery Systems

Multi-functional carriers are designed by integrating bioactive glass materials with multiple therapeutic agents, such as growth factors, antibiotics, anti-inflammatory drugs, and other bioactive molecules. The underlying principles involve:

- **Synthesis and Incorporation**: During the synthesis of bioactive glasses, therapeutic agents can be encapsulated within the glass matrix or adsorbed onto the surface. Techniques such as sol-gel processing, melt quenching, and ion exchange are commonly used to incorporate these agents without compromising the bioactivity of the glass.
- **Controlled Release Dynamics**: The release kinetics of each incorporated agent can be independently controlled by adjusting the composition, porosity, and degradation rate of the bioactive glass. This enables a sequential or simultaneous release of multiple agents, tailored to the specific needs of the treatment regimen.

5.6.3.3.2 Advantages of Multi-Functional Carriers

1. **Comprehensive Treatment Approach**: By delivering a combination of therapeutic agents, multi-functional carriers can address multiple aspects of a medical condition simultaneously. For example, in bone regeneration, growth factors can stimulate osteogenesis while antibiotics prevent infection.
2. **Synergistic Effects**: The co-delivery of growth factors and antimicrobial agents can have synergistic effects, enhancing the overall therapeutic outcome. Growth factors promote tissue repair and regeneration, while antibiotics ensure a sterile environment, preventing complications from infections.
3. **Localized and Sustained Release**: Multi-functional carriers ensure that therapeutic agents are released locally at the site of injury or disease,

maintaining effective concentrations over extended periods. This localized delivery minimizes systemic exposure and reduces the risk of side effects.

5.6.3.3.3 Applications of Multi-Functional Bioactive Glass Carriers

1. **Bone Tissue Engineering**: In bone regeneration, bioactive glasses can be loaded with growth factors such as bone morphogenetic proteins (BMPs) and antibiotics like gentamicin. The growth factors promote the proliferation and differentiation of osteoblasts, while the antibiotics prevent post-surgical infections, enhancing the overall success of bone grafts and implants.
2. **Wound Healing**: For chronic wounds, bioactive glass carriers can deliver a combination of anti-inflammatory drugs, antimicrobial agents, and growth factors. This multimodal approach accelerates wound closure, reduces inflammation, and prevents infection, facilitating faster and more effective healing.
3. **Dental Applications**: In periodontal therapy, bioactive glasses can release anti-inflammatory drugs and antimicrobial agents to manage gum disease while simultaneously delivering growth factors to promote the regeneration of periodontal tissues.
4. **Cancer Therapy**: Bioactive glass carriers can be engineered to deliver chemotherapeutic agents along with angiogenesis inhibitors and immunomodulatory drugs. This multi-pronged strategy can target tumour cells, inhibit blood vessel formation necessary for tumour growth, and modulate the immune response to attack cancer cells more effectively.

5.6.3.3.4 Summary

Multi-functional drug delivery systems based on bioactive glasses represent a significant advancement in medical therapeutics. By combining various therapeutic agents within a single platform, these systems offer a comprehensive approach to treatment, addressing multiple facets of disease simultaneously. The ability to tailor the release profiles of each agent further enhances their versatility and effectiveness, making bioactive glass-based multi-functional carriers a powerful tool in the fields of tissue engineering, wound healing, dental applications, and cancer therapy.

5.6 CONCLUSION

Bioactive glass materials have emerged as highly promising candidates for various biomedical applications due to their unique properties, including biocompatibility, bioactivity, and osteoconductivity. This chapter has explored the in vitro and in vivo behaviours of bioactive glasses, emphasizing the importance of these studies in understanding their performance in biological environments.

In vitro experiments, such as SBF immersion tests, provide initial insights into the bioactivity of these materials by analysing surface reactions and ion release kinetics. These studies are essential for evaluating the potential of bioactive glasses to form hydroxyapatite layers and support cellular functions. In vivo studies, on the other hand, offer a more comprehensive evaluation of bioactive glasses by examining their interactions with living tissues in animal models or clinical trials. These studies assess biocompatibility, tissue integration, and the formation of hydroxyapatite layers in a complex biological environment.

Understanding the correlation between in vitro and in vivo performance is crucial for optimizing bioactive glass compositions for specific biomedical applications. Consistencies between in vitro and in vivo data strengthen the confidence in the material's clinical efficacy, while discrepancies highlight areas needing further investigation and refinement.

The applications of bioactive glasses in bone regeneration, dental restoration, and drug delivery systems demonstrate their versatility and potential to revolutionize medical treatments. Advances in customization, nanotechnology, and multifunctional designs are paving the way for innovative solutions that address complex medical challenges.

However, several challenges must be addressed to fully realize the potential of bioactive glasses. These include standardization and quality control, long-term biocompatibility and safety, regulatory approval, and cost and accessibility. Interdisciplinary collaboration among material scientists, biologists, engineers, and clinicians is essential for overcoming these challenges and driving innovation.

In conclusion, bioactive glass materials hold significant promise for advancing regenerative medicine and tissue engineering. By continuing to explore their in vitro and in vivo behaviours, optimizing their compositions, and addressing the challenges in their development and application, we can unlock their full potential to improve patient outcomes and transform healthcare.

REFERENCES

1. C. Mocquot, N. Attik, N. Pradelle-Plasse, B. Grosgogeat, and P. Colon, 2020, "Bioactivity assessment of bioactive glasses for dental applications: a critical review," *Dental Materials Journal*, 36(9), 1116–1143. Elsevier, Accessed: May 21, 2024. [Online]. Available: https://www.sciencedirect.com/science/article/pii/S0109564120300750
2. H. Ylänen, 2017, *Bioactive glasses: materials, properties and applications*. Accessed: May 21, 2024. [Online]. Woodhead publications. Available: https://books.google.com/books?hl=en&lr=&id=pSYUDgAAQBAJ&oi=fnd&pg=PP1&dq=Bioactive+glasses+application&ots=UjYFUEoWFK&sig=Nche2LIJMTn6_ljCrd7eI2ydspc
3. A. J. Salinas, and M. Vallet-Regí, 2012, "Methods to study the mechanism of bioactivity," in L Rimondini (ed.), *Surface Tailoring of Inorganic Materials for Biomedical Applications*, pp. 359–375, Italy: Bentham books. doi: 10.2174/978160805462611 201010359.
4. F. Baino, and S. Yamaguchi, 2020, "The use of simulated body fluid (SBF) for assessing materials bioactivity in the context of tissue engineering: review and challenges," *Biomimetics*, 5, 57. doi: 10.3390/biomimetics5040057.
5. S. Ebrahimi, and C. S. Sipaut, 2022, "Synthesis of hydroxyapatite/bioglass composite nanopowder using design of experiments," *Nanomaterials*, vol. 12, no. 13, 2264. doi: 10.3390/NANO12132264.
6. A. A. El-Rashidy, J. A. Roether, L. Harhaus, U. Kneser, and A. R. Boccaccini, 2017, "Regenerating bone with bioactive glass scaffolds: a review of in vivo studies in bone defect models," *Acta biomaterialia*, 62. doi: 10.1016/j.actbio.2017.08.030.

7. P. A. Dash, S. Mohanty, and S. K. Nayak, 2023, "A review on bioactive glass, its modifications and applications in healthcare sectors," *Journal of Non-Crystalline Solids*, vol. 614, p. 122404, doi: 10.1016/J.JNONCRYSOL.2023.122404.
8. M. N. Rahaman et al., 2011, "Bioactive glass in tissue engineering," *Acta Biomater*, vol. 7, no. 6, p. 2355, doi: 10.1016/J.ACTBIO.2011.03.016.
9. A. M. P. Magri et al., 2017, "Osteoconductive properties of two different bioactive glass forms (powder and fiber) combined with collagen," *Applied Surface Science*, vol. 423, pp. 557–565, doi: 10.1016/J.APSUSC.2017.06.152.
10. M. Cannio, D. Bellucci, J. A. Roether, D. N. Boccaccini, and V. Cannillo, 2021, "Bioactive glass applications: a literature review of human clinical trials," *Materials*, vol. 14, no. 18, doi: 10.3390/MA14185440.
11. S. Ferraris et al., 2020, "Bioactive materials: in vitro investigation of different mechanisms of hydroxyapatite precipitation," *Acta Biomater*, vol. 102, pp. 468–480, doi: 10.1016/J.ACTBIO.2019.11.024.
12. H. E. Skallevold, D. Rokaya, Z. Khurshid, and M. S. Zafar, 2019, "Bioactive glass applications in dentistry," *International Journal of Molecular Sciences*, vol. 20, no. 23, 5960. doi: 10.3390/IJMS20235960.
13. H. R. Fernandes, A. Gaddam, A. Rebelo, D. Brazete, G. E. Stan, and J. M. F. Ferreira, 2018, "Bioactive glasses and glass-ceramics for healthcare applications in bone regeneration and tissue engineering," *Materials*, vol. 11, no. 12, 2530. doi: 10.3390/MA11122530.
14. G. Brunello, H. Elsayed, and L. Biasetto, 2019, "Bioactive glass and silicate-based ceramic coatings on metallic implants: open challenge or outdated topic?" *Materials (Basel)*, vol. 12, no. 18, 2929. doi: 10.3390/ma12182929.
15. P. K. Vallittu, T. O. Närhi, and L. Hupa, 2015, "Fiber glass-bioactive glass composite for bone replacing and bone anchoring implants," *Dental Materials*, vol. 31, no. 4, pp. 371–381, doi: 10.1016/j.dental.2015.01.003.
16. V. V. Välimäki, and H. T. Aro, 2006, "Molecular basis for action of bioactive glasses as bone graft substitute," *Scandinavian Journal of Surgery*, vol. 95, no. 2, pp. 95–102, doi: 10.1177/145749690609500204.
17. B. Ilharreborde et al., 2008, "Bioactive glass as a bone substitute for spinal fusion in adolescent idiopathic scoliosis: a comparative study with iliac crest autograft," *Journal of Pediatric Orthopaedics*, vol. 28, no. 3, pp. 347–351, doi: 10.1097/BPO.0B013E318168D1D4.
18. N. Jafari, M. S. Habashi, A. Hashemi, R. Shirazi, N. Tanideh, and A. Tamadon, 2022, "Application of bioactive glasses in various dental fields," *Biomaterials Research*, vol. 26, no. 1, pp. 1–15, doi: 10.1186/S40824-022-00274-6.
19. P. C. Yelick, and P. T. Sharpe, 2019, "Tooth bioengineering and regenerative dentistry," *Journal of Dental Research*, vol. 98, no. 11, pp. 1173–1182, doi: 10.1177/0022034519861903.
20. A. C. Profeta, and G. M. Prucher, 2017, "Bioactive-glass in endodontic therapy and associated microsurgery," *Open Dentistry Journal*, vol. 11, no. 1, pp. 164–170, doi: 10.2174/1874210601711010164.
21. A. Washio et al., 2020, "Effect of bioactive glass-based root canal sealer on the incidence of postoperative pain after root canal obturation," *International Journal of Environmental Research and Public Health*, vol. 17, no. 23, pp. 1–9, doi: 10.3390/ijerph17238857.
22. F. Abushahba, A. Algahawi, N. Areid, L. Hupa, and T. O. Närhi, 2023, "Bioactive glasses in periodontal regeneration: a systematic review," *Tissue Engineering, Part C: Methods*, vol. 29, no. 5, pp. 183–196, doi: 10.1089/ten.tec.2023.0036.
23. F. Zhao, Z. Yang, H. Xiong, Y. Yan, X. Chen, and L. Shao, 2023, "A bioactive glass functional hydrogel enhances bone augmentation via synergistic angiogenesis, self-swelling and osteogenesis," *Bioactive Materials*, vol. 22, pp. 201–210, doi: 10.1016/j.bioactmat.2022.09.007.

24. S. Gupta, S. Majumdar, and S. Krishnamurthy, 2021, "Bioactive glass: a multifunctional delivery system," *Journal of Controlled Release*, vol. 335, pp. 481–497, doi: 10.1016/J.JCONREL.2021.05.043.
25. J. Rivadeneira, and A. Gorustovich, 2017, "Bioactive glasses as delivery systems for antimicrobial agents," *Journal of Applied Microbiology*, vol. 122, no. 6, pp. 1424–1437, doi: 10.1111/jam.13393.
26. C. Wu, and J. Chang, 2014, "Multifunctional mesoporous bioactive glasses for effective delivery of therapeutic ions and drug/growth factors," *Journal of Controlled Release*, vol. 193, pp. 282–295, doi: 10.1016/j.jconrel.2014.04.026.

6 Mechanosensing Interactions of Bioactive Glasses

Y. B. Sudhir Sastry, Gebru Kiros Berhe, Riessom Weldegiorgis, Satish Jain, K. G. Prashanth, and Parthiban Ramaswamy

6.1 INTRODUCTION

6.1.1 Overview of Bioactive Glasses

Bioactive glasses (BGs), a class of materials developed by Larry Hench in the late 1960s, have emerged as pivotal entities in biomedical engineering. These glasses, primarily composed of silica (SiO_2), calcium oxide (CaO), and phosphorus pentoxide (P_2O_5), alongside varying amounts of oxides like sodium oxide (Na_2O) and magnesium oxide (MgO), possess a distinctive ability to bond with both bone and soft tissues. This characteristic renders them highly valuable in medical applications [1–3].

The composition of BGs is tailored to induce the controlled release of therapeutic ions upon dissolution. This controlled release mechanism plays a vital role in stimulating cellular responses and fostering tissue regeneration. For instance, calcium and phosphorus ions released from BGs facilitate the formation of hydroxyapatite (HA), a mineral component of bone, promoting bone integration. Similarly, other ions released contribute to various biological processes, further enhancing tissue healing and regeneration.

The bioactivity of BGs is a fundamental property attributed to their ability to form a HA layer on their surface upon exposure to bodily fluids. This HA layer closely mimics the mineral component of bone, facilitating robust interfacial bonding between the bioactive glass and surrounding biological tissues. The mechanism underlying this phenomenon involves a series of complex physicochemical interactions between the bioactive glass surface and the surrounding physiological environment.

6.1.1.1 Biomineralization Process

- **Nucleation and Growth**: Upon immersion in bodily fluids, such as simulated body fluid (SBF) or in vivo biological fluids, BGs undergo surface reactions that initiate the nucleation and growth of HA crystals on their surface.

DOI: 10.1201/9781003660781-6

- **Ion Exchange**: The dissolution of ions from the bioactive glass surface into the surrounding fluid environment triggers a series of ion exchange reactions, leading to the formation of calcium phosphate phases, including HA.
- **Silanol Formation**: Surface hydrolysis of silicate bonds on the bioactive glass surface generates silanol (Si-OH) groups, which serve as nucleation sites for HA crystal growth.

6.1.1.2 Biological Significance of HA Formation

- **Osteoconductivity**: The presence of a HA layer on the bioactive glass surface promotes osteoconduction, facilitating the migration and adhesion of osteogenic cells, such as osteoblasts and mesenchymal stem cells (MSCs), onto the material surface.
- **Cellular Response**: HA has been shown to enhance cellular adhesion, proliferation, and differentiation, thereby promoting tissue regeneration and integration.
- **Mineralization Cascade**: HA deposition on the bioactive glass surface initiates a cascade of mineralization events, leading to the formation of a biologically active interface conducive to bone bonding and tissue integration.

6.1.1.3 Interfacial Bonding and Tissue Integration

- **Strong Interfacial Bonding**: The formation of a HA layer on the bioactive glass surface facilitates strong interfacial bonding between the implant and surrounding biological tissues, promoting long-term stability and integration.
- **Biological Mimicry**: The chemical composition and crystalline structure of the HA layer closely resemble those of natural bone mineral, enabling seamless integration with the host tissue environment.

6.1.1.4 Applications of BGs

- **Bone Grafts**: BGs are widely used in bone grafting procedures to promote bone regeneration and facilitate the repair of bone defects and fractures.
- **Dental Implants**: In dental implantology, BGs enhance osseointegration, improving the success rate and longevity of dental implants.
- **Soft Tissue Repair**: BGs are also employed in soft tissue repair applications, where they promote wound healing and tissue regeneration.

In summary, the formation of a HA layer on the surface of BGs is a key determinant of their bioactivity and efficacy in biomedical applications. This process, driven by physicochemical interactions with bodily fluids, facilitates strong interfacial bonding and integration with biological tissues, making BGs versatile biomaterials for various clinical applications in bone and soft tissue repair [4, 5].

6.1.2 Mechanosensing in Biomedical Applications

Mechanosensing is a fundamental process by which cells detect and respond to mechanical signals from their environment. This capability is crucial for a myriad of physiological processes such as bone remodelling, wound healing, and immune responses. Mechanosensing involves a complex interplay between mechanical forces and cellular machinery, translating physical cues into biochemical signals through a process known as mechanotransduction [6, 7]. In the context of biomedical applications, mechanosensing plays a pivotal role in dictating the performance of biomaterials, including BGs. The mechanical properties of BGs, such as stiffness, elasticity, and surface roughness, can significantly influence cellular behaviour. For instance, the stiffness of a biomaterial can affect stem cell differentiation, with stiffer substrates promoting osteogenic differentiation while softer substrates may favour adipogenic or chondrogenic differentiation [8].

BGs can be engineered to provide specific mechanical stimuli that guide cellular processes. This is achieved by manipulating their composition and structural properties to tailor their mechanical characteristics. As a result, BGs can serve as potent tools in tissue engineering and regenerative medicine, offering both biochemical and mechanical cues to enhance tissue healing and regeneration [9]. Understanding the mechanosensing interactions of BGs is essential for optimizing their design and application. This involves studying how these materials influence cell proliferation, mechanotransduction, mechanical strength, and immune responses. Additionally, it is important to explore how BGs respond to mechanostimuli, which can further elucidate their role in guiding tissue regeneration and repair [10] and can be inferred in Figure 6.1. In the subsequent segments, we will conduct a comprehensive exploration into the mechanosensing mechanisms inherent in BGs, focusing on intricate analyses of cellular proliferation, mechanotransduction pathways, mechanical integrity, induction of T and B cell responses, and the role of mechanostimulation. These investigations aim to elucidate the fundamental interactions between BGs and biological systems, providing essential insights into the development of tailored compositions optimized for diverse biomedical applications.

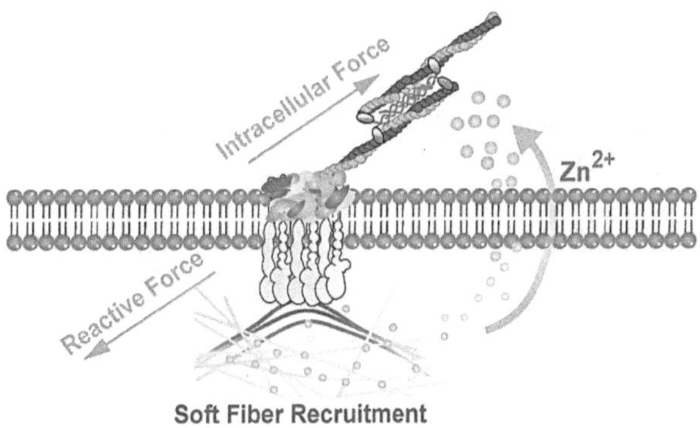

FIGURE 6.1 Mechanostimuli induced tissue generation and repair

6.2 CELL PROLIFERATION OF BGS

6.2.1 Cellular Response to BGs

In the realm of tissue engineering and regenerative medicine, BGs stand out for their exceptional capacity to promote cellular proliferation, a pivotal aspect in facilitating tissue regeneration and wound healing. Upon exposure to physiological fluids, BGs undergo surface reactions, liberating biologically active ions such as calcium, phosphate, and silicate [11]. These ions assume crucial roles in orchestrating cellular behaviour.

Of paramount importance are the calcium ions, which serve as indispensable mediators in a myriad of cellular functions, particularly in signal transduction pathways that foster cell proliferation. Additionally, phosphate ions contribute significantly to the formation of HA, a principal constituent of bone tissue, thereby creating an environment conducive to the proliferation and differentiation of osteoblasts, the cells responsible for bone formation. Conversely, silicate ions have been documented to exert a stimulating effect on the expression of genes associated with osteogenesis, thereby augmenting both cell proliferation and differentiation processes [11].

Moreover, empirical studies have underscored the profound impact of BGs on enhancing the proliferation rates of diverse cell types, including osteoblasts, fibroblasts, and endothelial cells [12]. This augmentation can be attributed, in part, to the establishment of a local microenvironment that mimics the natural extracellular matrix (ECM), thereby providing a milieu rich in both biochemical and mechanical cues crucial for optimal cell growth and proliferation. This elucidation of the mechanistic underpinnings behind the proliferative effects of BGs not only enhances our fundamental understanding of cellular interactions but also paves the way for the development of advanced biomaterial compositions tailored to meet the diverse demands of biomedical applications, as expounded upon in subsequent chapters of this book.

6.2.2 Mechanisms of Proliferation

The mechanisms underlying the pro-proliferative effects of BGs are intricate, involving a synergistic interplay of ionic release, alterations in pH, and osmotic pressure dynamics. Upon immersion in physiological fluids, BGs undergo dissolution, liberating ions that form a biologically active layer on their surface. Enriched in calcium and phosphate, this layer not only supplies the requisite constituents for HA formation but also elicits cellular responses, thereby stimulating cellular activity [12].

A notable consequence of the localized increase in calcium concentration is the activation of calcium-sensing receptors (CaSR) situated on cell surfaces. This activation instigates intracellular signalling cascades, notably the mitogen-activated protein kinase (MAPK) pathway, pivotal for cellular proliferation and survival. Furthermore, the presence of silicate ions has been demonstrated to augment collagen production, a fundamental component of the ECM, thereby bolstering cell adhesion and proliferation [13]. Concomitantly, changes in pH and osmotic pressure ensuing from bioactive glass dissolution exert significant influence on cellular responses. The slightly alkaline milieu generated by dissolution products fosters enhanced cell viability and proliferation, mimicking the physiological conditions conducive to bone healing and regeneration.

Moreover, the physical characteristics of BGs, including surface roughness and porosity, profoundly impact cellular behaviour. Surface roughness enhances cell attachment by augmenting available surface area for cellular adhesion, while porous structures facilitate superior nutrient and oxygen diffusion, thereby fostering a more favourable environment for cellular proliferation [12]. This comprehensive elucidation of the multifaceted mechanisms underpinning the proliferative effects of BGs not only advances our fundamental understanding of cellular interactions but also underscores the potential for tailored biomaterial design to optimize therapeutic outcomes in tissue engineering and regenerative medicine applications, as elaborated in subsequent chapters of this book.

6.3 MECHANOTRANSDUCTION OF BGS

6.3.1 Understanding Mechanotransduction

Mechanotransduction stands as a pivotal biological phenomenon wherein cells adeptly translate mechanical stimuli into biochemical signals, enabling them to dynamically respond to their physical milieu. This intricate process encompasses a diverse array of cellular constituents, including mechanoreceptors, ion channels, cytoskeletal components, and an array of signalling molecules [14]. Mechanotransduction assumes paramount significance in the maintenance of tissue homeostasis, exerting regulatory control over a myriad of cellular functions such as proliferation, differentiation, migration, and apoptosis [15]. At the crux of mechanotransduction lie mechanoreceptors, specialized cell surface proteins attuned to mechanical cues, which initiate signalling cascades upon sensing mechanical stimuli. These receptors can take various forms, including integrins, stretch-activated ion channels, and focal adhesions, each contributing to the transduction of mechanical signals into intracellular biochemical responses. Additionally, the intricate interplay between the cytoskeleton and ECM further facilitates the transmission of mechanical forces, with cytoskeletal elements such as actin filaments and microtubules serving as conduits for mechanical signals within the cell.

Upon activation, mechanotransduction pathways intricately modulate cellular behaviour through the orchestration of downstream signalling events. These signalling cascades culminate in the regulation of gene expression, cytoskeletal reorganization, and modulation of ion fluxes, ultimately dictating cellular responses such as proliferation, differentiation, migration, and programmed cell death (apoptosis). Notably, mechanotransduction not only facilitates cellular adaptation to mechanical cues but also plays a pivotal role in tissue remodelling and repair processes, thereby contributing to overall tissue homeostasis and physiological function. By comprehensively elucidating the intricate mechanisms of mechanotransduction, researchers can gain profound insights into the fundamental principles governing cellular behaviour and tissue dynamics. Moreover, an enhanced understanding of mechanotransduction holds immense promise for the development of novel therapeutic strategies aimed at manipulating cellular responses to mechanical stimuli, with implications spanning diverse fields such as tissue engineering, regenerative medicine, and the treatment of various pathological conditions characterized by aberrant mechanotransduction signalling.

Cells possess sophisticated mechanisms for sensing and responding to mechanical stimuli, a process mediated in part by specialized structures such as integrins. Integrins serve as transmembrane receptors that facilitate the physical linkage between the ECM and the cellular cytoskeleton. Upon exposure to mechanical forces, integrins undergo clustering, thereby initiating the recruitment of focal adhesion proteins to sites of contact between the cell and the ECM. This clustering event triggers a cascade of intracellular signalling events, culminating in the activation of various signalling pathways. Among the key players in these signalling cascades is focal adhesion kinase (FAK), a cytoplasmic tyrosine kinase that plays a pivotal role in transducing mechanical signals from integrins to intracellular signalling pathways. Additionally, Rho GTPases, a family of small GTP-binding proteins, are also implicated in mechanotransduction processes. Activation of Rho GTPases regulates cytoskeletal dynamics and cell contractility, thereby influencing cellular responses to mechanical cues.

Furthermore, the MAPK pathway represents another critical signalling axis involved in mechanotransduction. Activation of the MAPK pathway in response to mechanical stimuli leads to the phosphorylation and activation of downstream targets, ultimately influencing gene expression patterns and cellular behaviour. Collectively, these intracellular signalling pathways orchestrate a myriad of cellular responses to mechanical cues, ranging from alterations in gene expression to changes in cell morphology and motility. By deciphering the molecular mechanisms underlying mechanotransduction, researchers can gain valuable insights into how cells perceive and respond to their mechanical environment, with implications spanning various fields such as tissue engineering, regenerative medicine, and the treatment of mechanical-related pathologies.

6.3.2 Role of BGs in Mechanotransduction

BGs exert a notable influence on mechanotransduction mechanisms, primarily through their mechanical attributes and surface properties. Factors such as stiffness, elasticity, and surface topography of BGs are instrumental in dictating how cells sense and react to mechanical stimuli. The stiffness and elasticity of BGs directly impact cellular mechanosensitive, with cells exhibiting differential responses based on the substrate's mechanical properties. Furthermore, the surface topography of BGs modulates cell adhesion, spreading, and cytoskeletal organization, thereby influencing mechanotransduction pathways.

By altering the mechanical microenvironment and surface characteristics, BGs can effectively modulate cellular responses to mechanical cues, ultimately influencing processes such as cell proliferation, differentiation, and tissue regeneration. Understanding the role of BGs in mechanotransduction holds significant implications for the design of biomaterials tailored to optimize cellular interactions and therapeutic outcomes in tissue engineering and regenerative medicine applications.

6.3.2.1 Stiffness and Elasticity

The mechanical characteristics of BGs can be precisely engineered to closely mimic those of the desired target tissue, facilitating their effective integration into tissue engineering strategies. Specifically, BGs endowed with elevated stiffness levels offer crucial mechanical support necessary for applications in bone tissue engineering. Experimental evidence underscores the capacity of stiffer substrates to elicit favourable responses in MSCs, particularly promoting their osteogenic differentiation via mechanotransduction pathways [16, 17].

The heightened stiffness of BGs plays a pivotal role in modulating cellular behaviour through intricate mechanotransduction mechanisms. Notably, substrates with increased stiffness facilitate the clustering of integrin receptors and the formation of focal adhesions, pivotal events that culminate in the activation of signalling cascades regulating osteogenesis. These signalling pathways orchestrate a cascade of molecular events, ultimately influencing gene expression patterns and cellular fate determination towards osteogenic lineages. By precisely modulating the stiffness of BGs, researchers can effectively manipulate cellular responses to mechanical cues, thereby steering the trajectory of tissue regeneration and repair processes. This mechanistic understanding holds profound implications for the design and optimization of bioactive glass-based biomaterials tailored to enhance osteogenic outcomes in bone tissue engineering applications, underscoring the pivotal role of mechanical cues in dictating cellular behaviour and tissue development.

6.3.2.2 Surface Topography

The surface characteristics, encompassing both roughness and porosity, of BGs play pivotal roles in modulating mechanotransduction processes. Surface roughness is a critical determinant influencing cell adhesion, as it amplifies the available surface area for cellular attachment. This amplified adhesion not only fosters stronger cell-substrate interactions but also enhances the transmission of mechanical signals to the cells, thereby eliciting more robust mechanotransduction responses. Consequently, cells adhering to rough surfaces are subjected to heightened mechanical cues, which can profoundly impact their behaviour and fate.

Moreover, the porous nature of BGs imparts additional complexity to mechanotransduction dynamics. Porous substrates offer a three-dimensional (3D) architecture that closely resembles the natural ECM, facilitating cellular infiltration and nutrient diffusion within the material. This 3D microenvironment not only enhances cell viability but also influences mechanotransduction pathways by modulating the spatial distribution of mechanical forces experienced by the cells. Consequently, the intricate interplay between surface roughness and porosity dictates cellular responses to mechanical cues, thereby exerting profound effects on cellular behaviour and tissue regeneration processes. Understanding the interrelationship between surface topography and mechanotransduction is essential for the rational design of bioactive glass-based biomaterials optimized for tissue engineering applications. By tailoring surface characteristics to manipulate mechanotransduction responses, researchers can effectively modulate cellular behaviour and guide tissue development towards desired therapeutic outcomes. Thus, the elucidation of these mechanistic principles holds significant promise for advancing the field of biomaterials science and enhancing the efficacy of bioactive glass-based scaffolds in regenerative medicine [18-19].

6.3.2.3 Ionic Dissolution Products

The dissolution of BGs yields a spectrum of biologically active ions that intricately influence mechanotransduction pathways, thereby exerting profound effects on cellular behaviour. Among these ions, calcium ions emerge as key mediators in mechanotransduction-related signalling cascades. Calcium ions possess the capability to activate a plethora of calcium-dependent kinases and other signalling molecules implicated in mechanotransduction processes. By binding to specific receptors and channels, calcium ions elicit cellular responses that culminate in the modulation of gene expression patterns and cellular behaviour.

Furthermore, silicate ions released from BGs have garnered attention for their modulatory effects on mechanotransduction pathways. Silicate ions have been demonstrated to augment the expression of genes intricately involved in mechanotransduction processes, thereby potentiating cellular responses to mechanical stimuli. This augmentation of gene expression facilitates the transmission and integration of mechanical signals within the cellular milieu, ultimately influencing cellular behaviour and fate determination [20].

The interplay between the dissolution products of BGs and mechanotransduction pathways underscores the multifaceted mechanisms through which BGs regulate cellular responses to mechanical stimuli. By modulating the release kinetics of specific ions, researchers can tailor the mechanotransductive properties of BGs to optimize their therapeutic efficacy in tissue engineering and regenerative medicine applications. Thus, elucidating the intricate interplay between bioactive glass dissolution products and mechanotransduction pathways holds immense promise for advancing our understanding of cellular mechanobiology and harnessing these insights for the development of next-generation biomaterials [21].

6.3.2.4 Mechanotransduction Pathways

BGs are well-known for their ability to bond to bone and promote cellular responses beneficial for tissue regeneration. They influence several key mechanotransduction pathways, enhancing cellular responses to mechanical stimuli. The primary pathways affected by BGs include the FAK/Src pathway, MAPK pathway, and Rho/ROCK pathway. Here is an in-depth examination of how BGs interact with these pathways.

1. **FAK/Src Pathway**

   Activation Mechanism

   - **Integrin Engagement**: BGs can enhance integrin-mediated adhesion by providing a favourable surface for cell attachment. Integrins are transmembrane receptors that connect the ECM to the cytoskeleton.
   - **FAK Activation**: Upon integrin binding to ECM proteins, FAK is recruited and auto-phosphorylated. This activation leads to the formation of focal adhesion complexes.
   - **Src Kinase Activation**: Src family kinases are then recruited to these complexes, leading to further phosphorylation events and activation of downstream signalling cascades.

Impact on Cellular Functions

- **Focal Adhesions**: The formation and maturation of focal adhesions are critical for transmitting mechanical signals from the extracellular environment to the cell's interior.
- **Signal Transduction**: Activated FAK/Src complexes trigger downstream signalling pathways, including the activation of MAPK and other kinases.
- **Gene Expression**: This pathway influences gene expression by transmitting mechanical signals to the nucleus, regulating genes involved in cell proliferation, migration, and survival.

2. **MAPK Pathway**

Activation Mechanism

- **Mechanical Stress Response**: Bioactive glasses can induce mechanical stress in cells, activating the MAPK pathway.
- **MAPK Cascade**: The MAPK pathway comprises three main kinase families: ERK (extracellular signal-regulated kinases), JNK (c-Jun N-terminal kinases), and p38 MAPKs.
- **Upstream Activation**: Mechanical stimuli and integrin activation can lead to the recruitment and activation of small GTPases (e.g., Ras), which then activate the MAPK kinase kinase (MAP3K) levels.

Impact on Cellular Functions

- **ERK Pathway**: ERK is primarily involved in regulating cell proliferation and differentiation. BGs can enhance these processes, promoting tissue regeneration.
- **JNK Pathway**: JNK is activated by stress signals and is involved in apoptosis and inflammation. BGs can modulate JNK activity to control cell death and promote survival.
- **p38 Pathway**: p38 MAPKs are activated by stress stimuli and are involved in inflammatory responses and cell differentiation. BGs can influence p38 activity to regulate these processes.

3. **Rho/ROCK Pathway**

Activation Mechanism

- **Rho GTPases**: BGs can influence the activity of Rho GTPases, a family of small signalling G proteins. RhoA is a key member involved in cytoskeletal dynamics.
- **ROCK Activation**: RhoA activates Rho-associated kinase (ROCK), which is critical for actin filament organization and myosin light chain (MLC) phosphorylation.

Impact on Cellular Functions

- **Cytoskeletal Dynamics**: The Rho/ROCK pathway regulates the formation of stress fibres, focal adhesions, and cell contractility. This is essential for maintaining cell shape and enabling migration.
- **Cell Contractility**: ROCK influences cell contractility by modulating MLC phosphorylation, which controls the interaction between actin and myosin.
- **Cell Migration and Differentiation**: BGs enhance the cellular response to mechanical cues, promoting changes in cell shape, facilitating migration, and driving differentiation processes essential for tissue repair and regeneration.

6.3.2.4.1 Integrative Role of Bioactive Glasses

BGs serve as a multifunctional biomaterial that interacts with these mechanotransduction pathways to promote bone and tissue regeneration. They provide a conducive surface for cell adhesion, modulate mechanical stress responses, and activate key signalling pathways that drive cellular proliferation, differentiation, and migration. By influencing the FAK/Src, MAPK, and Rho/ROCK pathways, BGs enhance the mechanosensitivity of cells, facilitating effective tissue repair and regeneration.

In summary, the interaction of BGs with mechanotransduction pathways underscores their potential in biomedical applications, particularly in bone and tissue engineering, where the mechanical environment plays a crucial role in guiding cellular behaviour and tissue development.

6.4 IMMUNE RESPONSE: TRIGGERING T AND B ANTIGENS

6.4.1 BGs and the Immune System

BGs serve as versatile biomaterials capable of not only supporting tissue regeneration and healing but also actively interacting with the immune system. Understanding their ability to modulate immune responses is crucial for ensuring biocompatibility and promoting desired healing outcomes. When implanted in the body, BGs initiate a cascade of immune reactions that influence the overall success of the biomaterial [22].

6.4.1.1 Initial Immune Response

Recognition as Foreign Material

- Upon implantation, BGs are recognized by the immune system as foreign entities, triggering an immediate response.
- This recognition prompts the activation of innate immune cells, including macrophages and neutrophils, which play pivotal roles in the early inflammatory response.

Inflammatory Cascade

- Innate immune cells release pro-inflammatory cytokines and chemokines in response to bioactive glass implantation, orchestrating the recruitment of additional immune cells to the site of injury.
- Neutrophils are among the first responders, aiding in the clearance of debris and pathogens, while macrophages engulf and digest foreign particles, including bioactive glass debris.

6.4.1.2 Role of Adaptive Immune Cells

T and B Lymphocytes

- The subsequent interaction with adaptive immune cells, particularly T and B lymphocytes, is essential for shaping the long-term immune response to bioactive glass implants.

- T lymphocytes, including helper T cells (Th) and cytotoxic T cells (Tc), regulate immune responses and contribute to the orchestration of tissue repair processes.
- B lymphocytes produce antibodies that can recognize and target specific antigens associated with bioactive glass particles, influencing the immune response and tissue integration.

6.4.1.3 Modulation of Immune Responses

Immunomodulatory Properties

- BGs exhibit immunomodulatory properties that can modulate immune responses to promote tissue regeneration and integration.
- The release of ions from BGs, such as calcium, silicon, and phosphorus, can influence immune cell behaviour and cytokine production, thereby regulating inflammation and tissue healing processes.

Promotion of Regenerative Phenotypes

- BGs have been shown to promote the polarization of macrophages towards a regenerative phenotype, characterized by the secretion of anti-inflammatory cytokines and growth factors.
- This polarization facilitates tissue repair and regeneration by promoting angiogenesis, ECM deposition, and the recruitment of progenitor cells to the site of injury.

6.4.2 Mechanisms of Immune Activation

BGs exert profound effects on immune responses through intricate mechanisms involving the release of therapeutic ions, surface interactions, and activation of specific signalling pathways. A comprehensive understanding of these mechanisms is crucial for optimizing the design of BGs to elicit favourable immune responses, promoting tissue regeneration and integration [23].

6.4.2.1 Release of Therapeutic Ions

Calcium, Silicon, and Phosphorus Ions

- BGs release therapeutic ions, including calcium (Ca), silicon (Si), and phosphorus (P), into the surrounding tissue environment.
- These ions play pivotal roles in modulating immune responses by interacting with immune cells and influencing cytokine production and signalling pathways.

Immunomodulatory Effects

- Calcium ions have been shown to regulate macrophage polarization towards anti-inflammatory phenotypes, promoting tissue repair and regeneration.
- Silicon ions enhance the expression of anti-inflammatory cytokines while suppressing pro-inflammatory mediators, contributing to a more favourable immune microenvironment.

6.4.2.1.1 *Surface Interactions*

Cell-Material Interactions

- Bioactive glass surfaces interact with immune cells upon implantation, triggering cellular responses and immune activation.
- Surface properties, such as roughness, chemistry, and topography, influence the degree and nature of immune activation, impacting tissue integration and healing outcomes.

6.4.2.1.2 *Activation of Immune Cells*

- Immune cells, such as macrophages and dendritic cells, recognize bioactive glass surfaces as foreign entities, leading to cellular activation and cytokine secretion.
- Surface interactions can induce phenotypic changes in immune cells, influencing their polarization and cytokine production profiles.

6.4.2.1.3 *Activation of Signalling Pathways*

MAPK and NF-κB Signalling

- BGs activate intracellular signalling pathways, including MAPK and nuclear factor-κB (NF-κB) pathways.
- Activation of these signalling cascades regulates immune cell function, cytokine production, and inflammatory responses, shaping the immune microenvironment.

Gene Expression Regulation

- BGs modulate gene expression profiles in immune cells, leading to the upregulation of anti-inflammatory mediators and downregulation of pro-inflammatory factors.
- This gene expression modulation contributes to the resolution of inflammation and promotion of tissue regeneration and repair processes.

6.5 OPTIMIZATION OF BIOACTIVE GLASS DESIGN

Tailoring Ion Release Profiles

- Optimization of bioactive glass composition allows for precise control over ion release kinetics, influencing immune activation and tissue response.
- Fine-tuning the release of therapeutic ions can promote immunomodulation while minimizing adverse inflammatory reactions.

Surface Modification Strategies

- Surface engineering techniques enable the modification of bioactive glass surfaces to enhance immune compatibility and promote regenerative responses.
- Functionalization with bioactive molecules or polymers can modulate surface interactions with immune cells, influencing immune activation and tissue integration.

BGs modulate immune responses through the release of therapeutic ions, surface interactions, and activation of specific signalling pathways. Understanding these mechanisms is critical for optimizing the design of BGs to achieve favourable immune responses and promote tissue regeneration and integration. By tailoring ion release profiles, optimizing surface properties, and employing surface modification strategies, BGs can be engineered to elicit desired immune responses, facilitating their therapeutic applications in regenerative medicine and tissue engineering. Continued research in this field will further elucidate the complex interactions between BGs and the immune system, driving advancements in biomaterial design and therapeutic efficacy.

6.5.1 Ionic Dissolution Products

BGs, upon implantation, undergo partial dissolution, releasing ions such as calcium (Ca), phosphorus (P), and silicon (Si) into the surrounding tissue. These ions play crucial roles in modulating immune responses, influencing the behaviour of immune cells and the overall immune microenvironment. Understanding the immunomodulatory effects of these ions is essential for elucidating the mechanisms underlying the interaction between BGs and the immune system.

6.5.1.1 Calcium Ions (Ca^{2+})

Role in Immune Cell Functions

- Calcium ions are integral to various immune cell functions, including activation, differentiation, and cytokine production.
- Intracellular calcium signalling regulates processes such as T cell activation, B cell receptor signalling, and phagocytosis by macrophages.

Immunomodulatory Effects

- Elevated levels of extracellular calcium can influence immune cell behaviour, promoting T cell proliferation, cytokine secretion, and effector functions.
- Calcium signalling pathways regulate immune responses, with dysregulation implicated in autoimmune diseases and inflammatory disorders.

6.5.1.2 Phosphorus Ions (P)

Enhancement of Immune Cell Proliferation

- Phosphorus ions released from BGs can enhance the proliferation and activation of immune cells, including T lymphocytes and macrophages.
- Phosphorus-containing compounds are involved in intracellular signalling pathways that regulate cell growth, proliferation, and survival.

Immunomodulatory Effects

- Phosphorus ions can modulate immune cell functions by influencing gene expression, cytokine production, and immune cell signalling pathways.
- Phosphorus-containing molecules play roles in immune cell metabolism, energy production, and cellular homeostasis.

6.5.1.3 Silicon Ions (Si^{4+})

Anti-inflammatory Properties

- Silicon ions released from BGs exhibit anti-inflammatory properties, suppressing pro-inflammatory cytokine production and immune cell activation.
- Silicon-containing compounds have been shown to attenuate inflammatory responses and promote tissue regeneration in various biological contexts.

Immunomodulatory Effects

- Silicon ions regulate immune cell functions by modulating intracellular signalling pathways involved in inflammation and immune responses.
- Silicon-based biomaterials have been investigated for their potential therapeutic applications in immune-mediated diseases and inflammatory conditions.

6.5.2 Surface Interactions

The surface properties of BGs, including roughness, porosity, and chemical composition, can directly interact with immune cells. Macrophages, which are key players in the immune response, can adhere to the surface of BGs and become activated. The activation of macrophages can lead to the release of pro-inflammatory cytokines such as interleukin-1 (IL-1), interleukin-6 (IL-6), and tumour necrosis factor-alpha (TNF-α), which are crucial for the initial inflammatory response and subsequent tissue healing. The surface chemistry of BGs can also influence the polarization of macrophages. Depending on the surface cues, macrophages can adopt different phenotypes, such as the pro-inflammatory M1 phenotype or the anti-inflammatory and tissue-repairing M2 phenotype. The ability to modulate macrophage polarization is essential for controlling the immune response and promoting a regenerative environment [24].

The surface properties of BGs, including roughness, porosity, and chemical composition, play pivotal roles in mediating interactions with immune cells, particularly macrophages. Macrophages, as key regulators of the immune response, adhere to the surface of BGs upon implantation and undergo activation, leading to the release of pro-inflammatory cytokines essential for the initial inflammatory response and subsequent tissue healing.

6.5.2.1 Macrophage Activation and Cytokine Release

Surface Adhesion and Activation

- Macrophages recognize and adhere to the surface of BGs, initiating cellular responses.
- Surface properties such as roughness and porosity influence the extent of macrophage adhesion and activation.

Pro-inflammatory Cytokine Production

- Activated macrophages release pro-inflammatory cytokines such as IL-1, IL-6, and TNF-α.

- These cytokines play critical roles in initiating and amplifying the inflammatory response, recruiting additional immune cells to the site of injury, and stimulating tissue repair processes.

6.5.2.2 Influence of Surface Chemistry on Macrophage Polarization

Macrophage Phenotypic Plasticity

- Macrophages exhibit phenotypic plasticity and can adopt distinct functional phenotypes in response to environmental cues.
- Surface chemistry of BGs influences macrophage polarization, shaping the immune response and tissue healing outcomes.

M1 and M2 Phenotypes

- Depending on surface cues, macrophages can polarize towards pro-inflammatory M1 phenotype or anti-inflammatory and tissue-repairing M2 phenotype.
- M1 macrophages produce pro-inflammatory cytokines and promote tissue destruction, while M2 macrophages secrete anti-inflammatory cytokines and support tissue regeneration.

6.5.2.3 Modulation of Immune Responses for Regenerative Environment

Controlled Immune Activation

- The ability of BGs to modulate macrophage polarization is essential for controlling the immune response and promoting a regenerative environment.
- Surface modifications can be employed to tailor the immune response, favouring M2 polarization and tissue repair processes.

Surface Modification Strategies

- Surface functionalization with bioactive molecules or polymers can modulate surface interactions with immune cells, influencing macrophage phenotype and cytokine production.
- Optimizing surface chemistry and topography can promote favourable immune responses, facilitating tissue integration and regeneration.

The surface properties of BGs directly interact with immune cells, particularly macrophages, influencing their activation, cytokine production, and polarization towards distinct phenotypes. Surface chemistry plays a critical role in mediating these interactions, with implications for the immune response and tissue healing outcomes. By understanding and manipulating surface interactions, BGs can be designed to modulate immune responses effectively, promoting a regenerative environment conducive to tissue integration and repair in biomedical applications. Continued research in this area will further elucidate the complex interplay between BGs and the immune system, driving advancements in biomaterial design and therapeutic efficacy.

6.5.3 Activation of T and B Cells

BGs exert influence on the adaptive immune response by interacting with T and B lymphocytes, key players in orchestrating immune responses. T cells, comprising Th cells and Tc cells, are pivotal in regulating immune reactions. BGs can promote the activation and proliferation of T cells through various mechanisms, including ion release and antigenic signalling presentation.

6.5.3.1 T Cell Activation and Proliferation

Bioactive Glass-Mediated Stimulation

- BGs release ions such as calcium, phosphorus, and silicon, which can stimulate T cell activation and proliferation.
- Interaction with bioactive glass surfaces can also provide antigenic signals that trigger T cell responses.

Helper T Cells

- Activated T cells, particularly helper T cells, produce a diverse array of cytokines that regulate the activity of other immune cells.
- Th cells play crucial roles in coordinating immune responses by stimulating the proliferation and differentiation of other immune cells.

6.5.3.2 B Cell Activation and Antibody Production

Role of B Cells

- B cells are responsible for antibody production and play essential roles in adaptive immunity.
- Upon activation by BGs, B cells differentiate into plasma cells, which produce specific antibodies against the material.

Antibody Production

- Antibodies generated in response to BGs can bind to the material's surface, influencing its long-term biocompatibility and integration within the host tissue.
- The specificity of antibodies may impact the immune response and determine the persistence of the material in the body.

6.5.4 Influence on Long-Term Biocompatibility

Regulation of Immune Memory

- The activation of T and B cells by BGs can contribute to the development of immune memory against the material.
- Memory T and B cells retain information about the material, facilitating a rapid and robust immune response upon subsequent exposures.

Impact on Integration and Biocompatibility

- The immune memory established against BGs can influence their long-term integration and biocompatibility within the host tissue.
- Understanding and controlling the adaptive immune response are critical for designing BGs with optimal performance and long-term durability in biomedical applications.

BGs interact with T and B lymphocytes, activating and modulating the adaptive immune response. T cell activation and proliferation, driven by bioactive glass-mediated stimulation, influence immune cell functions and cytokine production. B cell activation leads to antibody production against the material, impacting its long-term biocompatibility and integration within the host tissue. By elucidating the mechanisms underlying T and B cell interactions with BGs, researchers can optimize the design of these materials to promote favourable immune responses and enhance their performance in biomedical applications. Continued research in this area will further advance our understanding of the complex interplay between BGs and the adaptive immune system, driving innovations in biomaterial design and therapeutic efficacy.

6.6 CYTOKINE PRODUCTION AND IMMUNE MODULATION

The interaction between BGs and immune cells elicits the production of various cytokines, critical signalling molecules that regulate immune responses. This cytokine milieu plays a pivotal role in orchestrating the immune response to bioactive glass implants, influencing inflammation, tissue repair, and integration. BGs can be tailored to modulate the cytokine profile, promoting a balanced immune response conducive to tissue regeneration while minimizing chronic inflammation and fibrosis. This modulation can be achieved through optimization of the composition, surface properties, and dissolution kinetics of the BGs [22].

6.6.1 Pro-Inflammatory Cytokines

Early Inflammatory Response

- BGs induce the secretion of pro-inflammatory cytokines such as IL-1, IL-6, and TNF-α upon interaction with immune cells.
- These cytokines play crucial roles in the early stages of inflammation, recruiting other immune cells to the site of implantation and initiating tissue repair processes.

Recruitment of Immune Cells

- Pro-inflammatory cytokines stimulate the recruitment and activation of immune cells, including macrophages, neutrophils, and T lymphocytes, to the site of bioactive glass implantation.
- This influx of immune cells is essential for clearing debris, resolving infections, and initiating tissue regeneration.

6.6.2 Anti-Inflammatory Cytokines

Resolution of Inflammation

- BGs can also induce the production of anti-inflammatory cytokines, such as interleukin-10 (IL-10) and transforming growth factor-beta (TGF-β).
- These cytokines play pivotal roles in resolving inflammation, suppressing excessive immune responses, and promoting tissue repair and regeneration.

Tissue Repair and Regeneration

- Anti-inflammatory cytokines promote the transition from the inflammatory phase to the proliferative and remodelling phases of tissue repair.
- They facilitate the recruitment of reparative cells, ECM deposition, and angiogenesis, contributing to the restoration of tissue architecture and function.

6.6.3 Modulation of Cytokine Profile

Tailoring Immune Response

- BGs can be designed to modulate the cytokine profile, promoting a balanced immune response that supports tissue regeneration.
- Optimization of the composition, surface properties, and dissolution kinetics of BGs enables precise control over cytokine production and immune modulation.

Minimization of Chronic Inflammation

- By promoting the secretion of anti-inflammatory cytokines and suppressing excessive pro-inflammatory responses, BGs mitigate the risk of chronic inflammation and fibrosis.
- This balanced immune response fosters an environment conducive to tissue regeneration and integration, enhancing the long-term biocompatibility of the material.

6.7 MECHANOSTIMULUS AND BGS

6.7.1 Concept of Mechanostimulus

Mechanostimulus denotes the application of mechanical forces or stresses that exert influence on cellular behaviour and function. In the realm of biomaterials, particularly BGs, mechanostimulus plays a pivotal role in regulating cellular activities such as proliferation, differentiation, and migration. The ability of BGs to impart mechanical stimuli is fundamental to their efficacy in tissue engineering and regenerative medicine, where they are often required to emulate the mechanical environment of native tissues.

6.7.1.1 Mechanotransduction: Sensing and Responding to Mechanical Forces

Mechanosensitive Structures

- Cells possess mechanosensitive structures, including integrins, ion channels, and the cytoskeleton, which enable them to detect mechanical forces and convert them into biochemical signals.
- These structures act in concert to sense and respond to mechanical changes in the extracellular environment, initiating a process known as mechanotransduction.

Integrins

- Integrins are cell surface receptors that bind to ECM components and transmit mechanical signals from the external environment to the cell interior.
- Upon activation by mechanical forces, integrins initiate signalling cascades that regulate cellular functions such as adhesion, migration, and gene expression.

Ion Channels

- Mechanosensitive ion channels in the cell membrane respond to mechanical stimuli by altering ion fluxes across the membrane.
- These changes in ion fluxes modulate cellular signalling pathways and gene expression, influencing cell behaviour and function.

Cytoskeleton

- The cytoskeleton, composed of actin filaments, microtubules, and intermediate filaments, serves as a structural scaffold and dynamic machinery for cellular mechanics.
- Mechanical forces induce rearrangements in the cytoskeletal architecture, transmitting signals from the cell membrane to the nucleus.

6.7.1.2 Cellular Response to Mechanostimuli

Regulation of Cellular Activities

- The cellular response to mechanostimuli is multifaceted, encompassing alterations in gene expression, cytoskeletal dynamics, and intracellular signalling pathways.
- Mechanostimulation regulates cellular activities such as proliferation, differentiation, migration, and ECM remodelling.

Maintenance of Tissue Homeostasis

- Mechanostimuli play a crucial role in maintaining tissue homeostasis by modulating cell phenotype and function in response to changes in mechanical cues.

- Perturbations in mechanotransduction pathways can disrupt tissue integrity and contribute to pathological conditions.

Promotion of Tissue Repair and Regeneration

- Proper mechanostimulation is essential for promoting tissue repair and regeneration by facilitating the recruitment and activation of progenitor cells, enhancing matrix deposition, and orchestrating tissue remodelling processes.

6.7.1.3 Implications for Biomaterial Design and Tissue Engineering

Mimicking Native Mechanical Environment

- Biomaterials, including BGs, must be designed to provide appropriate mechanostimulation to cells within the engineered tissue construct.
- Tailoring the mechanical properties and microstructure of biomaterials enables them to mimic the native mechanical environment of target tissues, promoting cellular responses conducive to tissue regeneration.

Integration of Mechanobiology Principles

- Incorporating mechanobiology principles into biomaterial design facilitates the development of advanced tissue engineering strategies that harness the regenerative potential of mechanostimulation.
- By understanding and exploiting the mechanotransduction pathways, biomaterials can be optimized to enhance tissue repair and regeneration outcomes.

In conclusion, mechanostimulus is a fundamental concept in biomaterials science, particularly in the context of BGs and tissue engineering. The ability of biomaterials to provide mechanical cues to cells through mechanotransduction pathways is essential for regulating cellular behaviour and promoting tissue regeneration. Incorporating mechanobiology principles into biomaterial design holds promise for advancing the field of regenerative medicine and achieving therapeutic outcomes in tissue engineering applications. Continued research in this area will deepen our understanding of mechanostimulation and its implications for biomaterial design and tissue regeneration strategies.

6.7.2 Role of BGs in Providing Mechanostimulus

BGs can indeed be engineered to impart specific mechanical cues that govern cellular responses. The mechanical properties of BGs, such as stiffness, elasticity, and surface topography, play critical roles in modulating cellular behaviour and influencing tissue regeneration processes. By tailoring these properties, BGs can provide appropriate mechanostimuli to cells, facilitating tissue regeneration. Let's delve into this in a more scientific manner.

(a) **Stiffness and Elasticity**

The stiffness and elasticity of a bioactive glass substrate play crucial roles in modulating cellular behaviour by impacting integrin clustering and focal adhesion formation. Cells cultured on substrates with varying stiffness levels demonstrate distinct responses, affecting adhesion, spreading, and proliferation dynamics. Notably, osteoblasts, the primary bone-forming cells, exhibit favourable responses to stiffer environments, leading to enhanced differentiation and matrix production. Through precise tuning of stiffness properties, researchers can engineer BGs to provide optimal mechanical cues tailored to specific cell types and applications.

6.7.2.1 Mechanisms of Cellular Response to Stiffness

Integrin Clustering and Focal Adhesion Formation

- Integrins, transmembrane receptors linking the ECM to the cell cytoskeleton, play pivotal roles in sensing and transmitting mechanical cues.
- On stiffer substrates, integrin clustering is enhanced, facilitating focal adhesion assembly and strengthening cell-substrate interactions.

Enhanced Adhesion and Spreading

- Cells grown on stiffer substrates typically exhibit increased adhesion and spreading due to enhanced integrin-mediated interactions with the substrate.
- The rigid mechanical environment promotes stable focal adhesion formation, allowing for robust cell attachment and spreading.

Proliferation and Differentiation

- Stiffer substrates often promote higher rates of cell proliferation, attributed to enhanced cell-substrate interactions and signalling cascades initiated by integrin engagement.
- Osteoblasts, in particular, demonstrate a preference for stiffer environments, as they stimulate osteogenic differentiation pathways and matrix production, crucial for bone formation and mineralization.

6.7.2.2 Impact of Stiffness on Cellular Functions

Matrix Remodelling and Tissue Formation

- The mechanical properties of the substrate influence cellular remodelling of the ECM and tissue formation processes.
- Stiffer substrates promote matrix deposition and organization, facilitating the formation of functional tissue structures.

Cellular Mechanotransduction Pathways

- Stiffness-mediated cellular responses are governed by mechanotransduction pathways, where mechanical signals are converted into biochemical responses.

- Integrin-mediated signalling pathways, such as the FAK/ Src pathway, play pivotal roles in transducing mechanical cues into intracellular signalling cascades that regulate cell behaviour and gene expression.

6.7.2.3 Engineering BGs with Tunable Stiffness

Material Composition and Processing Parameters

- The stiffness of BGs can be precisely controlled through adjustments in composition and processing parameters, such as sintering temperature and duration.
- Altering the ratio of network modifiers and glass formers can influence the rigidity of the glass network, thereby modulating substrate stiffness.

Applications in Tissue Engineering

- Tailoring the stiffness of BGs is essential for creating biomaterials that mimic the mechanical properties of native tissues and provide optimal environments for cell growth and tissue regeneration.
- For bone tissue engineering applications, BGs with stiffness resembling that of bone tissue are particularly desirable, as they promote osteoblastic differentiation and mineralization.

(b) **Surface Topography**

The surface topography of BGs, encompassing features such as roughness and patterning, exerts significant influence on cellular behaviours and functions. Surface roughness enhances cell attachment and spreading by augmenting the surface area available for cell adhesion. Moreover, micro- and nanoscale surface features play pivotal roles in directing cell alignment, migration, and differentiation. For instance, nanoscale roughness has been demonstrated to promote osteogenic differentiation of MSCs, while microscale grooves can guide cell orientation and migration. By meticulously designing bioactive glass surfaces with specific topographical features, it becomes feasible to provide targeted mechanostimuli that enhance cellular responses.

6.7.2.4 Mechanisms of Cellular Response to Surface Topography

Enhanced Cell Adhesion and Spreading

- Surface roughness increases the surface area available for cell adhesion, thereby promoting initial attachment and spreading of cells.
- Micro- and nanoscale surface features create focal points for cell adhesion, facilitating robust cell-substrate interactions.

Cell Alignment and Migration

- Surface patterning with microscale grooves or nanoscale ridges can induce directional cues that guide cell alignment and migration along specific orientations.

- Cells align and migrate along the direction of surface features, aligning their cytoskeletal elements and enhancing tissue organization.

Regulation of Cell Differentiation

- Surface topography influences cell fate decisions and lineage commitment by modulating intracellular signalling pathways.
- Nanoscale roughness and patterning have been shown to promote osteogenic differentiation of MSCs through activation of mechanotransduction pathways and regulation of gene expression.

6.7.2.5 Impact of Surface Topography on Tissue Engineering

Promotion of Tissue Regeneration

- Surface topography of BGs plays a critical role in promoting tissue regeneration by guiding cellular behaviours essential for tissue formation and remodelling.
- Engineered surface features facilitate cell adhesion, migration, proliferation, and differentiation, contributing to the development of functional tissue constructs.

(c) **Osteogenesis and Bone Tissue Engineering**

- BGs with specific surface topographies are particularly beneficial for bone tissue engineering applications.
- Nanoscale roughness enhances osteogenic differentiation of MSCs, while microscale grooves facilitate alignment of osteoblasts and deposition of mineralized matrix.

(d) **Dynamic Mechanical Loading**

Dynamic mechanical loading plays a crucial role in bone tissue engineering applications, where BGs serve as versatile biomaterials capable of withstanding and transmitting these dynamic loads. Through the application of cyclic mechanical loading, BGs can enhance bone formation and remodelling processes, mimicking the natural mechanical environment of bone tissue and promoting more effective and rapid tissue healing [25]

6.7.2.6 Importance of Dynamic Mechanical Loading

Stimulation of Bone Formation

- Dynamic mechanical loading induces mechanical strains within bone tissue, which serve as potent stimuli for osteogenesis.
- Cyclic loading promotes the activation and differentiation of osteoblasts, the bone-forming cells, leading to increased bone matrix deposition and mineralization.

Regulation of Bone Remodelling

- Mechanical loading regulates bone remodelling processes by modulating the activities of osteoblasts and osteoclasts.
- Properly applied dynamic loading promotes a balance between bone formation and resorption, resulting in the maintenance of bone integrity and strength.

6.7.3 Role of BGs in Dynamic Loading

Mechanical Resilience of BGs

- BGs are engineered to possess suitable mechanical properties, including strength, stiffness, and elasticity, to withstand dynamic loading conditions.
- The structural integrity of BGs allows them to effectively transmit mechanical loads to surrounding tissues, facilitating cellular responses and tissue regeneration.

Transmission of Mechanical Stimuli

- BGs act as intermediaries for transmitting dynamic mechanical stimuli to resident cells within the tissue-engineered construct.
- Mechanical signals generated by cyclic loading are transferred through the bioactive glass scaffold to osteogenic cells, stimulating their activity and promoting bone formation.

6.7.3.1 Mimicking the Natural Bone Environment

Mimicry of Bone Mechanics

- BGs, in combination with dynamic loading, mimic the mechanical properties and loading patterns observed in native bone tissue.
- This mimicry creates a more physiologically relevant microenvironment for osteogenic cells, enhancing their responsiveness to mechanical cues and facilitating tissue regeneration.

Accelerated Tissue Healing

- The synergistic effects of BGs and dynamic loading accelerate tissue healing processes by promoting enhanced osteogenic differentiation, matrix deposition, and tissue integration.
- The combination of mechanical stimuli and bioactive glass properties creates an environment conducive to rapid and effective bone regeneration.

Dynamic mechanical loading, when applied in conjunction with BGs, represents a powerful strategy for enhancing bone tissue engineering outcomes. By mimicking the natural mechanical environment of bone tissue, dynamic loading stimulates osteogenic responses within tissue-engineered constructs, leading to accelerated bone formation and remodelling. BGs serve as robust scaffolds capable of withstanding dynamic loads and transmitting mechanical stimuli to resident cells, thereby promoting tissue healing and regeneration. Continued research in this area holds promise for further optimizing the synergy between dynamic loading and BGs, advancing the field of bone tissue engineering towards improved clinical outcomes.

6.8 MECHANOTRANSDUCTION PATHWAYS

Mechanotransduction pathways play pivotal roles in cellular responses to mechanical stimuli provided by BGs. Upon interaction with these biomaterials, cells activate various signalling cascades to translate mechanical signals into biochemical responses. Integrin-mediated signalling emerges as a central pathway involved in sensing and responding to mechanical forces. When cells adhere to bioactive glass surfaces, integrins undergo clustering and form focal adhesions, which serve as mechanosensitive complexes that transmit mechanical information to the cell nucleus. This initiates a cascade of intracellular signalling events, including activation of the MAPK and Rho/ROCK pathways, which modulate gene expression and cellular behaviour.

6.8.1 Integrin-Mediated Signalling

Formation of Focal Adhesions

- Integrins, transmembrane receptors that bind to ECM components, cluster upon cell adhesion to bioactive glass surfaces, leading to the assembly of focal adhesions.
- Focal adhesions serve as mechanosensitive complexes that link the ECM to the cell cytoskeleton, enabling the transmission of mechanical signals across the plasma membrane.

Activation of Intracellular Signalling

- Integrin engagement initiates intracellular signalling cascades, including activation of FAK and Src kinases.
- FAK and Src phosphorylation events trigger downstream signalling pathways involved in gene expression regulation and cellular responses to mechanical cues.

6.8.2 MAPK Signalling Pathway

Regulation of Gene Expression

- The MAPK pathway, comprising extracellular signal-regulated kinase (ERK), c-Jun N-terminal kinase (JNK), and p38 kinases, is activated in response to mechanical stimulation.

- Activation of MAPK signalling leads to phosphorylation of transcription factors and modulation of gene expression profiles associated with cell proliferation, differentiation, and matrix remodelling.

6.8.3 Rho/ROCK Signalling Pathway

Regulation of Cytoskeletal Dynamics

- Rho GTPases, key regulators of cytoskeletal dynamics and cell contractility, play crucial roles in cellular responses to mechanical cues.
- Activation of the Rho/ROCK pathway leads to actin cytoskeleton reorganization, focal adhesion maturation, and cellular contractility, influencing cell shape, migration, and differentiation processes.

Mechanotransduction pathways are integral to cellular responses elicited by BGs, facilitating the translation of mechanical stimuli into biochemical signals that regulate gene expression and cellular behaviour. Integrin-mediated signalling serves as a primary mechanism for sensing and transducing mechanical forces, initiating downstream signalling cascades such as the MAPK and Rho/ROCK pathways. Understanding these mechanotransduction pathways is essential for elucidating the mechanisms underlying cellular responses to BGs and optimizing their design for enhanced tissue regeneration and biomedical applications.

6.9 SYNERGY WITH BIOCHEMICAL SIGNALS

The mechanical stimuli provided by BGs synergize with biochemical signals to amplify cellular responses, fostering enhanced tissue regeneration outcomes. Through the release of therapeutic ions, BGs complement mechanical cues, thereby promoting cell proliferation, differentiation, and ECM production. This synergistic interplay between mechanical and biochemical stimuli creates a holistic and effective microenvironment conducive to tissue regeneration.

6.9.1 Mechanotransduction and Biochemical Signalling

Integration of Mechanical and Biochemical Cues

- BGs release therapeutic ions, such as calcium, phosphorus, and silicon, into the local microenvironment, modulating cellular responses.
- These ions act as biochemical signals that regulate cellular functions, including proliferation, differentiation, and matrix synthesis.

Complementary Effects on Cellular Responses

- Mechanical stimuli provided by BGs, such as substrate stiffness and surface topography, initiate mechanotransduction pathways that influence cell behaviour.

- Concurrently, therapeutic ions released from BGs activate intracellular signalling cascades, further modulating cellular responses and tissue regeneration processes.

6.9.2 Promotion of Cellular Activities

Enhanced Cell Proliferation and Differentiation

- The combination of mechanical and biochemical stimuli synergistically promotes cell proliferation and differentiation.
- Mechanical cues facilitate cell adhesion, spreading, and cytoskeletal remodelling, while therapeutic ions regulate gene expression profiles associated with cell fate determination and tissue-specific differentiation.

Stimulation of Extracellular Matrix Production

- Mechanical and biochemical signals cooperate to enhance ECM production and remodelling.
- Mechanical cues stimulate ECM synthesis and assembly by promoting cell-matrix interactions and facilitating matrix deposition, while biochemical signals regulate ECM composition and organization.

6.10 APPLICATIONS OF MECHANOSENSING INTERACTIONS OF BGS

Mechanosensing interactions in BGs have profound implications across various biomedical applications, leveraging the ability of cells to perceive and respond to mechanical cues for tissue regeneration and therapeutic interventions.

6.10.1 Bone Tissue Engineering

Bone tissue engineering stands as a flagship application where the mechanosensing interactions of BGs play a pivotal role. By harnessing the ability of cells to perceive and respond to mechanical cues, BGs offer promising solutions for promoting bone regeneration and healing. Let's delve into the scientific intricacies of bone tissue engineering with BGs:

6.10.1.1 Scaffold Design

Scaffold design is a critical aspect of bone tissue engineering, and bioactive glass scaffolds offer versatile platforms with tailored mechanical properties and surface characteristics to mimic the natural bone environment. Through the integration of tailored stiffness, porosity, and surface topography, bioactive glass scaffolds provide mechanical cues that enhance osteoblast proliferation, differentiation, and matrix production, ultimately promoting bone regeneration and healing. Let's delve into the scientific intricacies of scaffold design in bone tissue engineering with BGs:

6.10.1.2 Tailored Mechanical Properties

Stiffness and Elasticity

- Bioactive glass scaffolds are engineered to exhibit stiffness and elasticity resembling that of native bone tissue, ensuring compatibility with the surrounding environment.
- The stiffness of the scaffold influences mechanotransduction pathways, affecting osteoblastic behaviour and bone regeneration processes.

Mechanical Support and Structural Integrity

- Scaffold designs optimize mechanical support and structural integrity to withstand physiological loads and provide a conducive microenvironment for cell attachment and tissue ingrowth.
- Mechanical stability is crucial for supporting osteogenic differentiation and matrix deposition by providing appropriate mechanical cues to resident cells.

6.10.1.3 Controlled Porosity

Enhanced Nutrient Transport

- Porous bioactive glass scaffolds facilitate nutrient and oxygen transport throughout the scaffold, supporting cell viability and metabolic activity.
- Controlled porosity enhances cell infiltration and tissue integration, promoting uniform distribution of cells and matrix deposition within the scaffold.

Mechanical Cues from Pore Structure

- Interconnected pores within the scaffold serve as channels for mechanical cues, influencing cell behaviour and tissue regeneration processes.
- The size, shape, and distribution of pores can be tailored to modulate mechanical stimuli and optimize cellular responses for enhanced bone regeneration.

6.10.1.4 Surface Topography

Promotion of Cell Adhesion and Spreading

- Surface topography of bioactive glass scaffolds, including roughness and patterning, enhances cell adhesion and spreading by providing increased surface area for cell attachment.

- Micro- and nanoscale surface features direct cell alignment, migration, and differentiation, further facilitating tissue regeneration processes.

Guidance of Osteogenic Differentiation

- Nanoscale surface roughness promotes osteogenic differentiation of MSCs by modulating cell-matrix interactions and signalling pathways.
- Microscale surface grooves guide the orientation and migration of osteoblasts, influencing matrix deposition and bone tissue formation within the scaffold.

6.10.1.5 Release of Therapeutic Ions

Support for Bone Mineralization

- Bioactive glass scaffolds release therapeutic ions, such as calcium and phosphate, into the local microenvironment, supporting bone mineralization and healing.
- These ions act as biochemical signals that regulate osteogenic differentiation, matrix mineralization, and bone tissue regeneration processes.

6.11 DESIGN AND LOADING CHARACTERISTICS

Scaffold design is a crucial aspect of bone tissue engineering with BGs, enabling the creation of biomimetic platforms that mimic the natural bone environment and promote enhanced bone regeneration and healing. By integrating tailored mechanical properties, controlled porosity, surface topography, and release of therapeutic ions, bioactive glass scaffolds offer versatile solutions for addressing bone defects and injuries, driving advancements in regenerative medicine and orthopaedic healthcare. Continued research in scaffold design and optimization will further enhance the efficacy of bioactive glass scaffolds in bone tissue engineering applications, leading to improved clinical outcomes and patient care.

6.11.1 Dynamic Loading

Dynamic loading, particularly when combined with BGs, represents a promising strategy to enhance bone formation and tissue development in bone tissue engineering applications. By subjecting BGs to cyclic mechanical loading within dynamic loading environments like bioreactors, researchers can stimulate osteogenic differentiation and accelerate bone tissue development. This approach harnesses the mechanosensing capabilities of BGs to optimize bone regeneration processes. Let's delve into the scientific underpinnings of dynamic loading in bone tissue engineering with BGs:

1. **Mechanosensitive Response of Cells**
   Osteogenic Differentiation

   - Mechanosensitive cells within bone tissue, including osteoblasts and MSCs, respond to mechanical cues by initiating osteogenic differentiation pathways.

- Cyclic mechanical loading triggers mechanotransduction mechanisms, activating signalling pathways involved in osteogenic gene expression and matrix mineralization.

Enhanced Cellular Activities

- Dynamic loading stimulates cellular activities essential for bone formation, including cell proliferation, ECM synthesis, and mineralization.
- Mechanosensitive cells exhibit increased metabolic activity and upregulation of osteogenic markers in response to cyclic mechanical stimulation.

2. **Optimization of Scaffold Integration**
   Improved Tissue Ingrowth

- Dynamic loading promotes tissue ingrowth and scaffold integration by enhancing cell migration, proliferation, and matrix deposition within bioactive glass scaffolds.
- Mechanical stimulation facilitates the infiltration of osteogenic cells into the scaffold, leading to more uniform distribution and enhanced tissue development.

Enhanced Vascularization

- Cyclic mechanical loading stimulates angiogenic responses within the engineered tissue, promoting the formation of functional blood vessels and improving nutrient transport and waste removal.
- Enhanced vascularization supports cell survival and metabolic activity, contributing to the overall success of bone tissue regeneration.

3. **Accelerated Bone Remodelling**
   Facilitation of Bone Remodelling Processes

- Dynamic loading accelerates bone remodelling processes by modulating the activities of osteoblasts and osteoclasts.
- Mechanical stimulation promotes the resorption of old bone tissue and the formation of new bone, leading to enhanced bone turnover and remodelling within the engineered tissue.

Optimization of Bone Quality

- Cyclic mechanical loading optimizes bone quality by promoting the alignment and organization of collagen fibres and the deposition of mineralized matrix.
- Mechanical cues from dynamic loading environments contribute to the development of structurally sound and functionally competent bone tissue.

Dynamic loading in combination with BGs offers a promising approach to optimize bone tissue engineering outcomes by harnessing the mechanosensitive nature of bone cells. By subjecting bioactive glass scaffolds to cyclic mechanical stimulation within dynamic loading environments, researchers can stimulate osteogenic differentiation, enhance scaffold integration, and accelerate bone remodelling processes. Continued research in this area will further elucidate the mechanisms underlying the synergistic effects of dynamic loading and BGs on bone regeneration, paving the way for innovative strategies in regenerative medicine and orthopaedic healthcare.

Successfully navigating the regulatory approval process for BGs requires a comprehensive and strategic approach. By conducting rigorous preclinical and clinical studies, adhering to quality assurance standards, and engaging with regulatory authorities, developers can demonstrate the safety and efficacy of bioactive glass products. Overcoming these regulatory hurdles is essential for bringing innovative bioactive glass technologies to clinical practice and improving patient outcomes.

Looking ahead, the versatility of BGs holds immense potential for addressing a spectrum of medical needs across diverse therapeutic areas. From bone tissue engineering to wound healing and drug delivery systems, BGs offer versatile platforms for tailored solutions to complex medical challenges. Through sustained interdisciplinary collaboration and concerted efforts to overcome technological barriers, BGs are poised to revolutionize medical interventions, enhancing human health and well-being on a global scale. As such, continued commitment to research, innovation, and collaboration will be paramount in unlocking the full potential of BGs and realizing their transformative impact in healthcare.

REFERENCES

1. M. V. Thomas, D. A. Puleo, and M. Al-Sabbagh, "Bioactive glass three decades on," *Journal of Long-Term Effects of Medical Implants,* vol. 15, no. 6, pp. 585–597, 2005, doi: 10.1615/JLongTermEffMedImplants.v15.i6.20.
2. F. Baino, "Bioactive glasses and glass-ceramics," *Encyclopaedia of Materials: Technical Ceramics and Glasses*, vol. 3, no. 2, pp. V3-614-V3-623, Jan. 2021, doi: 10.1016/B978-0-12-803581-8.12088-0.
3. L. L. Hench, "Bioceramics: from concept to clinic," *Journal of the American Ceramic Society*, vol. 74, no. 7, pp. 1487–1510, 1991, doi: 10.1111/j.1151-2916.1991.tb07132.x.
4. L. L. Hench, "The story of Bioglass®," *Journal of Materials Science: Materials in Medicine*, vol. 17, no. 11, pp. 967–978, 2006, doi: 10.1007/s10856-006-0432-z.
5. S. Gupta, S. Majumdar, and S. Krishnamurthy, "Bioactive glass: a multifunctional delivery system," *Journal of Controlled Release*, vol. 335, pp. 481–497, 2021, doi: 10.1016/j.jconrel.2021.05.043.
6. P. Fratzl and F. G. Barth, "Biomaterial systems for mechanosensing and actuation," *Nature 2009 462:7272*, vol. 462, no. 7272, pp. 442–448, 2009, doi: 10.1038/nature08603.
7. P. Fratzl, "Biomimetic materials research: what can we really learn from nature's structural materials?," *Journal of the Royal Society Interface*, vol. 4, no. 15, pp. 637–642, 2007, doi: 10.1098/rsif.2007.0218.
8. M. H. Kaou, M. Furkó, K. Balázsi, and C. Balázsi, "Advanced bioactive glasses: the newest achievements and breakthroughs in the area," *Nanomaterials*, vol. 13, no. 16, p. 2287, 2023, doi: 10.3390/NANO13162287.

9. M. Cannio, D. Bellucci, J. A. Roether, D. N. Boccaccini, and V. Cannillo, "Bioactive glass applications: a literature review of human clinical trials," *Materials (Basel)*, vol. 14, no. 18, 5440. 2021, doi: 10.3390/ma14185440.
10. H. Guo, X. Peng, X. Dong, J. Li, C. Cheng, and Q. Wei, "Promoting stem cell mechanosensing and osteogenesis by hybrid soft fibers," *ACS Applied Materials & Interfaces*, vol. 15, no. 41, pp. 47880–47892, 2023, https://doi.org/10.1021/acsami.3c07999.
11. S. Banijamali, M. Heydari, and M. Mozafari, "Cellular response to bioactive glasses and glass–ceramics," In Masoud Mozafari (ed), *Handbook of Biomaterials Biocompatibility*, pp. 395–421, Woodhead Publishing Series in Biomaterials. 2020, doi: 10.1016/B978-0-08-102967-1.00019-0.
12. G. Kaur, V. Kumar, G. R. Pickrell, J. C. Mauro, Y. Lin, and S. K. Arya, "Bioactive glasses in gene regulation and proliferation," *Biomedical, Therapeutic and Clinical Applications of Bioactive Glasses*, pp. 175–200, 2019, doi: 10.1016/B978-0-08-102196-5.00006-9.
13. K. Kajander, S. V. Sirkiä, P. K. Vallittu, T. J. Heino, and J. A. Määttä, "Bioactive glasses promote rapid pre-osteoblastic cell migration in contrast to hydroxyapatite, while carbonated apatite shows migration inhibiting properties," *Scientific Reports*, vol. 13, no. 1, pp. 1–14, 2023, doi: 10.1038/s41598-023-47883-2.
14. D. F. Williams, "Biocompatibility pathways and mechanisms for bioactive materials: The bioactivity zone," *Bioactive Materials*, vol. 10, pp. 306–322, 2022, doi: 10.1016/J.BIOACTMAT.2021.08.014.
15. L. Azizi, P. Turkki, N. Huynh, J. M. Massera, and V. P. Hytönen, "Surface modification of bioactive glass promotes cell attachment and spreading," *ACS Omega*, vol. 6, no. 35, pp. 22635–22642, 2021, https://doi.org/10.1021/acsomega.1c02669.
16. D. Bellucci et al., "Human mesenchymal stem cell combined with a new strontium-enriched bioactive glass: an ex-vivo model for bone regeneration," *Materials*,vol. 12, no. 21, 3633. 2019, doi: 10.3390/MA12213633.
17. P. Naruphontjirakul, O. Tsigkou, S. Li, A. E. Porter, and J. R. Jones, "Human mesenchymal stem cells differentiate into an osteogenic lineage in presence of strontium containing bioactive glass nanoparticles," *Acta Biomaterialia*, vol. 90, pp. 373–392, 2019, doi: 10.1016/J.ACTBIO.2019.03.038.
18. G. Kaur et al., "Mechanical properties of bioactive glasses, ceramics, glass-ceramics and composites: state-of-the-art review and future challenges," *Materials Science and Engineering C*, vol. 104, 109895.2019, doi: 10.1016/j.msec.2019.109895.
19. A. Mohammadkhah and D. E. Day, "Mechanical properties of bioactive glass/polymer composite scaffolds for repairing load bearing bones," *International Journal of Applied Glass Science*, vol. 9, no. 2, pp. 188–197, 2018, doi: 10.1111/IJAG.12339.
20. M. S. El-khooly, A. S. Abdraboh, A. M. Bakr, and K. H. T. Ereiba, "Bioactivity and mechanical properties characterization of bioactive glass incorporated with graphene oxide," *Silicon*, vol. 15, no. 3, pp. 1263–1271, 2023, doi: 10.1007/S12633-022-02088-6.
21. E. Pirhonen, L. Moimas, and M. Brink, "Mechanical properties of bioactive glass 9-93 fibres," *Acta Biomaterialia*, vol. 2, no. 1, pp. 103–107, 2006, doi: 10.1016/j.actbio.2005.08.008.
22. H. Abreu et al., "Human T-cell responses to metallic ion-doped bioactive glasses," *International Journal of Molecular Sciences*, vol. 25, no. 8, 4501. 2024, https://doi.org/10.3390/ijms25084501.

23. K. Zheng, W. Niu, B. Lei, and A. R. Boccaccini, "Immunomodulatory bioactive glasses for tissue regeneration," *Acta Biomaterialia*, vol. 133, pp. 168–186, 2021, doi: 10.1016/j.actbio.2021.08.023.
24. J. Park and D. Kim, "Advanced immunomodulatory biomaterials for therapeutic applications," *Advanced Healthcare Materials*, 2024, doi: 10.1002/ADHM.202304496.
25. J. Bobo, A. Garg, P. Venkatraman, M. Puthenveedu, and P. R. LeDuc, "3D in vitro neuron on a chip for probing calcium mechanostimulation," *Advanced Biosystems*, vol. 4, no. 10, 2000080. 2020, doi: 10.1002/ADBI.202000080.

7 Recent Advances in Additive Manufacturing for Printing Biological Tissues

Vishnu Vijay Kumar, S. Shiva,
R. G. Asuwin Prabu, P. Navaneetha Krishnan,
Shrishail B. Sollappur, M. Sharan Chandran
and Muhammad Akhsin Muflikhun

7.1 INTRODUCTION

Biomaterials have become indispensable in the fields of regenerative medicine, dentistry, and infection treatment, playing a crucial role in the restoration and enhancement of biological functions [1–6]. In the field of regenerative medicine, they are used to create scaffolds that guide cellular growth and tissue regeneration [3]. Among the various biomaterials, bioactive glasses (BGs) are considered a group of reactive ceramic materials with attractive properties (Field [7]). Primarily composed of silica, calcium, sodium, and phosphorus [8], BGs are designed to interact positively with biological tissues, making them particularly suitable for medical applications. One of its key properties is the ability to bond with living tissues through the formation of a hydroxyapatite layer on its surface that mimics the mineral composition of bone. This bioactivity facilitates its integration with the surrounding tissues, promoting bone regeneration and healing. Furthermore, BG exhibits excellent mechanical strength, making it an ideal candidate for various biomedical applications, such as bone grafts, dental implants, and tissue engineering scaffolds. Its controlled degradation over time allows for the gradual release of essential ions, promoting cell growth and enhancing the overall healing process.

Bioactive glass was first developed by Larry Hench and colleagues at the University of Florida [1] and was the first reported material to form an interfacial bond with host tissue after implantation. The composition of the first BG was 46.1% SiO_2, 24.4% NaO, 26.9% CaO, and 2.6% P_2O_5, in mol%, trademarked as 45S5 Bioglass®. Since then, several types of BGs have been developed primarily centred around Hench's original formulation, with the classic 45S5 Bioglass® composition offering remarkable advantages due to its high bioactivity and osteoconductivity. The S53P4 BG, commercially known as BonAlive® was developed in the early 1990s

DOI: 10.1201/9781003660781-7

at Åbo Akademi University and University of Turku and was the first BG having a composition different from 45S5 [8]. They deteriorated slowly and had stronger network connectivity and sintering range than Bioglass®. Another type of BG material was borate-based 13-93B, which replaced SiO_2 with B_2O_3 and included additional K_2O and MgO as network modifiers. They were widely utilized to create scaffolds for tissue engineering [2, 9, 10].

A plethora of scientific literature is available for research on various types of BG materials targeting specific properties and applications [11–17]. However, it is to be noted that despite achieving desired properties, bioactive materials for medical/biological applications require adequate mechanical strength to bear loads and must be shaped for specific requirements, necessitating careful manufacturing. The conventional manufacturing methods are the melt-quench and sol-gel methods [18, 19]. The melt-quench technique involves melting raw materials at high temperatures followed by rapid cooling to form glass [20–22]. In contrast, the sol-gel process requires lower temperatures. The sol-gel method is a wet-chemical process where a solution undergoes gelation and is subsequently heat-treated to form glass [23–25]. However, these approaches have inherent limitations. The melt-quench technique faces limitations in design complexity and time efficiency primarily due to its reliance on molds and subtractive manufacturing processes. Creating molds for intricate designs is a time-consuming process, with each unique design requiring new molds. This contributes to longer lead times and increased costs. Additionally, the subtractive machining methods that involve the removal of excess material to achieve the final shape further limit the intricacy of designs that can be realized. Also, the batch processing methods commonly employed for conventional manufacturing pose challenges for customizing each product to specific design requirements, particularly in applications requiring individualized components such as patient-specific implants. Furthermore, the setup and changeover time for machinery as well as the need for skilled labour, contribute to the perceived limitations in time efficiency and design flexibility [26, 27].

On the other hand, the sol-gel method, despite its distinctive advantages, presents certain drawbacks. A notable challenge is the difficulty in achieving consistent and reproducible products on a large scale. Variations in precursor concentrations and processing conditions can potentially undermine the uniformity of the final product, posing challenges in maintaining quality and reliability across production batches. Scalability is another concern associated with the sol-gel method. The precision achieved in the smaller-scale production encounters obstacles when attempting to scale up to industrial levels. This transition introduces difficulties in maintaining the same level of control and uniformity, impacting the efficiency and reliability of the manufacturing process. In this context, the role of additive manufacturing (AM), also widely known as three-dimensional (3D) printing, emerges as a promising technique (Field [28–30]). The foremost advantage of 3D printing in BG production lies in its unparalleled design flexibility. The layer-by-layer additive approach allows for the creation of intricate and customized structures, making it particularly advantageous for applications requiring patient-specific implants and complex designs.

Recent research is focused on the 3D printing of BGs for a variety of applications, including orthopaedic and dental implants, scaffolds for tissue engineering, wound healing dressings, and much more [31–35]. Bone healing is a complex process influenced by various factors, such as mechanical, chemical, and electrical signals. Recent work by Polley et al. [36] demonstrated the 3D printing of bioactive and piezoelectric barium titanate (BT) and BG scaffolds for bone tissues [37]. Recent works by Zhou et al. [38], on the other hand, show the development of a novel 3D-printed bi-layer brain patch that promotes repair from brain injury. The technique uses high concentrations of mesoporous BG nanoparticles in the first layer, followed by a second layer of methacrylate silk fibroin hydrogel, providing the necessary mechanical support. While Kohestani and Pishbin employed hydrogel-based nanocomposite inks, consisting of alginate/gelatin matrix with mesoporous BG and zeolite-imidazole nanoparticles for 3D printing of bone scaffolds, Hu et al. [39] carried out melt-extrusion 3D printing to prepare biodegradable porous composite scaffolds containing BG , calcium sulphate hemihydrate (CSH), and polylactic acid (PLA) for bone defect repair.

3D printing has also been used for wound healing. Fayyazbakhsh et al. [40] developed 3D-printed dressings using gelatin, alginate, and bioactive borate glass (BBG) for the treatment of second-degree burn wounds. The inclusion of 20 wt.% BBG enhanced mechanical properties, lowered degradation rates, and allowed for continuous water flow for up to 10 days, solving issues with extended healing and pain associated with standard hydrogel dressings. A 3D-printed wound dressing was also developed by Monavari et al. [41] using an alginate dialdehyde–gelatin (ADA-GEL) hydrogel together with astaxanthin (ASX) and BBG microparticles (70B). Furthermore, the studies by Sánchez-Salcedo et al. [42] showed 3D-printed mesoporous BG scaffolds with hierarchical pore structures to have higher antimicrobial capacity. All of these highlight the recent advances in AM for printing biological tissues.

7.2 BIOACTIVE GLASS MATERIALS: PROPERTIES AND APPLICATIONS

A comprehensive overview of the properties and applications of BG materials follows. The discussion encompasses their bioactivity, biocompatibility, and osteogenic potential, highlighting their role in promoting cellular activity and tissue regeneration. Properties that make them highly suitable for tissue engineering and regenerative medicine applications. This section provides an in-depth exploration of the properties and diverse applications of BG materials in general.

7.2.1 Bioactivity

Bioactive glass is characterized by its ability to form a hydroxyapatite layer on its surface when in contact with biological fluids, such as blood or interstitial fluid [43]. This hydroxyapatite layer mimics the composition of natural bone minerals, facilitating the bonding of the material with living tissues [44]. The formation of this layer is a dynamic process involving the exchange of ions between the BG and the surrounding environment. This bioactivity promotes osteoconduction, the growth of bone tissue into and around the material, fostering strong and lasting integration with the host bone. The hydroxyapatite layer not only enhances the mechanical stability of implants but also accelerates the healing process by providing a biologically favourable environment for cell attachment and proliferation [29].

7.2.2 Biocompatibility

Biocompatibility refers to the ability of a material to interact with biological systems without causing adverse reactions. BG materials demonstrate excellent biocompatibility, making them well suited for use in various biomedical applications. When implanted, BG does not elicit an immune response or toxicity, ensuring that it is well tolerated by the body. This property is crucial for the long-term success of implants and other medical devices [45]. Moreover, BG promotes cell adhesion and proliferation, supporting the formation of new tissue. The surface properties of BG can be tailored to encourage specific cellular responses, making it versatile for applications ranging from bone implants to tissue engineering scaffolds. The controlled release of ions during the bioactive process also contributes to the activation of signalling pathways that promote tissue regeneration and healing [46].

Compared to other materials used in biomedical applications, BG stands out for its unique combination of bioactivity and biocompatibility [37]. Traditional inert materials may lack the ability to stimulate tissue growth, while more reactive materials might induce excessive inflammation. BG strikes a balance, fostering a harmonious interaction with the body by actively participating in the biological processes, ultimately leading to improved patient outcomes and reduced risk of complications. The precise control over the composition and structure of BG further enhances its suitability for tailored biomedical solutions, such as patient-specific implants and regenerative medicine approaches. This layer facilitates osseointegration and promotes bone regeneration. Furthermore, BG materials exhibit excellent biocompatibility, minimizing adverse immune responses and facilitating cell adhesion and proliferation.

7.2.3 Osteogenic Potential

One of the hallmark features of BG materials is their osteogenic potential [45]. BG, with its inherent osteogenic potential, has emerged as a promising material for promoting bone regeneration and integration in biomedical applications. The unique composition of BG, which is also tailorable, facilitates the formation of a hydroxyapatite layer upon contact with biological fluids, mimicking the mineral structure of natural bone. This bioactivity not only enhances the material's osseointegration but also stimulates osteogenic activity. The released ions, such as silicon and calcium, play a pivotal role in activating signalling pathways that promote the differentiation of osteoprogenitor cells into osteoblasts, the cells responsible for bone formation. This activation of osteogenic processes accelerates the healing of bone defects and supports the successful incorporation of BG implants within the host tissue. Furthermore, BG scaffolds, manufactured using advanced AM techniques, provide 3D structures conducive to cell attachment and proliferation, fostering a favourable microenvironment for new bone tissue formation. The osteogenic potential of BG positions it as a versatile and effective material in regenerative medicine, particularly in orthopaedic and dental applications where bone healing and integration are critical for long-term success.

7.2.4 Controlled Release of Bioactive Ions

Bioactive glass materials can be engineered to release bioactive ions such as calcium, silicon, and phosphate ions, which play crucial roles in tissue regeneration processes, as already discussed in the above section. The controlled release of these ions from the glass matrix promotes angiogenesis, stimulates cell proliferation, and enhances tissue remodelling at the site of implantation [47]. Figure 7.1 depicts the application of bioglass using controlled release of bioactive ions.

7.2.5 Versatility in Formulation and Processing

Bioactive glass materials offer versatility in formulation and processing, allowing for customization to meet specific application requirements [2]. They can be synthesized using various techniques, including sol-gel processing, melt-quenching, and spray-drying, enabling precise control over composition, morphology, and surface properties. Customization of implants in accordance with the needs of the patient is also possible with AM technology, where control over the scaffold processing on the porosity can be advantageous for cell attachment, regeneration of tissue, and molecular movement. The personalization also allows the integration of drug delivery by controlled release of therapeutic agents, which shall be discussed subsequently.

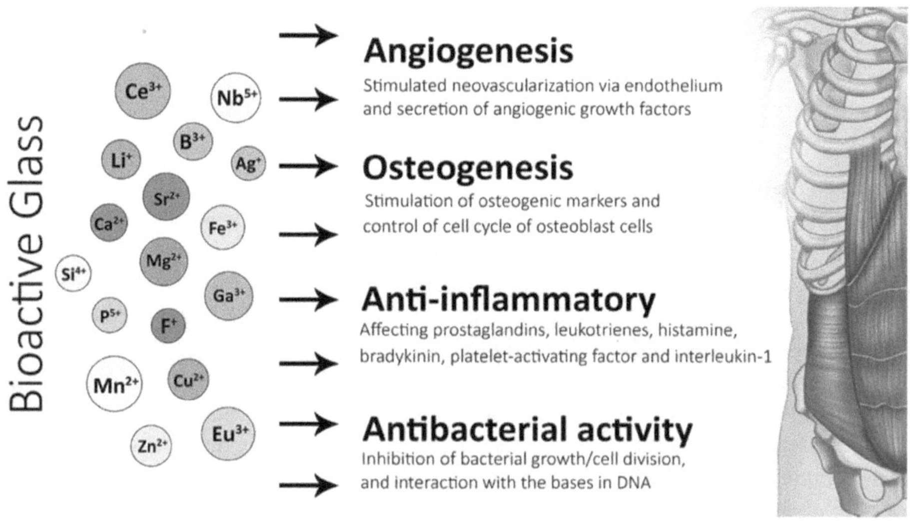

FIGURE 7.1 Depicting the prospects of controlled release of bioactive ions [48]. Under CC license

7.2.6 Applications in Tissue Engineering

The unique properties of BG materials make them well-suited for a wide range of tissue engineering applications. They are commonly used as scaffold materials for bone regeneration, dental implants, and cartilage repair [49]. Additionally, BG nanoparticles are incorporated into hydrogels and composite materials to enhance their bioactivity and mechanical properties [50].

3D-printed BG varieties have shown tremendous promise in bone tissue engineering, addressing challenges in bone defects and fractures. Customized implants and scaffolds, created through AM, offer precise control over the architecture and porosity of the structures. For instance, a BG scaffold designed with a composition like 13-93 provides an excellent framework for cell attachment and bone regeneration [51]. The scaffold acts as a temporary support, gradually degrading over time and being replaced by newly formed bone tissue. This approach has been applied in cases of critical-sized bone defects, trauma, or orthopaedic surgeries, facilitating enhanced bone healing and integration.

In the field of dentistry, 3D-printed BG materials have found applications in creating patient-specific dental implants, crowns, and bridges (Field [52]). The ability to precisely tailor the composition and structure of BGs allows for the development of dental implants that promote osseointegration and exhibit favourable biomechanical properties. This is particularly beneficial in cases of tooth loss or dental trauma arising from accidents, where the customization of implants ensures optimal fit and functionality. BG compositions, such as those containing strontium or zinc, may also contribute to improved dental implant outcomes by promoting bone regeneration and preventing bacterial infections [53].

Bioactive glass varieties, especially those designed for tissue engineering applications, are being explored for cartilage regeneration. 3D printing techniques enable the fabrication of scaffolds with specific porosity and mechanical properties conducive to cartilage growth [54]. By incorporating BG with tailored compositions, researchers aim to create implants that can support chondrogenesis and integrate seamlessly with the surrounding cartilaginous tissue. This approach holds promise for addressing cartilage defects, osteoarthritis, and other joint-related issues, offering a potential solution for improving joint function and reducing pain in patients. BG materials, when 3D printed into porous structures, have been investigated for their application in wound healing and skin regeneration. These scaffolds can support the attachment and proliferation of skin cells, facilitating the regeneration of dermal tissue [55]. The controlled release of ions from BG may also contribute to antibacterial properties, reducing the risk of infections in chronic wounds. This approach holds the potential for treating burns, chronic wounds, and skin injuries, providing a supportive matrix for tissue regeneration and minimizing scarring.

7.2.7 Drug Delivery Systems

Bioactive glass materials serve as effective carriers for the controlled release of therapeutic agents such as growth factors, antibiotics, and anti-inflammatory drugs [56]. The porous structure of BG scaffolds facilitates drug loading and release, enabling localized delivery to the target tissue while minimizing systemic side effects [56]. The versatility of preparing the formulations allows the customization of drugs based on the patient's specific needs, including the case of delivery of strontium or zinc ions to enhance the regeneration, which provides an enhanced therapeutic efficacy, especially in the case of bone-related disorders and in post-surgical recovery. The drug delivery system integrated into the BG-based implants also allows targeted delivery at the site, aiding in immediate treatment strategy, ensuring a localized release of drug for reducing inflammation or to prevent bacterial infection. Bacterial infections of even the minute degrees are to be completely prevented with the possible comorbidities that can cause and eventually lead to the need for the consumption of antibiotics. Consumption of antibiotics is also to be reduced, foreseeing the patient's health condition, which would be impaired, and the emerging antibiotic resistance exhibited by the microorganisms [57]. Thus, an antibacterial environment within the implant aids in a complete recovery process.

7.2.8 Antibacterial Properties

Certain formulations of BG materials exhibit inherent antibacterial properties, making them promising candidates for combating implant-associated infections. The release of bioactive ions disrupts bacterial cell membranes and inhibits microbial growth, contributing to improved implant success rates and patient outcomes [58]. Different BG compositions incorporate various antibacterial ions, and a comparative analysis sheds light on their efficacy in preventing infections. For instance, 45S5 Bioglass, enriched with sodium (Na) ions, has demonstrated antimicrobial activity against a broad spectrum of bacteria, including *Staphylococcus aureus, Staphylococcus epidermidis*, and *E. coli* [59]. S53P4 glass ceramic, which incorporates silver (Ag) ions, exhibits potent antibacterial effects and is commonly utilized in orthopaedic and dental applications (Field [60]). In contrast, BGs containing zinc (Zn) ions, such as those used in the 13-93 composition, showcase antimicrobial capabilities while also promoting tissue regeneration [61]. The choice of antibacterial ions influences the spectrum of pathogens targeted and the duration of antimicrobial activity. While silver ions are broadly effective, zinc ions contribute to both antibacterial and tissue-regenerative properties. Understanding the nuanced differences in antibacterial ion incorporation allows for the strategic selection of BG compositions tailored to specific biomedical applications, where preventing infections is a critical factor in the success of implants and regenerative therapies.

Overall, BG materials represent a versatile platform with immense potential for advancing regenerative medicine and tissue engineering. Their unique combination of properties makes them indispensable for a wide range of biomedical applications, from bone regeneration to controlled drug delivery systems. Continued research and innovation in BG materials hold promise for addressing complex clinical challenges and improving patient care outcomes.

7.3 INTEGRATING BIOACTIVE GLASS WITH ADDITIVE MANUFACTURING

The core of this chapter explores recent advances in integrating BG materials with AM technologies. It discusses advancements in material formulations, printing techniques, and post-processing strategies aimed at enhancing the bioactivity and structural integrity of printed tissues. BG is a type of glass that bonds with living tissues, encouraging bone regeneration and healing when implanted in the body [49]. The integration of AM and BG creates novel opportunities for the creation of personalized scaffolds, implants, and medical equipment with improved bioactivity and specific characteristics. This section explores recent developments and strategies for incorporating BG into AM processes:

7.3.1 Material Formulation and Optimization

In the realm of AM, the formulation of BG materials plays a critical role in determining printability, mechanical properties, and bioactivity. Researchers are actively exploring novel compositions and processing techniques to tailor BG formulations for specific printing applications. BGs often contain silicon, calcium, and phosphorus oxides, as well as other trace elements that promote bone repair and tissue integration [62]. Polymers, ceramics, and other materials in the nanoscale that are compatible with the AM process may be considered additives [45].

7.3.2 Printability and Scaffold Design

Additive manufacturing enables the precise fabrication of complex tissue scaffolds with customizable architectures. BG's printability and scaffold design with AM entails streamlining the manufacturing process to create intricate structures with precise mechanical strength, porosity, and bioactivity [63]. In order to optimize printing settings for uniform deposition and layer adhesion, it evaluates elements, including nozzle diameter, printing speed, and layer thickness. Reinforcements or additives to improve printability, mechanical strength, and biological responsiveness, such as polymers, ceramics, or nanoparticles. BG materials can be 3D printed into intricate scaffold designs that mimic the native extracellular matrix of target tissues [64]. Techniques such as fused deposition modelling (FDM), stereolithography (SLA), and selective laser sintering (SLS) offer precise control over scaffold geometry and porosity. Table 7.1 shows the various techniques employed for 3D printing of biotissues.

7.3.3 Surface Modification and Functionalization

Surface modification techniques are employed to enhance the bioactivity and cell-interaction properties of BG scaffolds [65]. Functionalization with bioactive molecules, growth factors, or peptides promotes cell adhesion, proliferation, and differentiation, facilitating tissue regeneration processes. Improved surface qualities of printed structures are necessary for surface modification and functionalization of BG via AM. This improves bioactivity, biocompatibility, and interaction with biological tissues. Modifying printing parameters or post-processing methods is done to impart surface roughness to the surface of BG objects at the micro- or nanoscale [28]. To encourage cell adhesion and tissue integration, thinly coating the surface of printed BG scaffolds with bioactive chemicals or biomolecules is also done.

TABLE 7.1
Description of the techniques

Printing technique	Description	Diagram
Material jetting	Entails utilizing a print head to deposit bioactive glass material droplets onto the build substrate. By precisely controlling the mix and distribution of materials, this approach makes it possible to create hybrid constructions with desired properties.	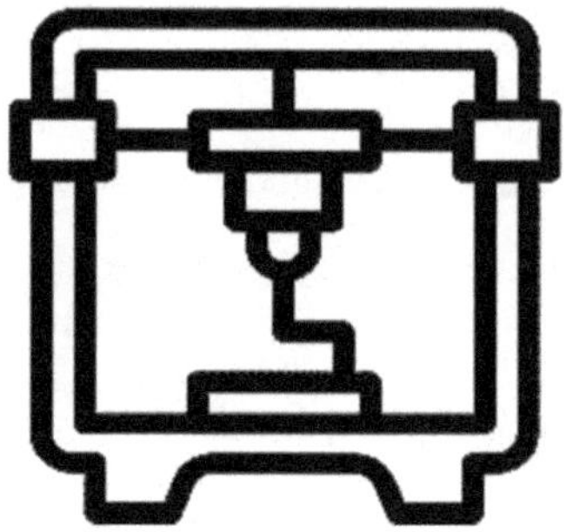
Binder jetting	It uses a binder to layer-by-layer selectively link bioactive glass particles together. This method works well for printing complex geometries, and it can be mixed with different materials to give the finished printed objects certain characteristics.	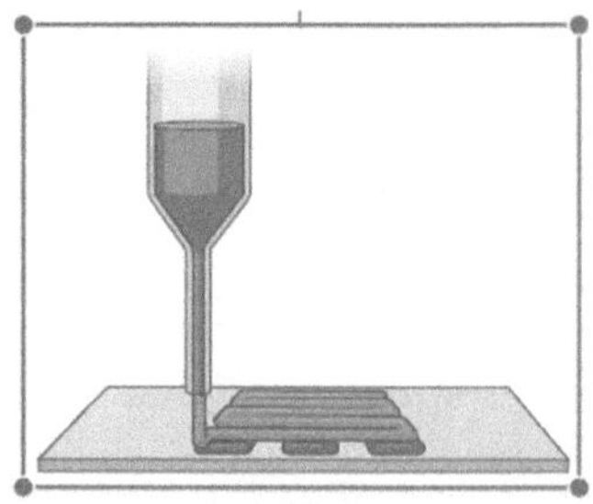
Nozzle based deposition	This method involves extruding bioactive glass material through a nozzle and depositing it onto the build surface. It allows for material selection freedom and allows for the creation of multi-material structures with customized properties for a range of biomedical applications.	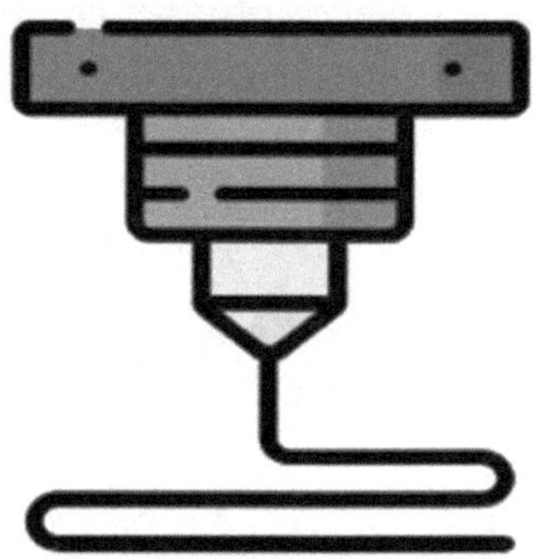

7.3.4 Incorporation of Bioactive Glass Nanoparticles

Bioactive glass nanoparticles combined with additive printing present a viable way to create innovative biomedical devices, implants, and scaffolds that have improved mechanical and bioactive capabilities. BG nanoparticles are increasingly utilized as additives in composite materials for AM. Advanced biomaterials with customized qualities and functionalities for orthopaedics, dentistry, tissue engineering, and regenerative medicine can be created by combining BG nanoparticles with AM. This method has a lot of potential for producing customized implants and medical equipment that encourage quicker healing and better clinical results. Their high surface area-to-volume ratio and bioactivity augment the mechanical properties and osteogenic potential of printed scaffolds [52]. Nanoparticle incorporation strategies aim to improve BG dispersion and homogeneity within the matrix [66].

7.3.5 Post-Processing and Surface Finishing

Post-processing techniques such as sintering, annealing, and surface polishing are employed to optimize the mechanical and bioactive properties of printed constructs. Heat treatments promote densification and crystallization of BG, enhancing its mechanical strength and bioactivity [67]. Surface finishing methods improve scaffold biocompatibility and minimize surface roughness, facilitating cell attachment and tissue ingrowth. BG's surface layers can be selectively removed by chemical etching using acids or alkaline solutions, resulting in textured or roughened surfaces that encourage tissue integration and cell adhesion [68]. It is possible to adjust etching parameters, including solution concentration, temperature, and time, to get the required surface shape and bioactivity [69]. Ion-exchange solutions can be used to alter the surface chemistry of printed BG structures in order to improve their bioactivity [30]. Ion exchange processes have the ability to introduce ions into the glass surface, such as strontium, calcium, or phosphate, which can stimulate osteogenic activity and promote the production of apatite. These surface finishing and post-processing methods allow us to improve the performance, quality, and usefulness of BG structures made with AM, which makes them suitable for use in a range of biomedical applications like scaffolds, implants, and medical equipment. Recent innovations integrating BG materials and critical ion release profiles in bioprinting technologies showcase remarkable progress towards realizing complex, viable tissue constructs, and organoids for regenerative medicine and pharmacological applications as shown in Figure 7.2.

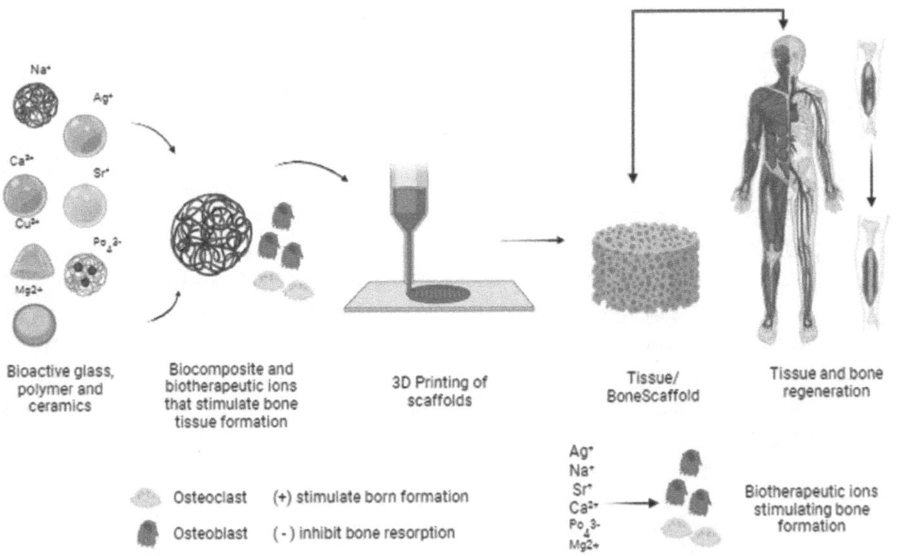

FIGURE 7.2 Image depicting the advances in achieving biomedical prospects by the integration of bioactive glass also aided by essential ions

7.3.6 Multi-Material Printing and Hybrid Constructs

Advances in multi-material printing enable the fabrication of hybrid constructs comprising BG materials and other biocompatible polymers or ceramics. Various materials can be deposited concurrently or sequentially using multi-material printing techniques, including material jetting, binder jetting, or nozzle-based deposition [70]. With the use of these procedures, hybrid structures can be precisely controlled in terms of material distribution and composition. Gradually switch between materials to attain desirable gradients in stiffness, porosity, or bioactivity for tissue engineering or regenerative medicine applications. Through the utilization of hybrid constructs and multi-material printing, we may design novel biomedical devices, implants, and scaffolds that exhibit improved functionality and performance [71]. These methods make it possible to create tailored solutions for medication delivery, tissue engineering, regenerative medicine, and personalized healthcare.

7.3.7 In Vitro and In Vivo Evaluation

The integration of BG with AM necessitates rigorous in vitro and in vivo evaluation to assess scaffold biocompatibility, bioactivity, and tissue regeneration potential. Preclinical studies involving cell culture assays, histological analysis, and animal models provide valuable insights into scaffold performance and guide translational research efforts. In vitro, assessment examines the cytocompatibility of BG scaffolds by culturing appropriate cell types on the scaffold surface, such as mesenchymal stem cells and osteoblasts. It uses assays like MTT, Alamar Blue, or live/dead staining to measure the morphology, proliferation, and viability of the cells [72]. Using microscopy methods like scanning electron microscopy (SEM) or fluorescence microscopy, it assesses cell adherence and dissemination on BG surfaces [73]. In vitro evaluation also analyses cellular interactions with the scaffold material and analyses cell shape, focal adhesions, and cytoskeletal architecture. In vivo assessment examines implantation studies in animal models (e.g., rats, rabbits, sheep) to evaluate the biocompatibility and tissue response to BG scaffolds. It assesses host tissue integration, inflammation, and immune response following implantation using histological analysis and immunohistochemistry [74]. Monitoring bone regeneration and remodelling around implanted BG scaffolds using imaging techniques such as X-ray, micro-computed tomography, or magnetic resonance imaging. Quantify bone formation, defect healing, and scaffold degradation rates to evaluate the effectiveness of the scaffold in promoting tissue regeneration. Evaluating the long-term biocompatibility and safety of BG scaffolds by monitoring host responses and tissue interactions over extended periods. Assess potential adverse effects, such as chronic inflammation, fibrosis, or foreign body reactions, to ensure the stability and compatibility of the scaffold in vivo [75].

Overall, the integration of BG materials with AM holds immense promise for the development of advanced tissue engineering scaffolds with enhanced bioactivity and functionality. Continued research efforts are aiming to optimize printing parameters, refine scaffold design strategies, and elucidate the mechanistic basis of tissue-material interactions for future clinical translation.

7.4 CHALLENGES AND FUTURE DIRECTIONS

Bioglass can be used as substrates for cells to support themselves since they can attach to living bone and soft tissues. Adopting bioglass materials for bioprinting successfully, however, presents a number of difficulties. Cell survival and function may be jeopardized by the severe processing temperatures required to melt and shape bioglasses into print-ready inks. More delicate techniques for preparing bio-ink are needed. Second, under some conditions, tissue maturation processes may be hampered by poor bioglass dissolving rates brought on by subpar paste chemistries. Optimizing ion release and degradation profiles to bolster cellular proliferation is still an unresolved research concern. Furthermore, the intentional building of complicated developmental paradigms required to mimic genuine tissue microstructures is hampered by our inadequate understanding of how bioglass surface reactions guide cell destiny processes. Enhancing architectural control may be elucidated by developments in high-resolution cell imaging and analysis during bioglass-supported cultures.

Up the future, bioglass AM presents intriguing opportunities for customized tissue implants with geometries that are therapeutically relevant for filling up bone deficiencies or supporting soft tissues that require restoration. We anticipate that advancements in multi-paste bioprinting will provide advanced compositional and microstructural control, enabling the creation of bioglasses that direct in vitro vascularization and innervation processes to maintain viability before implantation.

Furthermore, combining bioprinting with cutting-edge nanofabrication techniques may allow for precise topographical and biochemical patterning to guide stem cell development along certain lineages within printed tissues. Adoptive transfers of cells conditioned in this manner in vitro may help address host rejection problems, provided that immunological consequences are carefully taken into account. Bioglass provides special capabilities for quickening the translation of bioprinted tissues; nonetheless, to fully realize their potential, more fundamental research, along with supporting engineering advancements in print head technologies, bio-ink compositions, and multi-material control, is required.

7.5 CONCLUSION

Using cutting-edge multi-material 3D bioprinters, additive biomanufacturing provides ground-breaking potential for producing functioning, live tissue structures for medical applications and disease simulation. However, overcoming significant obstacles that current technologies are unable to address completely is necessary to realize the transformative medical potential of bioprinting. The current state of the art is not yet able to produce sustainable, higher-order tissues that replicate natural organ complexity due to difficulties with vascularization, innervation, biocompatibility, and controlled resorption rates. Moreover, regulatory advancement is hindered by vagueness in standards and benchmarks.

Nonetheless, the topic shows great potential as it quickly accumulates synergies across crossing fields like materials science, stem cell biology, microfluidics, imaging, biomechanics, and machine learning. Combined progress in enhancing technology capabilities and better mimicking developmental processes can result in a new generation of bioprinted tissues with hitherto unmatched complexity.

Moving forward, multi-disciplinary interactions between engineering and biological sciences will accelerate the pace of discovery, bringing bioprinting closer to clinical and commercial reality. Navigating the remaining hurdles will need patience and perseverance, but the results will be tremendously beneficial to medicine and people's lives. The impact is increasingly increasing with each incremental breakthrough as researchers transform it into practical applications.

REFERENCES

1. L. L. Hench, R. J. Splinter, W. C. Allen, and T. K. Greenlee, "Bonding mechanisms at the interface of ceramic prosthetic materials," *J. Biomed. Mater. Res.*, vol. 5, no. 6, pp. 117–141, 1971, doi: 10.1002/jbm.820050611.
2. M. Cannio, D. Bellucci, J. A. Roether, D. N. Boccaccini, and V. Cannillo, "Bioactive glass applications: a literature review of human clinical trials," *Materials (Basel)*, vol. 14, no. 18, pp. 1–25, 2021, doi: 10.3390/ma14185440.
3. X. Zhao, J. M. Courtney, and H. Qian, *Bioactive materials in medicine: design and applications*. India: Woodhead publishing. 2011. doi: 10.1533/9780857092939.
4. A. R. Boccaccini and J. J. Blaker, "Bioactive composite materials for tissue engineering scaffolds," *Expert Rev. Med. Devices*, vol. 2, no. 3, pp. 303–317, 2005, doi: 10.1586/17434440.2.3.303.
5. A. C. Profeta and G. M. Prucher, "Bioactive-glass in periodontal surgery and implant dentistry," *Dent. Mater. J.*, vol. 34, no. 5, pp. 559–571, 2015, doi: 10.4012/dmj.2014-233.
6. M. Vollenweider et al., "Remineralization of human dentin using ultrafine bioactive glass particles," *Acta Biomater.*, vol. 3, no. 6, pp. 936–943, 2007, doi: 10.1016/j.actbio.2007.04.003.
7. D. S. Brauer, "Bioactive glasses - structure and properties," *Angew. Chemie - Int. Ed.*, vol. 54, no. 14, pp. 4160–4181, 2015, doi: 10.1002/anie.201405310.
8. P. Sinitsyna, O. Karlström, and L. Hupa, "In vitro dissolution of bioactive glass S53P4 microspheres," *J. Am. Ceram. Soc.*, vol. 105, no. 3, pp. 1658–1670, 2022, doi: 10.1111/jace.18014.
9. A. Dukle, D. Murugan, A. J. Nathanael, L. Rangasamy, and T. H. Oh, "Can 3D-printed bioactive glasses be the future of bone tissue engineering?," *Polymers (Basel)*, vol. 14, no. 8, pp. 1–20, 2022, doi: 10.3390/polym14081627.
10. K. C. R. Kolan, Y. W. Huang, J. A. Semon, and M. C. Leu, "3D-printed biomimetic bioactive glass scaffolds for bone regeneration in rat calvarial defects," *Int. J. Bioprinting*, vol. 6, no. 2, pp. 1–17, 2020, doi: 10.18063/ijb.v6i2.274.
11. J. R. Smith, Bone dynamics associated with the controlled loading of bioglass-coated aluminum oxide endosteal implants. *American Journal of Orthodontics, 76*(6), pp. 618–636, 1979.
12. K. Kudo and M. Miyasawa, "Clinical application of dental implant with root of coated bioglass: short-term results," *Oral Surgery, Oral Medicine, Oral Pathology, 70*(1), pp. 18–23., 1990.
13. I. Allan, H. Newman, and M. Wilson, "Antibacterial activity of particulate bioglass® against supra- and subgingival bacteria," *Biomaterials*, vol. 22, pp. 1683–1687, 2001.
14. K. P. Ananth, S. Suganya, D. Mangalaraj, J. M. F. Ferreira, and A. Balamurugan, "Electrophoretic bilayer deposition of zirconia and reinforced bioglass system on Ti6Al4V for implant applications: an in vitro investigation," *Mater. Sci. Eng. C*, vol. 33, no. 7, pp. 4160–4166, 2013, doi: 10.1016/j.msec.2013.06.010.

15. S. Jebahi *et al.*, "Chitosan-based bioglass composite for bone tissue healing: oxidative stress status and antiosteoporotic performance in a ovariectomized rat model," *Korean J. Chem. Eng.*, vol. 31, no. 9, pp. 1616–1623, 2014, doi: 10.1007/s11814-014-0072-9.
16. L. Wang *et al.*, "Multi-functional bismuth-doped bioglasses: combining bioactivity and photothermal response for bone tumor treatment and tissue repair," *Light Sci. Appl.*, pp. 1–13, 2018, doi: 10.1038/s41377-018-0007-z.
17. P. Eshghinejad, H. Farnoush, M. S. Bahrami, X. B. Chen, H. Farnoush, and M. S. Bahrami, "Electrophoretic deposition of bioglass/graphene oxide composite on Ti-alloy implants for improved antibacterial and cytocompatible properties," *Mater. Technol.*, vol. 35, no. 2, pp. 69–74, 2020, doi: 10.1080/10667857.2019.1648740.
18. F. Baino *et al.*, "Processing methods for making porous bioactive glass-based scaffolds—A state-of-the-art review," *Int. J. Appl. Ceram. Technol.*, vol. 16, no. 5, pp. 1762–1796, 2019, doi: 10.1111/ijac.13195.
19. M. Maximov, O. C. Maximov, L. Craciun, D. Ficai, A. Ficai, and E. Andronescu, "Bioactive glass—an extensive study of the preparation and coating methods," *Coatings*, vol. 11, no. 11, pp. 1–28, 2021, doi: 10.3390/coatings11111386.
20. G. Koller, Æ. R. J. Cook, Æ. I. D. Thompson, T. F. Watson, and Æ. L. Di, "Surface modification of titanium implants using bioactive glasses with air abrasion technologies," *J. Mater. Sci. Mater. Med.*, vol. 18, pp. 2291–2296, 2007, doi: 10.1007/s10856-007-3137-z.
21. J. Chakraborty *et al.*, "Surface & coatings technology multifunctional gradient coatings of phosphate-free bioactive glass on SS316L biomedical implant materials for improved fi xation," *Surf. Coat. Technol.*, vol. 240, pp. 437–443, 2014, doi: 10.1016/j.surfcoat.2013.12.072.
22. T. Tite *et al.*, "Applied surface science phosphate bioglass thin-films: cross-area uniformity, structure and biological performance tailored by the simple modification of magnetron sputtering gas pressure," *Appl. Surf. Sci.*, vol. 541, no. November 2020, p. 148640, 2021, doi: 10.1016/j.apsusc.2020.148640.
23. P. Zhang, K. Yang, Z. Zhou, X. Zhu, and W. Li, "Customized borosilicate bioglass scaffolds with excellent biodegradation and osteogenesis for mandible reconstruction," *Front. Bioeng. Biotechnol.*, vol. 8, pp. 1–9, 2020, doi: 10.3389/fbioe.2020.610284.
24. M. Haftbaradaran-esfahani, M. Ahmadian, and A. H. Nassajpour-esfahani, "Applied surface science fabrication and characterization of porous biomedical vitallium alloy with 58S bioglass coating prepared by sol-gel method," *Appl. Surf. Sci.*, vol. 506, no. August 2019, p. 144959, 2020, doi: 10.1016/j.apsusc.2019.144959.
25. A. Anand, V. Lalzawmliana, V. Kumar, P. Das, and K. B. Devi, "Journal of the mechanical behavior of biomedical materials preparation and in vivo biocompatibility studies of di ff erent mesoporous bioactive glasses," *J. Mech. Behav. Biomed. Mater.*, vol. 89, no. July 2018, pp. 89–98, 2019, doi: 10.1016/j.jmbbm.2018.09.024.
26. V. Vijay Kumar, S. Ramakrishna, J. L. Kong Yoong, R. Esmaeely Neisiany, S. Surendran, and G. Balaganesan, "Electrospun nanofiber interleaving in fiber reinforced composites—recent trends," *Mater. Des. Process. Commun.*, vol. 1, no. 1, pp. 1–8, 2019, doi: 10.1002/mdp2.24.
27. V. V. Kumar, G. Balaganesan, J. K. Y. Lee, R. E. Neisiany, S. Surendran, and S. Ramakrishna, "A review of recent advances in nanoengineered polymer composites," *Polymers (Basel)*, vol. 11, no. 4, 2019, doi: 10.3390/polym11040644.
28. S. Simorgh *et al.*, "Additive manufacturing of bioactive glass biomaterials," *Methods*, vol. 208, no. November 2022, pp. 75–91, 2022, doi: 10.1016/j.ymeth.2022.10.010.
29. G. Turnbull et al., "3D bioactive composite scaffolds for bone tissue engineering," *Bioact. Mater.*, vol. 3, no. 3, pp. 278–314, 2018, doi: 10.1016/j.bioactmat.2017.10.001.
30. M. H. Kaou, M. Furkó, K. Balázsi, and C. Balázsi, "Advanced bioactive glasses: the newest achievements and breakthroughs in the area," *Nanomaterials*, vol. 13, no. 16, pp. 1–33, 2023, doi: 10.3390/nano13162287.

31. J. J. Chung, H. Im, S. H. Kim, J. W. Park, and Y. Jung, "Toward biomimetic scaffolds for tissue engineering: 3D printing techniques in regenerative medicine," *Front. Bioeng. Biotechnol.*, vol. 8, no. November, pp. 1–12, 2020, doi: 10.3389/fbioe.2020.586406.
32. H. N. Chia and B. M. Wu, "Recent advances in 3D printing of biomaterials," *J. Biol. Eng.*, vol. 9, no. 1, pp. 1–14, 2015, doi: 10.1186/s13036-015-0001-4.
33. M. Singh and S. Jonnalagadda, "Advances in bioprinting using additive manufacturing," *Eur. J. Pharm. Sci.*, vol. 143, no. August 2019, p. 105167, 2020, doi: 10.1016/j.ejps.2019.105167.
34. M. Javaid and A. Haleem, "3D printed tissue and organ using additive manufacturing: an overview," *Clin. Epidemiol. Glob. Heal.*, vol. 8, no. 2, pp. 586–594, 2020, doi: 10.1016/j.cegh.2019.12.008.
35. M. Rothbauer *et al.*, "Recent advances in additive manufacturing and 3D bioprinting for organs-on-a-chip and microphysiological systems," *Front. Bioeng. Biotechnol.*, vol. 10, no. February, pp. 1–14, 2022, doi: 10.3389/fbioe.2022.837087.
36. C. Polley *et al.*, "3D printing of piezoelectric and bioactive barium titanate-bioactive glass scaffolds for bone tissue engineering," *Mater. Today Bio.*, vol. 21, no. July, p. 100719, 2023, doi: 10.1016/j.mtbio.2023.100719.
37. S. Shiva *et al.*, "A review on the recent applications of synthetic biopolymers in 3D printing for biomedical applications," *J. Mater. Sci. Mater. Med.*, vol. 34, no. 12, 2023, doi: 10.1007/s10856-023-06765-9.
38. L. Zhou, H. Liu, B. Zhang, C. Wei, S. Zhou, and X. Huang, "A novel 3D-printed bi-layer cranial-brain patch promotes brain injury repair and bone tissue regeneration," *Adv. Funct. Mater.*, vol. 2314330, pp. 1–14, 2024, doi: 10.1002/adfm.202314330.
39. H. Hu *et al.*, "3D printing of porous degradable scaffolds with polylactic acid-loaded bioactive glass and calcium sulfate hemihydrate for bone defect repair," *Adv. Mater. Technol.*, vol. 8, no. 15, pp. 1–13, 2023, doi: 10.1002/admt.202300061.
40. F. Fayyazbakhsh, M. J. Khayat, C. Sadler, D. Day, Y. W. Huang, and M. C. Leu, "3D-printed hydrogels dressings with bioactive borate glass for continuous hydration and treatment of second-degree burns," *Int. J. Bioprinting*, vol. 9, no. 6, pp. 132–150, 2023, doi: 10.36922/IJB.0118.
41. M. Monavari *et al.*, "A 3D-printed wound-healing material composed of alginate dialdehyde-gelatin incorporating astaxanthin and borate bioactive glass microparticles," *ACS Appl. Mater. Interfaces*, vol. 15, no. 44, pp. 50626–50637, 2023, doi: 10.1021/acsami.2c23252.
42. S. Sánchez-Salcedo, A. García, A. González-Jiménez, and M. Vallet-Regí, "Antibacterial effect of 3D printed mesoporous bioactive glass scaffolds doped with metallic silver nanoparticles," *Acta Biomater.*, vol. 155, pp. 654–666, 2023, doi: 10.1016/j.actbio.2022.10.045.
43. M. N. Rahaman *et al.*, "Bioactive glass in tissue engineering," *Acta Biomater.*, vol. 7, no. 6, pp. 2355–2373, 2011, doi: 10.1016/j.actbio.2011.03.016.
44. S. M. Lee *et al.*, "Physical, morphological, and wound healing properties of a polyurethane foam-film dressing," *Biomater. Res.*, vol. 20, no. 1, pp. 1–11, 2016, doi: 10.1186/s40824-016-0063-5.
45. H. R. Fernandes, A. Gaddam, A. Rebelo, D. Brazete, G. E. Stan, and J. M. F. Ferreira, "Bioactive glasses and glass-ceramics for healthcare applications in bone regeneration and tissue engineering," *Materials (Basel)*, vol. 11, no. 12, pp. 1–54, 2018, doi: 10.3390/ma11122530.
46. N. L. Nechaeva *et al.*, "Multiscale flaked silver SERS-substrate for glycated human albumin biosensing," *Anal. Chim. Acta*, vol. 1100, pp. 250–257, 2020, doi: 10.1016/j.aca.2019.11.072.
47. Y. Gao, M. A. Seles, and M. Rajan, "Role of bioglass derivatives in tissue regeneration and repair: a review," *Rev. Adv. Mater. Sci.*, vol. 62, no. 1, 2023, doi: 10.1515/rams-2022-0318.

48. N. Al-Harbi *et al.*, "Silica-based bioactive glasses and their applications in hard tissue regeneration: a review," *Pharmaceuticals*, vol. 14, no. 2, pp. 1–20, 2021, doi: 10.3390/ph14020075.
49. L. C. Gerhardt and A. R. Boccaccini, "Bioactive glass and glass-ceramic scaffolds for bone tissue engineering," *Materials (Basel)*, vol. 3, no. 7, pp. 3867–3910, 2010, doi: 10.3390/ma3073867.
50. E. Zeimaran *et al.*, "Advances in bioactive glass-containing injectable hydrogel biomaterials for tissue regeneration," *Acta Biomater.*, vol. 136, pp. 1–36, 2021, doi: 10.1016/j.actbio.2021.09.034.
51. Q. Fu, M. N. Rahaman, B. Sonny Bal, R. F. Brown, and D. E. Day, "Mechanical and in vitro performance of 13-93 bioactive glass scaffolds prepared by a polymer foam replication technique," *Acta Biomater.*, vol. 4, no. 6, pp. 1854–1864, 2008, doi: 10.1016/j.actbio.2008.04.019.
52. N. Jafari, M. S. Habashi, A. Hashemi, R. Shirazi, N. Tanideh, and A. Tamadon, "Application of bioactive glasses in various dental fields," *Biomater. Res.*, vol. 26, no. 1, pp. 1–15, 2022, doi: 10.1186/s40824-022-00274-6.
53. H. E. Skallevold, D. Rokaya, Z. Khurshid, and M. S. Zafar, "Bioactive glass applications in dentistry," *Int. J. Mol. Sci.*, vol. 20, no. 23, pp. 1–24, 2019, doi: 10.3390/ijms20235960.
54. S. Stratton, N. B. Shelke, K. Hoshino, S. Rudraiah, and S. G. Kumbar, "Bioactive polymeric scaffolds for tissue engineering," *Bioact. Mater.*, vol. 1, no. 2, pp. 93–108, 2016, doi: 10.1016/j.bioactmat.2016.11.001.
55. P. E. Antezana *et al.*, "The 3D bioprinted scaffolds for wound healing," *Pharmaceutics*, vol. 14, no. 2, pp. 1–46, 2022, doi: 10.3390/pharmaceutics14020464.
56. S. Gupta, S. Majumdar, and S. Krishnamurthy, "Bioactive glass: a multifunctional delivery system," *J. Control. Release*, vol. 335, no. May, pp. 481–497, 2021, doi: 10.1016/j.jconrel.2021.05.043.
57. L. Z. Yamani and N. Elhadi, "Virulence characteristics, antibiotic resistance patterns and molecular typing of enteropathogenic producing *Escherichia coli* (EPEC) isolates in eastern province of Saudi Arabia: 2013–2014," *Infect. Drug Resist.*, vol. 15, no. November, pp. 6763–6772, 2022, doi: 10.2147/IDR.S388956.
58. A. Vaishampayan and E. Grohmann, "Antimicrobials functioning through ros-mediated mechanisms: current insights," *Microorganisms*, vol. 10, no. 1, 2022, doi: 10.3390/microorganisms10010061.
59. S. Hu, J. Chang, M. Liu, and C. Ning, "Study on antibacterial effect of 45S5 Bioglass®," *J. Mater. Sci. Mater. Med.*, vol. 20, no. 1, pp. 281–286, 2009, doi: 10.1007/s10856-008-3564-5.
60. L. Drago *et al.*, "In vitro antibiofilm activity of bioactive glass S53P4," *Future Microbiol.*, vol. 9, no. 5, pp. 593–601, 2014, doi: 10.2217/fmb.14.20.
61. D. Ege, K. Zheng, and A. R. Boccaccini, "Borate bioactive glasses (BBG): bone regeneration, wound healing applications, and future directions," *ACS Appl. Bio Mater.*, vol. 5, no. 8, pp. 3608–3622, 2022, doi: 10.1021/acsabm.2c00384.
62. A. J. Salinas and P. Esbrit, "Mesoporous bioglasses enriched with bioactive agents for bone repair, with a special highlight of María vallet-Regí's contribution," *Pharmaceutics*, vol. 14, no. 1, 2022, doi: 10.3390/pharmaceutics14010202.
63. M. H. Mobarak *et al.*, "Recent advances of additive manufacturing in implant fabrication – a review," *Appl. Surf. Sci. Adv.*, vol. 18, no. October, p. 100462, 2023, doi: 10.1016/j.apsadv.2023.100462.
64. A. Martelli, D. Bellucci, and V. Cannillo, "Additive manufacturing of polymer/bioactive glass scaffolds for regenerative medicine: a review," *Polymers (Basel)*, vol. 15, no. 11, 2023, doi: 10.3390/polym15112473.

65. S. Kargozar *et al.,* "Functionalization and surface modifications of bioactive glasses (BGs): tailoring of the biological response working on the outermost surface layer," *Materials (Basel)*, vol. 12, no. 22, 2019, doi: 10.3390/ma12223696.
66. C. Vichery and J. M. Nedelec, "Bioactive glass nanoparticles: from synthesis to materials design for biomedical applications," *Materials (Basel)*, vol. 9, no. 4, 2016, doi: 10.3390/ma9040288.
67. M.-V. K. and M. M. Friese C, Yang J, "乳鼠心肌提取 HHS public access," *Physiol. Behav.*, vol. 46, no. 2, pp. 248–256, 2019, https://doi.org/10.1016/j.pmatsci.2017.08.003.
68. L. Azizi, P. Turkki, N. Huynh, J. M. Massera, and V. P. Hytönen, "Surface modification of bioactive glass promotes cell attachment and spreading," *ACS Omega*, vol. 6, no. 35, pp. 22635–22642, 2021, doi: 10.1021/acsomega.1c02669.
69. P. Chauhan, V. Koul, and N. Bhatnagar, "Critical role of etching parameters in the evolution of nano micro sla surface on the ti6al4v alloy dental implants," *Materials (Basel)*, vol. 14, no. 21, 2021, doi: 10.3390/ma14216344.
70. H. Chen, L. Guo, W. Zhu, and C. Li, "Recent advances in multi-material 3d printing of functional ceramic devices," *Polymers (Basel)*, vol. 14, no. 21, pp. 1–32, 2022, doi: 10.3390/polym14214635.
71. N. Ashammakhi *et al.,* "Bioinks and bioprinting technologies to make heterogeneous and biomimetic tissue constructs," *Mater. Today Bio*, vol. 1, no. February, 2019, doi: 10.1016/j.mtbio.2019.100008.
72. M. Salètes *et al.,* "Mesoporous bioactive glasses cytocompatibility assessment: a review of in vitro studies," *Biomimetics*, vol. 6, no. 1, pp. 1–32, 2021, doi: 10.3390/biomimetics6010009.
73. Q. Nawaz *et al.,* "Comparison of microstructure, sintering behavior, and biological response of sol-gel and melt-derived 13–93 bioactive glass scaffolds," *Open Ceram.*, vol. 15, no. July, p. 100407, 2023, doi: 10.1016/j.oceram.2023.100407.
74. S. K. Mahmood *et al.,* "In vivo evaluation of the novel nanocomposite porous 3d scaffold in a rabbit model: Hematology and biochemistry analysis," *Iraqi J. Vet. Sci.*, vol. 32, no. 2, pp. 219–230, 2018, doi: 10.33899/ijvs.2019.153853.
75. A. Carnicer-Lombarte, S. T. Chen, G. G. Malliaras, and D. G. Barone, "Foreign body reaction to implanted biomaterials and its impact in nerve neuroprosthetics," *Front. Bioeng. Biotechnol.*, vol. 9, no. April, pp. 1–22, 2021, doi: 10.3389/fbioe.2021.622524.

8 Biodegradable Polymers-Based Bioactive Glasses Nanocomposite

Yugesh A. Kharche and Santosh R. Shekokar

8.1 INTRODUCTION

Bioactive glasses have attracted a lot of attention in the area of biomaterials because of their bioactive properties, osteoconductive properties, and the potential to stimulate bone regeneration [1, 2]. However, due to their inherent brittle nature and low mechanical strength, bioactive glasses have not been directly used in load bearing bone tissue engineering (BTE). To overcome these challenges, bioactive glass-based nanocomposites have become an active field of research [3, 4]. One promising approach is to incorporate bioactive glasses into BTE polymer matrices (BPMs) to form nanocomposite material(s). BPMs such as polylactic acid (PLA) and polyglycolic acid (PGA) copolymers have been shown to be highly biocompatible, have tunable mechanical properties and degrade over time, and are attractive candidates for BTE applications [5, 6]. In this chapter, we'll look at the development and characterization of BPMs based on bioactive glasses, as well as the potential applications of BPMs (BTEs). We'll also look at how synergistic effects can occur when bioactive glasses and BPMs are combined, how to fabricate these.

8.2 BIOACTIVE GLASSES: PROPERTIES AND CONSIDERATIONS

Bioactive glass is a type of inorganic material (see Figure 8.1) that can be implanted in the human body and can form a tight bond with surrounding bone tissue. The most common type of bioactive glass is SiO_2-Na_2O-CaO-P_2O_5, also known as the Quaternary System of Bioactive Glass. 45S5 Bioactive Glass is a quaternary structure of bioactive glass. The name "45S5" is derived from the molecule 45S5, which stands for "45s5-sodium-5-sorbate-3". Larry Hench developed this molecule in the 1960s [7].

Bioactive glasses have a number of desirable properties for use in BTE, such as bioactivity, osteoconductivity, osteoinductiveness, dissolution, and ion release. When bioactive glasses are exposed to bodily fluids, they can form a hydroxyapatite layer (HA) on their surface, which helps to attach, proliferate, and differentiate osteoblasts (bone-forming cells). In addition, some bioactive glass compositions have been found to stimulate osteoinductive mesenchymal stem cell differentiation

DOI: 10.1201/9781003660781-8

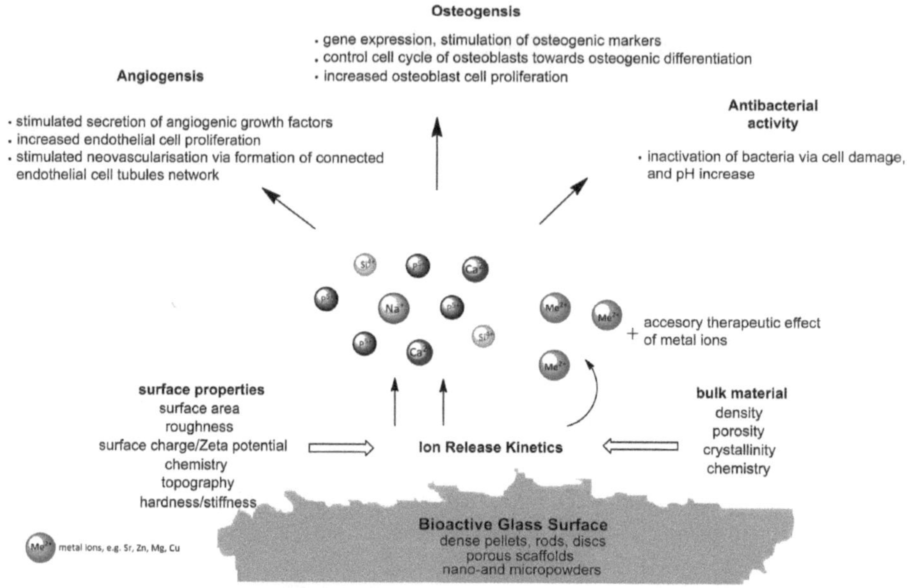

FIGURE 8.1 Visualizing biological reactions to ionic dissolution products from bioactive glasses [8]

(i.e., osteoblasts) and promote bone regeneration. However, bioactive glasses are naturally brittleness-prone and lack mechanical strength, making them unsuitable for direct application in BTE with load-bearing applications. To overcome these drawbacks, a promising approach has been developed, which is the development of biocompatible nanocomposites.

8.3 BIODEGRADABLE POLYMERS: VERSATILITY AND BIOCOMPATIBILITY

Polymers that are biodegradable have been extensively used in biomedical applications (see Figure 8.2 for BTE) due to their high biocompatibility properties, adjustable mechanical properties, and long-term degradation [5, 6].

Some of the regularly utilized biodegradable polymers in BTE are:

1. Polylactic acid (PLA): PLA is a synthetic aliphatic polyester made from renewable materials like corn flour or sugarcane. PLA has high mechanical qualities and is biodegradable and biocompatible [10].
2. Polyglycolic acid (PGA): Another synthetic aliphatic polyester, PGA is extremely crystalline and degrades quite quickly. It has been employed in a variety of biological applications, including sutures and bone fixation devices.
3. Polycaprolactone (PCL): PCL is a semi-crystalline, aliphatic polyester with a lower degradation rate than PLA and PGA. It is widely utilized in BTE because of its excellent mechanical characteristics and biocompatibility [11].

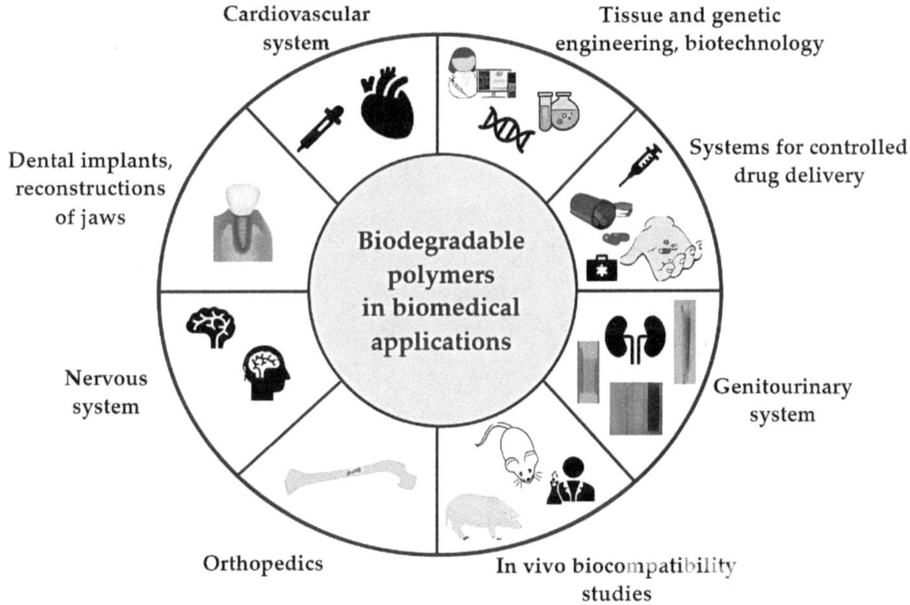

FIGURE 8.2 Application of biodegradable polymers in biomedical application [9]

4. Biodegradable Polymers: Copolymers, such as polylactic acid (PLA) or polylactic chloride (PL-PCL), can be formulated to have specific mechanical properties and degradation rates for particular uses [12].

Bioactive Glass in Biodegradable Polymer Matrices: Bioactive glasses can be used to create nanocomposite materials with enhanced biological and mechanical properties, making them attractive for BTE.

8.4 FABRICATION OF BIODEGRADABLE POLYMERS-BASED BIOACTIVE GLASSES NANOCOMPOSITES

Figure 8.3 presents two distinct methodologies (Strategy 1 and Strategy 2) for the synthesis of nanoparticles, specifically calcium/calcium oxide (Ca/CaO) nanoparticles, utilizing tetraethyl orthosilicate (TEOS) and an acid in either water or ethanol (ETOH) solution as initial components.

In Strategy 1, the process involves the formation of primary particles by combining TEOS and acid in water/ETOH solution. These primary particles are then mixed with calcium nitrate ($Ca(NO_3)_2$) to generate secondary particles, which are subsequently subjected to additional treatment, likely including heat treatment or annealing, resulting in the formation of the final Ca/CaO nanoparticles.

Strategy 2 comprises two sub-strategies, 2.I and 2.II.

In sub-strategy 2.I, primary particles formed from TEOS and acid in water/ETOH solution are blended with $Ca(NO_3)_2$ and undergo washing and annealing steps to yield the final Ca/CaO nanoparticles.

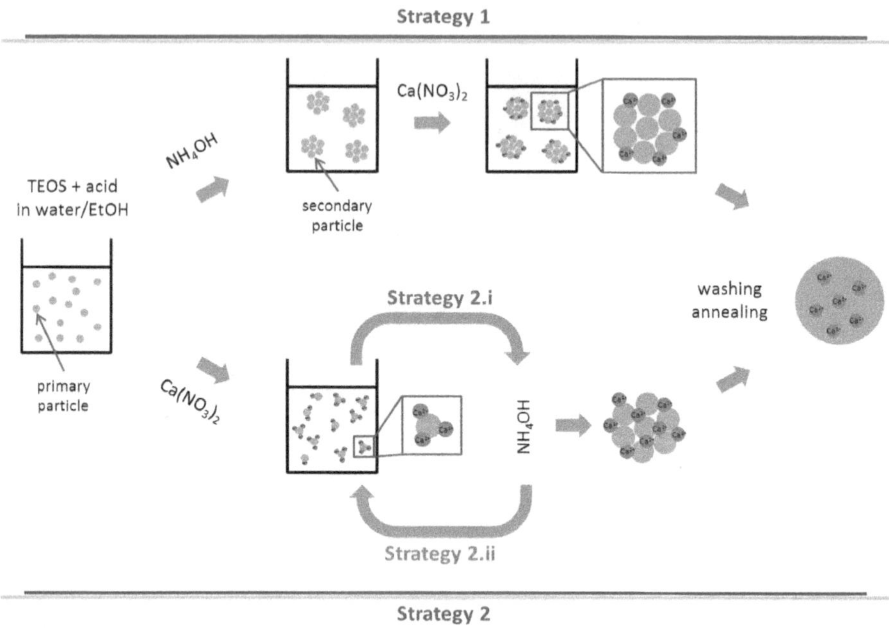

FIGURE 8.3 Schematic representation of the different strategies to synthesize binary bioactive glass nanoparticles [13]

Sub-strategy 2.II involves combining primary particles with $Ca(NO_3)_2$ initially, followed by treatment with sodium hydroxide (NaOH). Subsequent washing and annealing steps are then applied to obtain the final Ca/CaO nanoparticles.

These strategies, as shown in Figure 8.3, consist of sequential steps and additional reagents (e.g. $Ca(NO_3)_2$) and NaOH) to control the generation and properties of Ca/CaO nanoparticles. These strategies are likely intended to improve particle size, particle morphology, crystal structure, and purity.

The fabrication of nanocomposites based on biodegradable polymers and bioactive glasses typically involves several strategies:

1. **In Situ Polymerization**: In this process, the nanocomposite is synthesized concurrently with the polymer. It involves distributing bioactive glass particles in a monomer solution and then starting a polymerization process. This procedure produces a polymer matrix in which the bioactive glass particles are distributed. In situ polymerization has various advantages in the production of nanocomposites. It provides precise control over the dispersion of bioactive glass particles in the polymer matrix, resulting in improved mechanical, biological, and degrading characteristics. Furthermore, this approach allows for the integration of a broad range of bioactive glass compositions and particle sizes, providing flexibility in designing the nanocomposite for specific applications in tissue engineering, drug administration, or biomedical implants.
2. **Solvent Casting**: Bioactive glass particles are dispersed in a solvent, followed by dissolving the biodegradable polymer in the same solvent. The

resulting solution is then cast into a mold, with subsequent solvent evaporation yielding the nanocomposite. Solvent casting offers a relatively simple and versatile method for fabricating nanocomposites with controlled particle dispersion and composition. However, careful selection of solvent and process parameters is essential to ensure the desired properties and performance of the final nanocomposite material.

3. **Melt-Mixing**: Bioactive glass particles are blended with the biodegradable polymer in its molten state, then extruded or injection molded to create the nanocomposite.
4. **Electrospinning**: Bioactive glass particles are dispersed within a solution containing the biodegradable polymer. This composite solution undergoes electrospinning to produce nanofiber-based nanocomposites. Electrospinning is a method used to produce ultrafine fibers with diameters ranging from nanometers to micrometers. It involves the application of an electric field to a polymer solution or melt to draw out a thin fiber from a spinneret. In the context of nanocomposites, electrospinning is utilized to incorporate bioactive glass particles into nanofibers made of biodegradable polymers. Electrospinning is a powerful technology for manufacturing nanocomposites with regulated shape, content, and functionality, appropriate for a wide range of biomedical and tissue engineering applications.
5. **Freeze-Drying**: Bioactive glass particles are mixed into a polymer solution, which is then frozen and subjected to lyophilization, resulting in a porous nanocomposite scaffold.

The choice of fabrication method depends on several factors, including the specific composition of the biodegradable polymer and bioactive glass, the desired microstructure and porosity of the nanocomposite, and the intended application.

8.5 CHARACTERIZATION OF BIODEGRADABLE POLYMERS-BASED BIOACTIVE GLASSES NANOCOMPOSITES

The characterization of biodegradable polymers-based bioactive glasses nanocomposites typically involves the following techniques as shown in Figure 8.4.

1. Structural and Morphological Examination: Methods such as scanning electron microscopy (SEM), transmission electron microscopy (TEM), and X-ray diffraction (XRD) are employed for scrutinizing the microstructure, particle size, and dispersion of bioactive glass particles within the polymer matrix [14].
2. Analysis of Chemical Composition: Fourier-transform infrared spectroscopy (FTIR) and energy-dispersive X-ray spectroscopy (EDS) are employed to scrutinize the chemical composition and interplay between the bioactive glass and the biodegradable polymer.
3. Evaluation of Mechanical Characteristics: Tensile testing, compressive testing, and nanoindentation are utilized to assess the mechanical attributes of

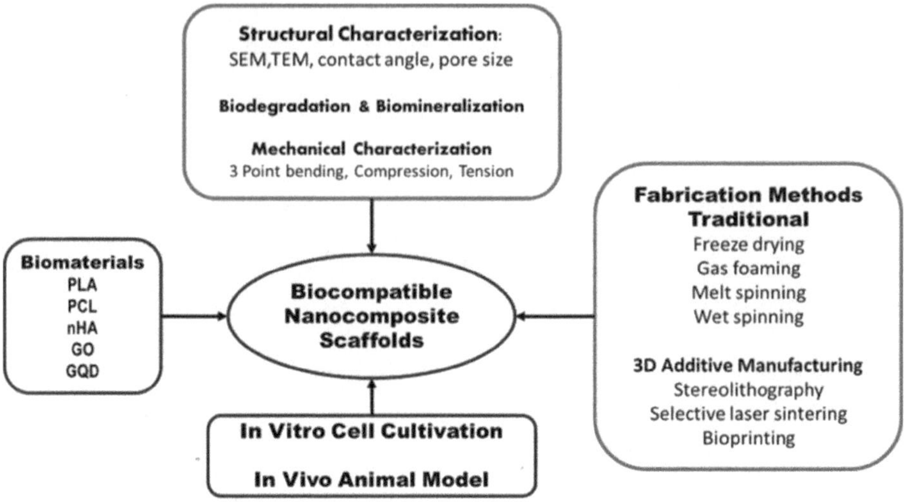

FIGURE 8.4 Different techniques for polymers-based bioactive glasses nanocomposites

the nanocomposites, encompassing Young's modulus, tensile strength, and compressive strength [8].

4. Thermal Property Assessment: Differential scanning calorimetry (DSC) and thermogravimetric analysis (TGA) are employed to probe the thermal attributes of the nanocomposites, including glass transition temperature, melting point, and degradation behavior [15, 16].
5. In Vitro Evaluation of Bioactivity: The bioactivity of the nanocomposites is typically gauged by immersing them in simulated body fluid (SBF) and observing the formation of a HA on their surface using techniques such as SEM and XRD [9].
6. In Vitro Cell Investigations: The biocompatibility and interactions of the nanocomposites with cells are examined using in vitro cell culture experiments, including assays for cell proliferation, viability, and differentiation [17].

The comprehensive characterization of these nanocomposites is essential for understanding their structure-property relationships and their suitability for various biomedical applications, particularly in the field of BTE.

8.6 APPLICATIONS OF BIODEGRADABLE POLYMERS-BASED BIOACTIVE GLASSES NANOCOMPOSITES

Biodegradable polymers-based bioactive glasses nanocomposites have been explored for a variety of biomedical applications as shown in Figure 8.5, including:

1. Bone Tissue Engineering: These nanocomposites can be used to fabricate scaffolds, bone grafts, and other implants for the repair and regeneration of bone tissue. The bioactive glass component enhances the osteoconductivity and osteoinductivity of the scaffold, while the biodegradable polymer

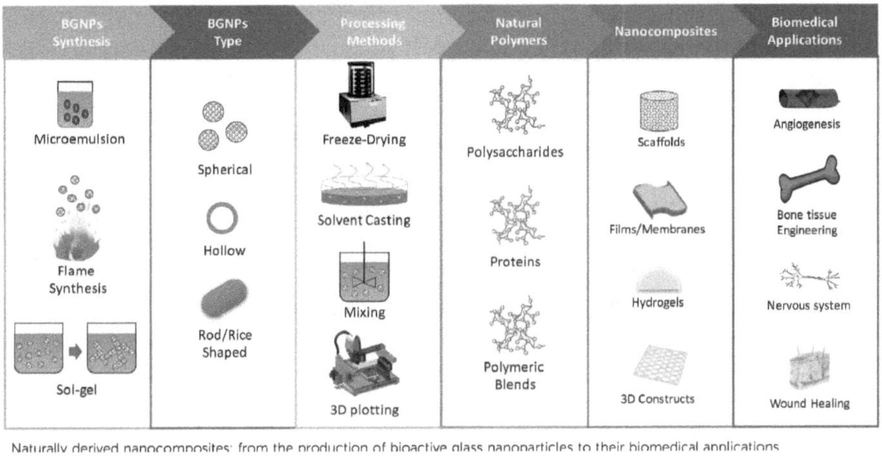

FIGURE 8.5 Application of biodegradable materials

provides the necessary mechanical support and allows for gradual replacement by new bone tissue.

2. Drug Delivery Systems: The bioactive glass component in the nanocomposites can be used to encapsulate and deliver therapeutic agents, such as antibiotics, growth factors, and stem cells, for the treatment of bone-related diseases or injuries [18].
3. Dental Applications: Biodegradable polymers-based bioactive glasses nanocomposites have been investigated for dental applications, such as dental fillings, root canal sealers, and bone grafting materials for dental implants.
4. Soft Tissue Engineering: In addition to BTE, these nanocomposites have also been explored for the regeneration of other soft tissues, such as cartilage and ligaments, due to their tunable mechanical properties and bioactive nature.

The successful integration of biodegradable polymers and bioactive glasses in nanocomposite materials has demonstrated promising results in various in vitro and in vivo studies, paving the way for their potential clinical translation and widespread application in the field of tissue engineering and regenerative medicine.

8.7 CHALLENGES AND OUTLOOK

8.7.1 Challenges

The development and application of biodegradable polymer-based bioactive glass nanocomposites present several challenges that need to be addressed to realize their full potential in biomedical applications.

8.7.1.1 Processing Challenges

Achieving a uniform dispersion of bioactive glass nanoparticles or fibers within the biodegradable polymer matrix is a significant challenge. Agglomeration and poor interfacial adhesion between the two components can lead to compromised mechanical properties and inconsistent biological performance. Various processing techniques, such as melt blending, solvent casting, and electrospinning, have been explored, but each method has its own limitations.

Melt blending, for instance, can induce thermal degradation of the polymer or bioactive glass components, while solvent casting may introduce residual solvents, which can be cytotoxic. Electrospinning, although promising for producing nanofiber-based composites, often requires the use of harsh solvents and can be challenging to scale up.

Additionally, achieving a homogeneous distribution of bioactive glass nanoparticles or fibers within the polymer matrix becomes increasingly difficult as the filler content increases, leading to potential agglomeration and compromised mechanical properties.

8.7.1.2 Degradation Control

Controlling the degradation rates of both the biodegradable polymer and bioactive glass components is crucial for ensuring the desired performance and longevity of the nanocomposites in vivo. The degradation rates of these materials can be influenced by various factors, such as polymer composition, molecular weight, crystallinity, and pH of the surrounding environment.

Ideally, the degradation rates of the polymer and bioactive glass components should be tailored to match the specific application and the desired rate of tissue regeneration or healing. For instance, in BTE applications, a slower degradation rate may be desirable to provide structural support until the new bone tissue has formed and matured.

However, achieving this precise control over degradation rates is challenging, as the degradation mechanisms of the polymer and bioactive glass components can interact in complex ways, leading to unpredictable degradation behaviors.

8.7.1.3 Bioactivity and Mechanical Property Balance

One of the main challenges in developing biodegradable polymer-based bioactive glass nanocomposites is balancing the bioactive properties, provided by the bioactive glass component, with the mechanical properties contributed by the polymer matrix. While bioactive glasses impart bioactivity and promote bone mineralization, their incorporation into the polymer matrix can compromise the mechanical properties, especially at higher filler concentrations.

Conversely, increasing the polymer content to enhance mechanical properties may reduce the overall bioactivity of the nanocomposite. Finding the optimal composition and processing conditions to achieve the desired balance between bioactivity and mechanical properties is a significant challenge.

8.7.1.4 Regulatory Challenges

The introduction of innovative biomaterials, such as biodegradable polymer-based bioactive glass nanocomposites, into clinical applications necessitates extensive testing and assessment to assure safety and efficacy [19]. Regulatory organizations, like the United States Food and Drug Administration (FDA) and the European Medicines

Agency (EMA), have created stringent criteria and procedures for the licensing of novel biomaterials.

Meeting these regulatory criteria can be time-consuming and costly since substantial in vitro and in vivo investigations are needed to establish the nanocomposites' biocompatibility, biodegradability, and long-term performance. In addition, the inclusion of nanoparticles or nanofibers in the composites may generate concerns about possible toxicity and environmental implications, complicating the regulatory clearance process.

8.7.1.5 Scale-Up and Cost-Effectiveness

While significant progress has been made in the development of biodegradable polymer-based bioactive glass nanocomposites at the laboratory scale, scaling up the production to industrial levels remains a challenge. The synthesis and processing of these nanocomposites often involve complex and multistep procedures, which can be difficult and costly to replicate on a larger scale.

Moreover, the raw materials used, such as high-purity bioactive glasses and specialized biodegradable polymers, can be expensive, further increasing the overall cost of production. Developing cost-effective and scalable manufacturing processes is crucial for the commercial viability of these nanocomposites and their widespread adoption in various biomedical applications.

8.7.2 Outlook

Despite the challenges faced in the development and application of biodegradable polymer-based bioactive glass nanocomposites, the field holds significant promise and potential for future advancements.

8.7.2.1 Novel Polymer and Bioactive Glass Combinations

Researchers are continuously exploring novel combinations of biodegradable polymers and bioactive glasses to tailor the properties and performance of the resulting nanocomposites for specific applications. For instance, the incorporation of bioactive glasses into natural polymers, such as chitosan or alginate, has shown promising results in terms of bioactivity and biodegradability.

Furthermore, the development of new bioactive glass compositions, such as mesoporous bioactive glasses or glasses doped with therapeutic ions (e.g., strontium, copper, or silver), can introduce additional functionalities to the nanocomposites, such as enhanced bioactivity, antimicrobial properties, or controlled drug release [3, 12].

8.7.2.2 Multifunctional Nanocomposites

Beyond their structural and bioactive properties, biodegradable polymer-based bioactive glass nanocomposites have the potential to be developed into multifunctional biomaterials by incorporating additional components, such as therapeutic agents, growth factors, or signaling molecules [20]. These multifunctional nanocomposites can simultaneously provide structural support, promote tissue regeneration, and deliver therapeutic agents in a controlled manner, offering potential solutions for various biomedical applications, such as bone and cartilage regeneration, wound healing, and cancer therapy [21].

8.7.2.3 Advanced Manufacturing Techniques

The combination of sophisticated manufacturing processes, such as 3D printing (also known as additive manufacturing), with biodegradable polymer-based bioactive glass nanocomposites has created new opportunities for developing complex and patient-specific implants or scaffolds [22]. 3D printing techniques, such as fused deposition modeling (FDM) or stereolithography (SLA), provide fine control over the architecture, porosity, and spatial distribution of the bioactive glass and polymer components inside the nanocomposite [23] (Figure 8.6).

Combining 3D printing technology with bioactive glass nanocomposites has transformed the area of osteology, with a concentration on bone research. Using synthetic polymers as a foundation material for 3D printing provides various benefits in this area. Reinforcing 3D-printed synthetic polymer scaffolds with bioactive glass nanoparticles allows for the replication of real bone's structural and mechanical capabilities. This replication creates a milieu that promotes bone cell adhesion, proliferation, and differentiation, therefore aiding bone tissue regeneration. These nanocomposites enable accurate 3D printing of customized implants and prostheses, providing enhanced biocompatibility, osseointegration, and mechanical strength. Furthermore, by integrating bioactive glass nanoparticles into 3D-printed polymer matrices, controlled drug delivery systems may be produced for the localized therapy of bone ailments or injuries with adjusted release kinetics.

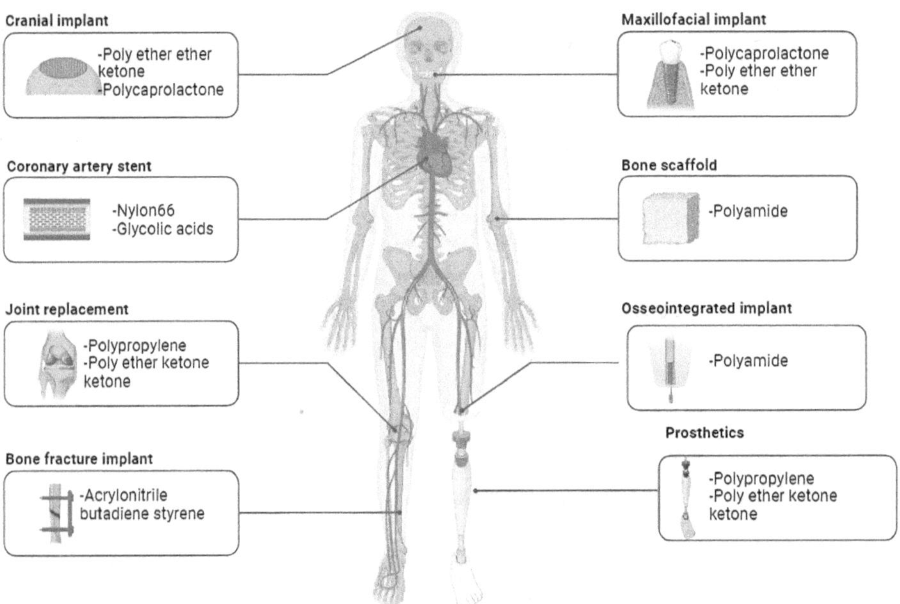

FIGURE 8.6 Applications of 3D-printed synthetic polymers in the area of osteology [14]

The design of 3D-printed nanocomposite scaffolds can include precisely regulated porosity, pore size, and interconnectivity, closely approaching real bone structure. These scaffolds can be used to fix bone flaws or gaps, therefore encouraging new bone production and tissue regeneration. The bioactive glass nanoparticles have an important function in increasing osteoblast activity and mineralization. Furthermore, 3D-printed polymer-based nanocomposite models might be extremely useful platforms for biomedical research. They allow for the study of bone biology, disease development, medication screening, and preclinical assessments, therefore minimizing reliance on animal research.

The introduction of novel printing processes, such as 3D bioprinting, has enabled the inclusion of living cells or biologics into nanocomposite structures. This breakthrough paves the path for the creation of bioactive and biomimetic tissue constructions, which offer significant potential for the future of regenerative medicine and tissue engineering.

8.7.2.4 In Vivo Performance and Biocompatibility Studies

While extensive research has been conducted on the in vitro properties and behavior of biodegradable polymer-based bioactive glass nanocomposites, their in vivo performance and long-term biocompatibility require further investigation. Preclinical animal studies are essential to evaluate the degradation kinetics, tissue integration, and potential adverse effects of these nanocomposites in a living system.

Furthermore, the long-term fate and potential accumulation of bioactive glass nanoparticles or fibers in the body need to be thoroughly investigated to ensure their safe and effective use in clinical applications. Collaborations between researchers, clinicians, and regulatory authorities will be crucial in addressing these concerns and facilitating the translation of these nanocomposites into clinical practice.

8.7.2.5 Clinical Translation and Commercialization

Ultimately, the success of biodegradable polymer-based bioactive glass nanocomposites will depend on their successful translation from the laboratory to clinical applications and their commercialization [13]. Collaboration between academic researchers, industry partners, and regulatory bodies will be essential to overcome the challenges associated with scaling up production, ensuring quality control, and navigating the regulatory approval processes.

Furthermore, the development of cost-effective manufacturing processes and business models will be crucial for the widespread adoption of these nanocomposites in various biomedical applications, such as orthopedic implants, tissue engineering scaffolds, and drug delivery systems.

Biodegradable polymer-based bioactive glass nanocomposites represent a promising class of biomaterials with tremendous potential for applications in regenerative medicine, tissue engineering, and drug delivery. While significant progress has been made in their development and characterization, several challenges remain to be addressed, including processing difficulties, degradation control, balancing bioactivity and mechanical properties, regulatory hurdles, and scalability.

8.8 CONCLUSION

Biodegradable polymer-based bioactive glass nanocomposites have emerged as an extremely promising class of biomaterials, notably for BTE and other biomedical applications. The combination of bioactive glasses' bioactivity and osteogenic capabilities with polymers' adjustable mechanical properties and biodegradability resulted in the development of innovative nanocomposite materials with dramatically improved biological and functional performance. Researchers used a variety of manufacturing approaches to create nanocomposites with specialized microstructures, compositions, and characteristics that successfully satisfy the unique needs of numerous biomedical applications. The comprehensive characterization of these nanocomposites has provided vital insights into their structure-property correlations, allowing for their effective translation from laboratory to clinical applications. As the field of biodegradable polymer-based bioactive glass nanocomposites progresses, advances in materials design, processing techniques, and in vivo evaluation methods will be critical in realizing their full potential in tissue engineering and regenerative medicine.

REFERENCES

1. Hench, L. L. (1998). Bioactive materials: the potential for tissue regeneration. *Journal of Biomedical Materials Research*, 41(4), 511–518.
2. Jones, J. R. (2013). Review of bioactive glass: from Hench to hybrids. *Acta Biomaterialia*, 9(1), 4457–4486.
3. Rezwan, K., Chen, Q. Z., Blaker, J. J., & Boccaccini, A. R. (2006). Biodegradable and bioactive porous polymer/inorganic composite scaffolds for bone tissue engineering. *Biomaterials*, 27(18), 3413–3431.
4. Shi, X., Zheng, Y., Wang, G., Browne, D. J., & Zhao, Q. (2017). Bioactive glass/polymer composite scaffolds for bone tissue engineering. *Regenerative Biomaterials*, 4(3), 167–177.
5. Puppi, D., Chiellini, F., Piras, A. M., & Chiellini, E. (2010). Polymeric materials for bone and cartilage repair. *Progress in Polymer Science*, 35(4), 403–440.
6. Nair, L. S., & Laurencin, C. T. (2007). Biodegradable polymers as biomaterials. *Progress in Polymer Science*, 32(8–9), 762–798.
7. Hench, L. L. (1991). Bioceramics: from concept to clinic. *Journal of the American Ceramic Society*, 74(7), 1487–1510.
8. Hoppe, A., Güldal, N. S., & Boccaccini, A. R. (2011). A review of the biological response to ionic dissolution products from bioactive glasses and glass-ceramics. *Biomaterials*, 32(11), 2757–2774.
9 Sollapur, S.B., Sharath, P.C., & Waghmare, P. (2024). Applications of additive manufacturing in biomedical and sports industry. In: Rajendrachari, S. (ed) *Practical Implementations of Additive Manufacturing Technologies. Materials Horizons: From Nature to Nanomaterials*. Springer, Singapore. https://doi.org/10.1007/978-981-99-5949-5_13.
10. Agrawal, C. M., & Ray, R. B. (2001). Biodegradable polymeric scaffolds for musculoskeletal tissue engineering. *Journal of Biomedical Materials Research: An Official Journal of The Society for Biomaterials, The Japanese Society for Biomaterials, and The Australian Society for Biomaterials and the Korean Society for Biomaterials*, 55(2), 141–150.

11. Woodruff, M. A., & Hutmacher, D. W. (2010). The return of a forgotten polymer—polycaprolactone in the 21st century. *Progress in Polymer Science*, 35(10), 1217–1256.
12. Venkate Gowda, C., Nagaraja, T. K., Yogesha, K. B., Prem Chand, R., Manjunatha, M. C., Sollapur, S., Manjunath, C. J., & Pushpa, N. (2024). Study on structural behavior of HVOF-sprayed NiCr/Mo coating. *Journal of The Institution of Engineers (India): Series D* (2024). https://doi.org/10.1007/s40033-024-00641-8.
13. Vichery, C., & Nedelec, J.-M. (2016). Bioactive glass nanoparticles: from synthesis to materials design for biomedical applications. *Materials*, 9, 288. https://doi.org/10.3390/ma9040288.
14. Shiva, S., Asuwin Prabu, R. G., Bajaj, G., John, A. E., Chandran, S., Kumar, V. V., & Ramakrishna, S.(2023). A review on the recent applications of synthetic biopolymers in 3D printing for biomedical applications. *Journal of Materials Science: Materials in Medicine*, 34, 62. https://doi.org/10.1007/s10856-023-06765-9.
15. Kumar, V. V., Narayanan, D., Chandran, S., Rajendran, S., & Ramakrishna, S. (2023). Lightweight and sustainable self-reinforced composites. In: S. M. Rangappa, S. M. Doddamani, S. Siengchin, & M. Doddamani (eds) *Lightweight and Sustainable Composite Materials*. India: Elsevier. pp. 19-46.
16. Nugraha, A. D., Vijay Kumar, V., Gautama, J. P., Wiranata, A., Mangunkusumo, K. G. H., Rasyid, M. I., Dzanzani, R., & Muflikhun, M. A. (2024). Investigating the characteristics of nano-graphite composites additively manufactured using stereolithography. *Polymers*, 16(8), 1021.
17. Li, Y., Liao, C., & Tjong, S. C. (2019). Synthetic biodegradable aliphatic polyester nanocomposites reinforced with nanohydroxyapatite and/or graphene oxide for bone tissue engineering applications. *Nanomaterials*, 9, 590. https://doi.org/10.3390/nano9040590.
18. Vijay Kumar, V., Balaganesan, G., Lee, J. K. Y., Neisiany, R. E., Surendran, S., & Ramakrishna, S. (2019). A review of recent advances in nanoengineered polymer composites. *Polymers*, 11(4), 644.
19. Kargozar, S., Montazerian, M., Fiume, E., & Baino, F. (2019). Multiple and promising applications of strontium (Sr)-containing bioactive glasses in bone tissue engineering. *Frontiers in Bioengineering and Biotechnology*, 7, 161.
20. Misra, S. K., Ansari, T. I., Valappil, S. P., Mohn, D., Philip, S. E., Stark, W. J., ... & Salih, V. (2010). Poly (3-hydroxybutyrate) multifunctional composites for tissue engineering applications. *Biomaterials*, 31(10), 2806–2815.
21. Sarker, B., Papageorgiou, D. G., Silva, R., Zehnder, T., Gul-E-Noor, F., Bertmer, M., ... & Boccaccini, A. R. (2014). Fabrication of alginate–gelatin crosslinked hydrogel microcapsules and evaluation of the microstructure and physico-chemical properties. *Journal of Materials Chemistry B*, 2(11), 1470–1482.
22. Chate, G. R., Kulkarni, R. M., Nikhil, R., Chate, V. R., Manjunath Patel, G. C., Sollapur, S., & Shettar, M. (2023). Ceramic material coatings: emerging future applications. *Advanced Ceramic Coatings for Emerging Applications*, 3–17. https://doi.org/10.1016/B978-0-323-99624-2.00007-3.
23. Reys, L. L., Silva, S. S., Pirraco, R. P., Marques, A. P., Mano, J. F., & Reis, R. L. (2017). Stem cell-based bone tissue engineering: a review. *Tissue Engineering Part B: Reviews*, 23(3), 211–224.

9 Bioinspired Synthesis-Based Bioactive Glasses

Laxmikanth Cherupally, Dheeraj Kumar Gara, Shakuntala Ojha, Satish Jain, Locherla Daloji, and P. Phani Prasanthi

9.1 INTRODUCTION

Bioactive glasses have emerged as a pivotal class of biomaterials due to their unique ability to interact with biological tissues, facilitating the regeneration and repair of bone and other tissues. Since their inception by Larry Hench in 1969, bioactive glasses have been extensively studied and utilized in various biomedical applications, including bone grafts, dental implants, and tissue engineering scaffolds. The inherent bioactivity of these materials stems from their ability to bond with bone and soft tissues through the formation of a hydroxyapatite layer on their surface upon implantation [1, 2].

Recent advancements in the synthesis of bioactive glasses have been inspired by natural processes, leading to the development of bioinspired synthesis techniques. These methods aim to mimic the sophisticated mechanisms found in nature to produce materials with enhanced properties and functionalities. Bioinspired synthesis leverages the principles of biomimicry, where natural materials, structures, and processes are replicated to create advanced biomaterials with superior performance [3].

This chapter delves into the various aspects of bioinspired synthesis-based bioactive glasses, focusing on the following key areas:

- Focus Materials: Natural and Synthetic: Exploring the use of natural materials such as collagen, chitosan, and alginate, as well as synthetic polymers like poly(lactic-co-glycolic acid) (PLGA) and polycaprolactone (PCL) in the development of bioactive glass composites.
- Surface Functionalization: Discussing the techniques used to functionalize the surfaces of bioactive glasses, including silanization, peptide grafting, and plasma treatment, and their applications in enhancing bioactivity and biocompatibility.
- Super Wettable Surfaces: Examining the fabrication and applications of superhydrophilic and superhydrophobic surfaces on bioactive glasses, which play a crucial role in modulating interactions with biological environments.

 DOI: 10.1201/9781003660781-9

- Supramolecular Chemistry: Highlighting the role of supramolecular chemistry in designing bioactive glasses with advanced properties such as self-healing, controlled degradation, and enhanced bioactivity.

Through these sections, we aim to provide a comprehensive understanding of the latest advancements in bioinspired synthesis-based bioactive glasses and their potential applications in the field of biomedical materials. By integrating natural and synthetic materials, advanced surface functionalization techniques, and the principles of supramolecular chemistry, these innovative materials hold the promise of revolutionizing tissue engineering and regenerative medicine [4].

9.2 FOCUS MATERIALS: NATURAL AND SYNTHETIC

In the development of bioactive glasses, the choice of materials plays a critical role in determining their properties and applications. Bioinspired synthesis often involves the integration of both natural and synthetic materials to create composite structures that mimic the complex architecture and functionality of biological tissues. This section explores the use of natural materials such as collagen, chitosan, and alginate, as well as synthetic polymers like PLGA and PCL in the development of bioactive glass composites [5].

9.2.1 Natural Materials

Natural materials are increasingly used in bioactive glass composites due to their biocompatibility, bioactivity, and ability to promote cell adhesion and proliferation. These materials are derived from biological sources and possess inherent properties that are beneficial for tissue engineering applications.

9.2.1.1 Collagen

Collagen is the most abundant protein in the extracellular matrix (ECM) of animals and plays a crucial role in maintaining the structural integrity of tissues. Its biocompatibility and ability to promote cell adhesion and proliferation make it an ideal candidate for bioactive glass composites.

- Properties: Collagen fibers provide mechanical strength and a natural scaffold that supports cell growth and differentiation.
- Applications: Collagen-bioactive glass composites are used in bone tissue engineering, where they promote the formation of new bone tissue and enhance the integration of implants with the surrounding bone [6].

9.2.1.2 Chitosan

Chitosan, derived from chitin found in the exoskeletons of crustaceans, is a biopolymer known for its antimicrobial properties and ability to promote wound healing.

- Properties: Chitosan is biodegradable, biocompatible, and has inherent antimicrobial activity, making it suitable for biomedical applications.

- Applications: Chitosan-bioactive glass composites are used in wound dressings and tissue engineering scaffolds, where they support tissue regeneration and prevent infections [7].

9.2.1.3 Alginate

Alginate, extracted from brown algae, is a natural polysaccharide that forms hydrogels in the presence of divalent cations.

- Properties: Alginate hydrogels are highly porous, which facilitates cell infiltration and nutrient exchange.
- Applications: Alginate-bioactive glass composites are used in soft tissue engineering and as carriers for bioactive glass particles in drug delivery systems [8–10].

9.2.2 Synthetic Materials

Synthetic polymers offer the advantage of controlled properties and tunability, making them ideal for tailoring bioactive glass composites to specific biomedical applications. These materials can be engineered to enhance the mechanical strength, degradation rate, and bioactivity of bioactive glasses.

9.2.2.1 Poly(Lactic-co-Glycolic Acid)

PLGA is a copolymer of lactic acid and glycolic acid, known for its biodegradability and biocompatibility.

- Properties: The degradation rate of PLGA can be controlled by adjusting the ratio of lactic acid to glycolic acid, allowing for tailored degradation profiles.
- Applications: PLGA-bioactive glass composites are used in controlled drug delivery systems and as scaffolds for tissue engineering, where they provide mechanical support while gradually degrading to allow for tissue regeneration [11, 12].

9.2.2.2 Polycaprolactone

PCL is a biodegradable polyester with a slow degradation rate and excellent mechanical properties.

- Properties: PCL provides long-term structural support and has a slow degradation rate, making it suitable for applications where prolonged support is required.
- Applications: PCL-bioactive glass composites are used in bone tissue engineering and as long-term implants, where they provide sustained support during the healing process [13, 14].

9.2.3 Composite Structures

The combination of natural and synthetic materials in bioactive glass composites aims to leverage the advantages of both types of materials. By integrating the biocompatibility and bioactivity of natural materials with the tunable properties of synthetic polymers, composite structures can be designed to meet the specific requirements of various biomedical applications [15].

9.2.3.1 Enhanced Mechanical Properties

Combining natural materials like collagen or chitosan with synthetic polymers such as PLGA or PCL can enhance the mechanical properties of bioactive glass composites. This synergy ensures that the composite structures are both strong and flexible, mimicking the mechanical behavior of natural tissues.

9.2.3.2 Controlled Degradation

The integration of synthetic polymers allows for precise control over the degradation rate of bioactive glass composites. By adjusting the composition and properties of the synthetic components, the degradation profile can be tailored to match the rate of tissue regeneration [16].

9.2.3.3 Improved Bioactivity

Natural materials inherently promote cell adhesion, proliferation, and differentiation. When combined with bioactive glasses, these materials enhance the overall bioactivity of the composites, leading to improved performance in tissue engineering applications [17].

9.3 SURFACE FUNCTIONALIZATION

Surface functionalization is a critical aspect of enhancing the bioactivity and biocompatibility of bioactive glasses. By modifying the surface properties of these materials, it is possible to improve their interactions with biological tissues, thereby promoting cell adhesion, proliferation, and differentiation. This section explores various surface functionalization techniques, including silanization, peptide grafting, and plasma treatment, and their applications in biomedical fields [18].

9.3.1 Functionalization Techniques

9.3.1.1 Silanization

Silanization involves the attachment of silane molecules to the surface of bioactive glasses. Silanes are organosilicon compounds that can form covalent bonds with the glass surface, introducing functional groups that enhance the material's interaction with biological molecules.

- Process: Silanization typically involves treating the bioactive glass surface with a silane solution, followed by a curing step to ensure the formation of stable covalent bonds.
- Functional Groups: Common silane molecules used for functionalization include aminopropyltriethoxysilane (APTES), which introduces amine groups, and mercaptopropyltrimethoxysilane (MPTS), which introduces thiol groups.

- Benefits: Silanized surfaces exhibit improved protein adsorption and cell adhesion, making them more effective for tissue engineering and regenerative medicine applications [19].

9.3.1.2 Peptide Grafting

Peptide grafting involves the covalent attachment of bioactive peptides to the surface of bioactive glasses. These peptides mimic natural cell signaling molecules, enhancing cellular interactions and promoting specific biological responses.

- Process: Peptides can be grafted onto the bioactive glass surface using chemical crosslinkers or direct coupling reactions. The choice of peptide and grafting method depends on the desired biological outcome.
- Examples: Commonly used peptides include the arginine-glycine-aspartic acid (RGD) sequence, which promotes cell adhesion, and bone morphogenetic protein (BMP) peptides, which induce osteogenic differentiation.
- Benefits: Peptide-grafted surfaces can specifically enhance cell adhesion, proliferation, and differentiation, leading to improved performance in applications such as bone regeneration and wound healing [20, 21].

9.3.1.3 Plasma Treatment

Plasma treatment is a surface modification technique that uses ionized gas to alter the surface properties of bioactive glasses. This method can introduce functional groups, increase surface roughness, and improve wettability.

- Process: Plasma treatment involves exposing the bioactive glass surface to a plasma generated by an electric field in a controlled atmosphere. The type of gas used (e.g., oxygen, nitrogen, or argon) determines the functional groups introduced.
- Effects: Plasma treatment can make the surface more hydrophilic, enhancing protein adsorption and cell adhesion. It can also introduce reactive functional groups that facilitate further surface modifications.
- Benefits: Plasma-treated surfaces show improved bioactivity and biocompatibility, making them suitable for various biomedical applications, including implants and tissue engineering scaffolds [22–24].

9.3.2 Applications of Surface Functionalization

Functionalized bioactive glasses have a wide range of applications in biomedical fields, where enhanced surface properties can lead to better clinical outcomes [25].

9.3.2.1 Bone Regeneration

Functionalized bioactive glasses are widely used in bone regeneration due to their ability to promote osteogenesis and enhance the integration of implants with surrounding bone tissue.

- Mechanisms: Surface functionalization techniques, such as peptide grafting and silanization, can introduce bioactive molecules that promote the adhesion and differentiation of osteoblasts, the cells responsible for bone formation.
- Applications: Functionalized bioactive glasses are used in bone grafts, coatings for orthopedic implants, and scaffolds for bone tissue engineering. These materials can accelerate bone healing and improve the mechanical stability of implants [26].

9.3.2.2 Wound Healing

The antimicrobial and bioactive properties of functionalized bioactive glasses make them ideal for wound healing applications.

- Mechanisms: Functionalized surfaces can release therapeutic agents, provide antimicrobial protection, and promote the migration and proliferation of fibroblasts and keratinocytes, the cells involved in wound closure and skin regeneration.
- Applications: Functionalized bioactive glasses are used in wound dressings, gels, and scaffolds for skin regeneration. They can accelerate the healing process and reduce the risk of infections.

9.3.2.3 Drug Delivery

Surface functionalization enables bioactive glasses to act as carriers for controlled drug delivery, providing localized and sustained release of therapeutic agents.

- Mechanisms: Functional groups introduced through silanization or peptide grafting can bind to drugs or therapeutic molecules, allowing for their controlled release as the bioactive glass degrades.
- Applications: Functionalized bioactive glasses are used in drug delivery systems for bone regeneration, cancer treatment, and antimicrobial therapies. They offer the advantage of targeted delivery and reduced systemic side effects [27].

9.3.3 Advanced Functionalization Techniques

9.3.3.1 Layer-by-Layer Assembly

Layer-by-layer (LbL) assembly is a technique that involves the sequential deposition of alternating layers of oppositely charged molecules, such as polyelectrolytes or nanoparticles, onto the bioactive glass surface.

- Process: LbL assembly is performed by immersing the bioactive glass in solutions of the desired molecules, allowing each layer to adsorb before rinsing and repeating the process with the next molecule.

- Benefits: This technique allows for precise control over the thickness and composition of the surface coatings, enabling the creation of multifunctional surfaces with tailored properties [28, 29].

9.3.3.2 Bioorthogonal Chemistry

Bioorthogonal chemistry involves reactions that occur in the presence of biological molecules without interfering with their normal functions. This approach is used to attach bioactive molecules to bioactive glass surfaces in a highly specific manner.

- Process: Bioorthogonal reactions, such as click chemistry, are employed to graft bioactive molecules onto the bioactive glass surface with high efficiency and specificity.
- Benefits: Bioorthogonal chemistry enables the creation of surfaces with complex and well-defined bioactive coatings, enhancing their interaction with biological tissues [30].

9.4 SUPER WETTABLE SURFACES

Super wettable surfaces, including superhydrophilic and superhydrophobic surfaces, have garnered significant attention in the field of bioactive glasses due to their ability to manipulate interactions with biological environments. These surfaces can profoundly influence cell behavior, protein adsorption, and bacterial adhesion, making them highly relevant for biomedical applications. This section explores the fabrication techniques, properties, and applications of super wettable surfaces on bioactive glasses.

9.4.1 Types of Super Wettable Surfaces

9.4.1.1 Superhydrophilic Surfaces

Superhydrophilic surfaces have a water contact angle of less than 10°, allowing water to spread rapidly across the surface. These surfaces are characterized by their high surface energy and excellent wettability.

- Properties: Superhydrophilic surfaces facilitate rapid water spreading and promote protein adsorption, which is crucial for cell adhesion and proliferation.
- Applications: These surfaces are particularly useful in applications where enhanced cell attachment and rapid integration with biological tissues are desired, such as in tissue engineering scaffolds and implants [31].

9.4.1.2 Superhydrophobic Surfaces

Superhydrophobic surfaces have a water contact angle greater than 150°, causing water to bead up and roll off the surface. These surfaces exhibit low surface energy and high repellency to water.

- Properties: Superhydrophobic surfaces are effective at preventing bacterial adhesion and biofilm formation, which is beneficial for reducing infections.
- Applications: These surfaces are ideal for applications where antimicrobial properties and the prevention of fouling are important, such as in medical devices and wound dressings [32].

9.4.2 Fabrication Techniques

Several techniques are used to create super wettable surfaces on bioactive glasses, each offering unique advantages in terms of surface morphology and functional properties.

9.4.2.1 Chemical Etching

Chemical etching involves treating the bioactive glass surface with acidic or basic solutions to create nanoscale roughness, which enhances wettability.

- Process: The bioactive glass is immersed in an etching solution (e.g., hydrofluoric acid for superhydrophilic surfaces or sodium hydroxide for superhydrophobic surfaces) for a specific duration, followed by thorough rinsing and drying.
- Advantages: Chemical etching is a straightforward and cost-effective method for creating nanoscale surface features that significantly alter wettability.

9.4.2.2 Sol-Gel Coating

The sol-gel process involves the deposition of thin films onto the bioactive glass surface to impart super wettable properties.

- Process: A sol containing metal alkoxides (e.g., silicon alkoxides) is applied to the bioactive glass surface and then undergoes gelation and curing to form a uniform coating.
- Advantages: Sol-gel coatings can be tailored to achieve both superhydrophilic and superhydrophobic properties by adjusting the composition and processing conditions [33].

9.4.2.3 Plasma Treatment

Plasma treatment uses ionized gas to modify the surface properties of bioactive glasses, introducing functional groups that enhance or reduce wettability.

- Process: The bioactive glass surface is exposed to plasma generated by an electric field in a controlled atmosphere, such as oxygen plasma for superhydrophilic surfaces or fluorine plasma for superhydrophobic surfaces.
- Advantages: Plasma treatment is a versatile and precise method for achieving desired surface properties without the need for chemical reagents.

9.4.2.4 Layer-by-Layer Assembly

Layer-by-layer (LbL) assembly involves the sequential deposition of alternating layers of materials to create structured coatings with tailored wettability.

- Process: The bioactive glass is alternately immersed in solutions containing oppositely charged polyelectrolytes or nanoparticles, allowing each layer to adsorb before rinsing and repeating the process.
- Advantages: LbL assembly allows for precise control over the thickness and composition of the coatings, enabling the fabrication of multifunctional super wettable surfaces.

9.4.3 Applications of Super Wettable Surfaces

The unique properties of super wettable surfaces on bioactive glasses make them suitable for a wide range of biomedical applications.

9.4.3.1 Tissue Engineering

Superhydrophilic surfaces are particularly advantageous for tissue engineering scaffolds as they enhance cell adhesion and proliferation.

- Benefits: These surfaces provide an optimal environment for cell attachment, spreading, and differentiation, leading to improved tissue regeneration and integration.
- Applications: Superhydrophilic bioactive glass scaffolds are used in bone and soft tissue engineering, where they support the formation and growth of new tissue.

9.4.3.2 Antimicrobial Coatings

Superhydrophobic surfaces are effective in preventing bacterial adhesion and biofilm formation, making them ideal for antimicrobial coatings.

- Benefits: By reducing bacterial colonization, these surfaces help prevent infections and extend the lifespan of medical devices.
- Applications: Superhydrophobic bioactive glass coatings are used in medical devices such as catheters, implants, and wound dressings to minimize the risk of infection.

9.4.3.3 Drug Delivery Systems

Super wettable surfaces can be used to control the release of drugs from bioactive glass-based delivery systems.

- Benefits: Superhydrophilic surfaces can enhance the adsorption and subsequent release of hydrophilic drugs, while superhydrophobic surfaces can provide sustained release of hydrophobic drugs.

- Applications: Bioactive glass drug delivery systems with tailored wettability are used for localized and controlled delivery of therapeutic agents in applications such as bone regeneration and cancer treatment [34, 35].

9.4.4 Future Directions

The development of super wettable surfaces on bioactive glasses is an evolving field with significant potential for innovation.

9.4.4.1 Multifunctional Surfaces

Research is ongoing to create multifunctional super wettable surfaces that combine superhydrophilic and superhydrophobic properties in a single material.

- Approaches: Techniques such as patterned surface fabrication and gradient coatings are being explored to achieve surfaces with spatially controlled wettability.
- Benefits: These multifunctional surfaces can offer combined benefits, such as enhanced cell adhesion and antimicrobial properties, in a single material.

9.4.4.2 Stimuli-Responsive Surfaces

The development of stimuli-responsive super wettable surfaces that can change their wettability in response to external stimuli (e.g., pH, temperature, or light) is a promising area of research.

- Mechanisms: Incorporating stimuli-responsive polymers or nanoparticles into bioactive glass surfaces can enable dynamic control over wettability.
- Applications: Stimuli-responsive surfaces can be used in smart drug delivery systems, where the release of therapeutic agents can be triggered by specific environmental conditions.

9.5 SUPRAMOLECULAR CHEMISTRY

9.5.1 Principles of Supramolecular Chemistry

Supramolecular chemistry focuses on the study of non-covalent interactions between molecules, such as hydrogen bonding, van der Waals forces, π-π stacking, and electrostatic interactions. These interactions govern the assembly and organization of molecules into well-defined structures. In the context of bioactive glasses, supramolecular chemistry can be harnessed to create materials with unique properties that are difficult to achieve through conventional covalent chemistry.

9.5.2 Applications in Bioactive Glasses

Utilizing supramolecular chemistry in the development of bioactive glasses offers innovative solutions to enhance their functionality. These applications include the creation of self-healing materials, controlled degradation rates, and enhanced bioactivity through precise molecular design.

9.5.2.1 Self-Healing Bioactive Glasses

Self-healing materials are designed to repair damage autonomously, extending their lifespan and functionality. In bioactive glasses, self-healing can be achieved by incorporating supramolecular motifs that respond to external stimuli, such as changes in pH or temperature, to trigger the repair process. For example, incorporating reversible hydrogen bonds or metal-ligand interactions can enable the material to reform its structure after being damaged, thus maintaining its integrity and performance over time.

9.5.2.2 Controlled Degradation

Controlled degradation is crucial for ensuring that bioactive glasses provide sustained support during tissue regeneration. Supramolecular interactions offer a precise method to tune the degradation rate of bioactive glasses. By designing molecules that interact through reversible non-covalent bonds, the degradation can be matched with the pace of tissue healing. This controlled degradation ensures that the material provides mechanical support and bioactivity only as long as needed, minimizing the risk of long-term foreign body reaction.

9.5.2.3 Enhanced Bioactivity

Supramolecular chemistry can significantly enhance the bioactivity of bioactive glasses by facilitating the incorporation of bioactive molecules and motifs. For instance, the inclusion of peptides or growth factors through non-covalent interactions can promote cell adhesion, proliferation, and differentiation. The spatial organization and density of these bioactive motifs can be precisely controlled using supramolecular strategies, leading to materials that more closely mimic the natural ECM and provide optimal environments for tissue regeneration.

9.5.3 Fabrication Techniques

The fabrication of bioactive glasses using supramolecular chemistry involves several advanced techniques to ensure the proper assembly and functionality of the materials.

9.5.3.1 Sol-Gel Process

The sol-gel process is a versatile method for creating bioactive glasses with supramolecular properties. By incorporating supramolecular building blocks during the sol-gel synthesis, it is possible to create materials with tailored pore structures and surface functionalities. This method allows for the homogeneous distribution of bioactive molecules and the formation of intricate networks of non-covalent interactions.

9.5.3.2 Layer-by-Layer Assembly

Layer-by-layer (LbL) assembly is a technique that involves the sequential deposition of thin layers of materials. This method can be used to construct bioactive glasses with precise control over the composition and functionality of each layer. By using supramolecular interactions to guide the assembly process, LbL can produce multilayered structures with enhanced bioactivity and tailored degradation rates.

9.5.3.3 3D Printing

3D printing is an emerging technique for fabricating complex bioactive glass structures with high precision. By incorporating supramolecular chemistry into the 3D printing process, it is possible to design materials with hierarchical structures that closely mimic natural tissues. This approach enables the creation of bioactive glasses with customized shapes and properties, making them suitable for personalized medical applications.

9.6 CONCLUSION

Bioinspired synthesis-based bioactive glasses signify a groundbreaking development in biomedical materials, offering a convergence of advanced functionalities that enhance their performance in medical applications. The exploration of both natural and synthetic materials has allowed for the creation of bioactive glasses that better mimic the natural ECM, improving their biocompatibility and bioactivity.

9.6.1 Advances in Material Composition

Incorporating natural materials like collagen, chitosan, and alginate has significantly improved the biological performance of bioactive glasses. These materials provide enhanced cellular interactions, antimicrobial properties, and support for tissue regeneration. On the synthetic front, polymers like PLGA and PCL have allowed for precise control over mechanical properties and degradation rates, making these composites highly versatile for various biomedical applications.

9.6.2 Surface Functionalization

Surface functionalization techniques such as silanization, peptide grafting, and plasma treatment have been pivotal in enhancing the interaction between bioactive glasses and biological tissues. These modifications improve protein adhesion, cell proliferation, and differentiation, which are crucial for applications in bone regeneration, wound healing, and drug delivery. The ability to tailor surface properties to specific medical needs ensures that bioactive glasses can provide targeted and efficient therapeutic outcomes.

9.6.3 Super Wettable Surfaces

The development of super wettable surfaces, including superhydrophilic and superhydrophobic coatings, has further expanded the potential applications of bioactive glasses. Superhydrophilic surfaces promote rapid cell adhesion and integration, making them ideal for tissue engineering. Conversely, superhydrophobic surfaces offer antimicrobial properties and resistance to biofouling, which are beneficial in preventing infections and enhancing the longevity of implants.

9.6.4 Supramolecular Chemistry

Supramolecular chemistry has introduced a new dimension to the design and functionality of bioactive glasses. By leveraging non-covalent interactions, researchers have developed self-healing materials, controlled degradation profiles, and enhanced bioactivity. These advanced properties ensure that bioactive glasses not only support tissue regeneration effectively but also maintain their performance over extended periods, reducing the need for replacements and further interventions.

9.6.5 Future Directions

The future of bioinspired synthesis-based bioactive glasses lies in the continuous exploration of new materials and techniques. Emerging fields such as nanotechnology, 3D printing, and bioprinting offer exciting possibilities for creating highly customized and efficient biomedical implants. Moreover, ongoing research into the molecular mechanisms of bioactivity and tissue interactions will provide deeper insights, allowing for the development of next-generation bioactive glasses with unprecedented capabilities.

9.6.6 Clinical Implications

The advancements in bioactive glass technology hold significant promise for improving patient outcomes in various medical fields. Enhanced bone regeneration materials can reduce recovery times and improve the success rates of orthopedic surgeries. Improved wound healing materials can lead to faster and more effective treatments for chronic wounds. Furthermore, the potential for controlled drug delivery systems can revolutionize the management of chronic diseases, providing sustained and localized therapy with minimal side effects.

In conclusion, bioinspired synthesis-based bioactive glasses are at the forefront of biomedical innovation, offering solutions that combine biocompatibility, bioactivity, and functionality. As research progresses, these materials are expected to play an increasingly vital role in enhancing the quality of healthcare and patient outcomes. Continued interdisciplinary collaboration and technological advancements will drive the evolution of bioactive glasses, making them indispensable tools in the arsenal of modern medicine.

REFERENCES

1. F. Baino, S. Hamzehlou, and S. Kargozar, "Bioactive glasses: where are we and where are we going?," *J Funct Biomater*, vol. 9, no. 1, 2018, doi: 10.3390/jfb9010025.
2. J. R. Jones, D. S. Brauer, L. Hupa, and D. C. Greenspan, "Bioglass and bioactive glasses and their impact on healthcare," *Int J Appl Glass Sci*, vol. 7, no. 4, pp. 423–434, 2016, doi: 10.1111/IJAG.12252.
3. M. M. Stevens and G. Mecklenburg, "Bio-inspired materials for biosensing and tissue engineering," *Polym Int*, vol. 61, no. 5, pp. 680–685, 2012, doi: 10.1002/PI.4183.
4. N. Dey, F. P. Mohny, G. Betsy Reshma, D. Rao, M. Ganguli, and D. Santhiya, "Bioinspired synthesis of bioactive glass nanocomposites for hyaluronic acid delivery to bone and skin," *Int J Biol Macromol*, vol. 253, p. 127262, 2023, doi: 10.1016/J.IJBIOMAC.2023.127262.

5. D. Dhinasekaran, S. Vimalraj, A. R. Rajendran, S. Saravanan, B. Purushothaman, and B. Subramaniam,, "Bio-inspired multifunctional collagen/electrospun bioactive glass membranes for bone tissue engineering applications," *Mater Sci Eng C*, 126, p. 111856. 2021. Accessed: May 22, 2024. [Online]. Available: https://www.sciencedirect.com/science/article/pii/S0928493120337759
6. J. Wu, S. Wang, Z. Zheng, and J. Li, "Fabrication of Biologically Inspired Electrospun Collagen/Silk fibroin/bioactive glass composited nanofibrous scaffold to accelerate the treatment efficiency of," *Regen Ther*, 21, pp. 122–1382022. Accessed: May 22, 2024. [Online]. Available: https://www.sciencedirect.com/science/article/pii/S2352320422000487
7. D. Vukajlovic, J. Parker, O. Bretcanu, and K. Novakovic, "Chitosan based polymer/bioglass composites for tissue engineering applications," *Mater Sci Eng C*, vol. 96, pp. 955–967, 2019, doi: 10.1016/J.MSEC.2018.12.026.
8. J. Zhu *et al.*, "Incorporation of ZnO/bioactive glass nanoparticles into alginate/chitosan composite hydrogels for wound closure," *ACS Publ*, vol. 2, no. 11, pp. 5042–5052, 2019, doi: 10.1021/acsabm.9b00727.
9. F. Zhao, W. Zhang, X. Fu, W. Xie, and X. Chen, "Fabrication and characterization of bioactive glass/alginate composite scaffolds by a self-crosslinking processing for bone regeneration," *RSC Adv*, 2016. pubs.rsc.org, pp. 91201–91208 doi: 10.1039/c6ra18309c.
10. B. Begines, C. Arevalo, C. Romero, Z. Hadzhieva, A. R. Boccaccini, and Y. Torres, "Fabrication and characterization of bioactive gelatin–alginate–bioactive glass composite coatings on porous titanium substrates," *ACS Publ*, vol. 14, no. 13, pp. 15008–15020, 2022, doi: 10.1021/acsami.2c01241.
11. J. Chen, X. Fan, Z. Zhou, J. Zou, and J. Ruan, "The preparation and properties of bioactive composites based on modification bioactive glass and poly (lactide-co-glycolide)," *Polym Plast Technol Eng*, vol. 49, no. 11, pp. 1155–1162, 2010, doi: 10.1080/03602551003664610.
12. E. Pamula *et al.*, "Preparation of a PLGA-coated porous bioactive glass scaffold with improved mechanical properties for bone tissue engineering approaches," *Regen Eng Transl Med*, vol. 39, no. 8, pp. 2114–2129, 2011, doi: 10.1007/s10439-011-0307-4.
13. A. Deliormanlı and R. Konyalı, "Bioactive glass/hydroxyapatite-containing electrospun poly (ε-caprolactone) composite nanofibers for bone tissue engineering," *Fiber Polym*, vol. 55, no. 1, pp. 247–256, 2019, doi: 10.1007/s41779-018-0229-9.
14. M. Dziadek, K. Dziadek, K. Checinska, B. Zagrajczuk, and K. Cholewa-Kowalska, "Bioactive glasses modulate anticancer activity and other polyphenol-related properties of polyphenol-loaded PCL/bioactive glass composites," *ACS Appl Mater Interfaces*, vol. 16, pp. 24261–24273, 2024, doi: 10.1021/acsami.4c02418.
15. M. Marcolongo, P. Ducheyne, J. Garino, and E. Schepers, "Bioactive glass fiber/polymeric composites bond to bone tissue," *J Biomed Mater Res*, vol. 39, pp. 161–170, 1998, https://doi.org/10.1002/(SICI)1097-4636(199801)39:1%3C161::AID-JBM18%3E3.0.CO;2-I .
16. P. Gentile *et al.*, "Bioactive glass/polymer composite scaffolds mimicking bone tissue," *J Biomed Mater Res Part A*, vol. 100 A, no. 10, pp. 2654–2667, 2012, doi: 10.1002/jbm.a.34205.
17. H. Lu, S. El-Amin, K. D. Scott, and C. T. Laurencin, "Three-dimensional, bioactive, biodegradable, polymer–bioactive glass composite scaffolds with improved mechanical properties support collagen synthesis and mineralization of human osteoblast-like cells *in vitro*" *J Biomed Mater Res Part A*, vol. 64, no. 3, pp. 465–474, 2003, doi: 10.1002/jbm.a.10399.
18. E. Verné, C. Vitale-Brovarone, E. Bui, C. L. Bianchi, and A. R. Boccaccini, "Surface functionalization of bioactive glasses," *J Biomed Mater Res Part A*, vol. 90, no. 4, pp. 981–992, 2008, doi: 10.1002/jbm.a.32153.

19. Q. Z. Chen *et al.*, "The surface functionalization of 45S5 Bioglass®-based glass-ceramic scaffolds and its impact on bioactivity," *J Mater Sci Mater Med*, vol. 17, no. 11, pp. 979–987, 2006, doi: 10.1007/s10856-006-0433-y.
20. R. Aluko, "Bioactive peptides," *Funct Food Nutraceu*, 37–61, 2012, doi: 10.1007/978-1-4614-3480-1_3.
21. E. Daliri, B. Lee, and D. H. Oh, "Current trends and perspectives of bioactive peptides," *Crit Rev Food Sci Nutr*, vol. 58, no. 13, pp. 2273–2284, 2017, doi: 10.1080/10408398.2017.1319795.
22. P. K. Chu, "Plasma-treated biomaterials," *IEEE Trans Plasma Sci*, *35*(2), pp. 181–187. 2007. Accessed: May 23, 2024. [Online]. Available: https://ieeexplore.ieee.org/abstract/document/4154851/
23. C. C. Lin *et al.*, "Enhancement of biocompatibility on bioactive titanium surface by low-temperature plasma treatment," *Japan J Appl Phys Part 1 Reg Paper Short Notes Rev Papers*, vol. 44, no. 12, pp. 8590–8598, 2005, doi: 10.1143/JJAP.44.8590.
24. F. Barbugian, F. Cadamuro, F. Nicotra, C. Riccardi, and L. Russo, "Plasma-treated collagen functionalized with chondroitin sulfate as bioactive and nanostructured extracellular matrix mimics," *Nanomedicine*, vol. 19, no. 9, pp. 799–810, 2024, doi: 10.2217/NNM-2023-0310.
25. K. Á. Magyari, L. Baia, A. Vulpoi, S. Simon, O. Popescu, and V. Simon, "Bioactivity evolution of the surface functionalized bioactive glasses," *J Biomed Mater Res B Appl Biomater*, vol. 103, no. 2, pp. 261–272, 2015, doi: 10.1002/JBM.B.33203.
26. X. Zhang *et al.*, "Functionalized mesoporous bioactive glass scaffolds for enhanced bone tissue regeneration," *Sci Rep*, *6*(1), p. 19361. 2015. nature.com, doi: 10.1038/srep19361.
27. M. Vallet-Regi, I. Izquierdo-Barba, and M. Colilla, "Structure and functionalization of mesoporous bioceramics for bone tissue regeneration and local drug delivery," *Phil Trans R Soc A, 370*(1963), pp. 1400–1421. 2012. Accessed: May 23, 2024. [Online]. Available: https://royalsocietypublishing.org/doi/abs/10.1098/rsta.2011.0258
28. B. N. Singh, and K. Pramanik, "Development of novel silk fibroin/polyvinyl alcohol/sol–gel bioactive glass composite matrix by modified layer by layer electrospinning method for bone tissue," *Biofabrication*, *9*(1), p. 015028. 2017, doi: 10.1088/1758-5090/aa644f.
29. C. Pontremoli *et al.*, "Polyelectrolyte-coated mesoporous bioactive glasses via layer-by-layer deposition for sustained co-delivery of therapeutic ions and drugs," *Pharmaceutics*, *13*(11), p. 19522021, doi: 10.3390/pharmaceutics13111952.
30. K. Hast, M. L. Rhia Stone, Z. Jia, M. Baci, T. Aggarwal, and E. Cagri Izgu, "Bioorthogonal functionalization of material surfaces with bioactive molecules," *ACS Publ*, vol. 15, no. 4, pp. 4996–5009, 2023, doi: 10.1021/acsami.2c20942.
31. J. J. Blaker, V. Maquet, A. R. Boccaccini, R. Jérôme, and A. Bismarck, "Wetting of bioactive glass surfaces by poly(α-hydroxyacid) melts: interaction between Bioglass® and biodegradable polymers," *E-Polymers*, *5*(1), p. 023. 2005, https://doi.org/10.1515/epoly.2005.5.1.248.
32. S. K. Misra *et al.*, "Effect of nanoparticulate bioactive glass particles on bioactivity and cytocompatibility of poly(3-hydroxybutyrate) composites," *J R Soc Interface*, vol. 7, no. 44, pp. 453–465, 2010, doi: 10.1098/RSIF.2009.0255.
33. K. Deshmukh *et al.*, "Recent advances and future perspectives of sol–gel derived porous bioactive glasses: a review," *RSC Adv*, vol. 10, no. 56, pp. 33782–33835, 2020, doi: 10.1039/D0RA04287K.
34. S. Shin, J. Seo, H. Han, S. Kang, H. Kim, and T. Lee, "Bio-inspired extreme wetting surfaces for biomedical applications," *Materials*, vol. 9, no. 2, 2016, doi: 10.3390/MA9020116.
35. A. Abbas *et al.*, "Recent developments in artificial super-wettable surfaces based on bioinspired polymeric materials for biomedical applications," *Polymers*, vol. 14, no. 2, p. 238, 2022, doi: 10.3390/POLYM14020238.

10 Challenges for Industrial Compliance and Life Cycle Analysis of Bioactive Glasses

P. Venkateswara Rao, P. Abdul Azeem, Shakuntala Ojha, Rakesh Kanakam, P. Gopinath Chowdary and Tan Fırat Eyüboğlu

10.1 INTRODUCTION

Bioactive glasses have remained a cornerstone of biomaterials research since their introduction in 1969 by Dr. Larry Hench [1, 2]. Unlike traditional inert implant materials, which do not interact with biological tissues, bioactive glasses represent a groundbreaking class of biomaterials that actively engage with the physiological environment to form strong, stable bonds with host tissues. This interaction facilitates the integration and regeneration of tissues, positioning bioactive glasses as superior alternatives in various medical applications.

The initial discovery of 45S5 Bioglass marked a pivotal moment in the field of biomaterials. Comprising a specific composition of silicon dioxide (SiO_2), sodium oxide (Na_2O), calcium oxide (CaO), and phosphorus pentoxide (P_2O_5), 45S5 Bioglass exhibits unique properties that promote biological activity. When implanted, this glass undergoes a series of surface reactions that lead to the formation of a hydroxycarbonate apatite (HCA) layer, closely resembling the mineral phase of bone. This HCA layer is critical for the material's ability to bond with bone and soft tissues, facilitating cellular attachment, proliferation, and differentiation. Initially utilized for bone repair and regeneration due to its osteoconductive properties, subsequent research expanded its use into other areas such as dental applications, tissue engineering, and wound healing. The ability of bioactive glasses to release therapeutic ions that can stimulate angiogenesis, antimicrobial activity, and overall tissue regeneration has further diversified their applicability.

By modifying the ratios of the constituent oxides or incorporating additional elements such as boron, zinc, or magnesium, researchers have developed specialized glasses with enhanced bioactivity, improved mechanical properties, and targeted

DOI: 10.1201/9781003660781-10

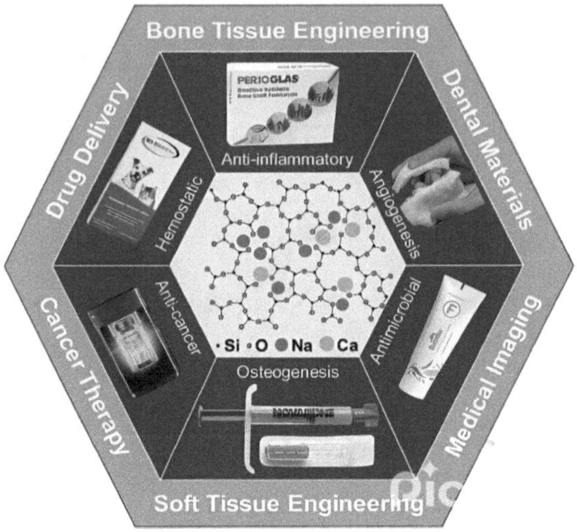

FIGURE 10.1 Bioactive glass applications [3]

therapeutic effects. This adaptability underscores the potential of bioactive glasses to address a wide array of medical challenges (Figure 10.1).

Despite their success, the journey from discovery to clinical and commercial use has not been without challenges. Industrial compliance and life cycle analysis (LCA) are two critical aspects that need to be thoroughly addressed to ensure the sustainable and responsible development of bioactive glasses. Industrial compliance involves navigating complex regulatory frameworks to ensure the safety and efficacy of bioactive glass products [3].

This chapter aims to explore the challenges associated with industrial compliance and LCA of bioactive glasses. It will provide an in-depth look at the regulatory hurdles that must be overcome to bring these materials to market, as well as the environmental considerations that must be addressed to ensure their sustainable production and use. By understanding these challenges, researchers and industry professionals can develop strategies to overcome them, paving the way for the continued innovation and application of bioactive glasses in various clinical settings.

10.2 DISCOVERY OF BIOACTIVE GLASSES

10.2.1 Historical Background

45S5 Bioglass® is composed of 45% silicon dioxide (SiO_2), 24.5% calcium oxide (CaO), 24.5% sodium oxide (Na_2O), and 6% phosphorus pentoxide (P_2O_5) by weight. This specific composition was found to exhibit unique bioactive properties, setting it apart from other materials used in medical implants. The significance of this discovery lay in its ability to form a stable bond with bone, a property that was revolutionary at the time [4].

10.2.2 Mechanism of Bioactivity

The bioactivity of glasses like 45S5 is primarily due to their ability to form a hydroxyapatite (HA) layer on their surface when in contact with physiological fluids. This process involves several stages [5]:

- **Ionic Exchange**: When bioactive glass comes into contact with body fluids, an ionic exchange occurs. Sodium ions (Na+) from the glass are exchanged with hydrogen ions (H+) from the solution, leading to the formation of a silica gel layer on the glass surface.
- **Silica Network Dissolution**: The continuous exchange of ions causes the dissolution of the silica network, releasing silicon (Si) ions into the solution.
- **Formation of Silica-Rich Layer**: A silica-rich layer is formed on the glass surface, which further undergoes condensation and repolymerization.
- **Calcium and Phosphate Deposition**: Calcium (Ca^{2+}) and phosphate (PO_4^{3-}) ions from the solution precipitate onto the silica-rich layer, leading to the formation of a calcium-phosphate (Ca-P) layer.
- **Hydroxyapatite Layer Formation**: The Ca-P layer crystallizes into HA, a mineral phase similar to natural bone. This HA layer is critical for bonding the bioactive glass to the bone.

10.2.3 Impact on Biomaterials Science

The paradigmatic shift towards bioactive materials has catalysed the development of a novel class of biomaterials with multifaceted applications extending beyond traditional implantable devices. Bioactive glasses, in particular, have emerged as integral components in tissue engineering and regenerative medicine, leveraging their inherent capacity to foster cellular processes such as attachment, proliferation, and differentiation. The antimicrobial properties inherent in bioactive glasses, stemming from the controlled release of biologically active ions, confer a dual benefit by both preventing microbial colonization and fostering tissue regeneration. This multifaceted functionality not only augments wound healing processes but also mitigates the risk of infection, thereby advancing therapeutic outcomes in soft tissue repair.

This pioneering work has spurred ongoing research endeavours aimed at refining and diversifying bioactive glass compositions to address specific medical requirements. A notable outcome of this research trajectory has been the creation of bioactive glasses with tailored properties, offering a spectrum of dissolution rates and bioactive ion release profiles finely tuned to distinct clinical applications.

Among the notable innovations emerging from this line of inquiry are borate-based and phosphate-based bioactive glasses. These variants exhibit distinct dissolution kinetics and ion release characteristics, thus presenting versatile platforms for addressing varied clinical needs. Borate-based bioactive glasses, for instance, are characterized by their accelerated dissolution rates, facilitating rapid release of bioactive ions. This property renders them particularly suitable for applications necessitating expedited tissue regeneration or targeted therapeutic interventions. Conversely, phosphate-based bioactive glasses feature more controlled dissolution kinetics, allowing for sustained release of bioactive ions over extended periods. This attribute lends itself to applications requiring prolonged tissue stimulation or modulation, such as in the context of chronic wound management or tissue engineering endeavours.

10.3 CLINICAL APPLICATIONS

10.3.1 Early Clinical Use

In the 1980s, the inception of clinical applications for bioactive glasses primarily centred on their utilization within orthopaedic and dental domains. Among the earliest applications was their deployment in bone grafting procedures, wherein bioactive glass particulates emerged as a promising adjunct to stimulate bone growth and facilitate repair processes. The osteoconductive attributes inherent in bioactive glasses, rooted in their capacity to form robust bonds with bone tissue and provide a supportive matrix for new bone formation, rendered them exceptionally well-suited for addressing bone defects and promoting healing in fractured regions.

Overall, the advent of bioactive glasses in the realm of orthopaedics and dentistry heralded a paradigm shift in bone grafting strategies, offering a biomimetic approach that capitalizes on the innate regenerative capacity of bone. By leveraging their osteoconductive properties, bioactive glasses continue to play a pivotal role in enhancing the outcomes of bone repair procedures, exemplifying the synergistic interface between materials science and clinical orthopaedics.

The success of 45S5 Bioglass in its early applications within orthopaedic and dental procedures can be attributed to its remarkable capacity to establish a robust bond with bone tissue. Upon implantation, the glass swiftly initiates the formation of a HA layer on its surface, a process facilitated by its inherent bioactivity. This HA layer exhibits a chemical composition akin to the mineral phase of natural bone, thereby endowing the bioactive glass with a biomimetic quality that enables it to function as a scaffold for new bone growth.

10.3.2 Expansion and Widespread Adoption

As the understanding of the bioactivity of glasses expanded, so did their clinical applications. Bioactive glasses began to be used in various forms, including granules, powders, and even as coatings for metallic implants. This versatility enabled their application in a wide range of medical fields, including:

- **Orthopaedics**: Bioactive glass has been used extensively in orthopaedic surgeries to repair bone defects, enhance bone fusion, and support the healing of fractures. Its ability to stimulate bone growth makes it an ideal material for spinal fusion surgeries, joint replacements, and the treatment of bone tumours.
- **Dentistry**: In dental applications, bioactive glass is used for bone grafting procedures, periodontal therapy, and as a component in dental composites and fillers. Its biocompatibility and bioactivity promote the regeneration of alveolar bone and periodontal tissues, supporting the long-term stability of dental implants.

- **Maxillofacial Surgery**: Bioactive glass has found applications in reconstructive surgery for the maxillofacial region, helping to repair and regenerate bone and soft tissues affected by trauma, congenital defects, or surgical resections [6].
- **Otorhinolaryngology (ENT)**: In the field of ENT, bioactive glasses are used in the reconstruction of middle ear ossicles and the repair of bony defects in the skull and sinuses.

10.3.3 Specific Case Studies and Clinical Outcomes

Several case studies and clinical trials have robustly demonstrated the efficacy of bioactive glasses across a spectrum of medical applications. In orthopaedic surgery, for instance, the application of bioactive glass granules in spinal fusion procedures has yielded promising outcomes. These granules enhance bone growth at the fusion site, promoting osteogenesis and improving the overall integration of the implant with the host bone. Patients undergoing these procedures have shown improved recovery times and better fusion rates, highlighting the potential of bioactive glasses to improve surgical outcomes in orthopaedic interventions.

In the realm of dental applications, bioactive glass-based materials have been effectively utilized to address periodontal defects and enhance the stability of dental implants. Clinical trials have shown that bioactive glasses can significantly improve the regeneration of periodontal tissues, including alveolar bone, cementum, and periodontal ligament. The bioactive glass particles stimulate the formation of new bone and connective tissue, providing a stable and durable support for dental implants. This not only enhances the longevity of the implants but also improves overall oral health and functionality for patients.

Bioactive glass particles incorporated into dental materials serve as osteoconductive scaffolds that promote tissue regeneration and osseointegration. Upon placement in periodontal defects, these particles initiate surface reactions that lead to the formation of a HA layer, facilitating the ingrowth of new bone tissue and the regeneration of periodontal ligament fibres. This process stimulates the formation of a stable and durable support structure around dental implants, enhancing their long-term stability and success rates.

Clinical trials evaluating the use of bioactive glass-based materials in periodontal therapy have consistently demonstrated significant improvements in tissue regeneration and clinical outcomes. Patients treated with these materials have shown enhanced periodontal tissue regeneration, reduced pocket depths, and improved attachment levels compared to conventional treatments.

A particularly notable application of bioactive glass is in the treatment of chronic osteomyelitis, a severe and persistent bone infection that is often resistant to conventional treatments. Bioactive glass granules, when introduced into the infected site, serve multiple functions. They fill the bone defect, providing a scaffold for new bone growth, and simultaneously release biologically active ions such as calcium, phosphate, and silicon. These ions exhibit antimicrobial properties, effectively helping to eradicate the infection. Additionally, the ions promote osteogenesis and angiogenesis, aiding in the regeneration of healthy bone tissue and the restoration of the affected area.

Upon introduction into the infected site, bioactive glass granules serve several key functions:

1. **Scaffold for Bone Growth**: Bioactive glass granules fill the bone defect created by osteomyelitis, providing a scaffold for new bone growth. The bioactivity of the glass initiates surface reactions, leading to the formation of a HA layer that mimics the mineral composition of natural bone. This layer facilitates the ingrowth of new bone tissue, promoting the repair and regeneration of the affected bone.
2. **Release of Biologically Active Ions**: Bioactive glass granules release biologically active ions such as calcium, phosphate, and silicon into the surrounding environment. These ions exhibit antimicrobial properties, effectively combating the infective agents responsible for osteomyelitis. By inhibiting microbial growth and promoting bacterial eradication, the release of biologically active ions helps to eliminate the source of infection and prevent its recurrence.
3. **Promotion of Osteogenesis and Angiogenesis**: The biologically active ions released from bioactive glass granules also play a pivotal role in promoting osteogenesis (bone formation) and angiogenesis (formation of new blood vessels). Calcium and phosphate ions provide essential mineral components for bone formation, while silicon ions stimulate osteogenic and angiogenic cellular responses. This dual action promotes the regeneration of healthy bone tissue and facilitates the restoration of the affected area, ultimately contributing to the resolution of chronic osteomyelitis.

10.3.4 Regulatory Approvals and Market Adoption

The clinical success of bioactive glasses has garnered approval from various regulatory bodies globally, including the U.S. Food and Drug Administration (FDA) and the European Medicines Agency (EMA). These regulatory endorsements have been pivotal in facilitating the widespread adoption of bioactive glass-based products in clinical practice, enabling their integration into standard medical treatments and procedures. The market for bioactive glasses has experienced substantial growth, driven by the increasing recognition of their therapeutic benefits and versatile applications. Numerous companies have emerged, focusing on the development and commercialization of bioactive glass products tailored for diverse medical applications. These products range from granules and scaffolds for bone regeneration to coatings for dental implants and components for wound healing. This market expansion is underpinned by continuous research and development efforts aimed at enhancing the properties of bioactive glasses [7]. Scientists are working on optimizing the composition and structure of bioactive glasses to improve their bioactivity, mechanical strength, and biocompatibility. For instance, modifications in the silica, calcium oxide, and phosphate content of bioactive glasses can fine-tune their dissolution rates and ion release profiles, thereby enhancing their ability to stimulate cellular responses and promote tissue regeneration.

Moreover, innovative approaches are being explored to extend the functionality of bioactive glasses. Researchers are investigating the incorporation of additional therapeutic agents, such as antibiotics, growth factors, and anti-inflammatory compounds, into bioactive glass matrices. These hybrid materials have the potential to offer multifaceted therapeutic effects, addressing infection, inflammation, and tissue repair simultaneously. The regulatory approvals and advancements in bioactive glass technology have led to their application in a broad range of clinical settings. In orthopaedics, bioactive glasses are used in bone grafts and spinal fusion procedures, where their osteoconductive properties facilitate bone healing and integration. In dentistry, bioactive glass-containing composites and cements are employed to repair periodontal defects and enhance the longevity of dental implants. Additionally, bioactive glasses are increasingly being utilized in wound care, where their antimicrobial properties and ability to promote angiogenesis contribute to faster and more effective healing.

Recent advancements in bioactive glass research have led to innovative approaches to enhance their functionality. Researchers are exploring the incorporation of therapeutic agents such as antibiotics, growth factors, and anti-inflammatory compounds into bioactive glass matrices. These hybrid materials aim to provide multifaceted therapeutic effects, addressing infection, inflammation, and tissue repair simultaneously.

10.3.4.1 Incorporation of Therapeutic Agents

Antibiotics: Embedding antibiotics in bioactive glass can help prevent or treat infections at the site of implantation. For example, bioactive glasses doped with silver or copper ions exhibit significant antimicrobial properties. These ions disrupt bacterial cell membranes and inhibit bacterial growth, making the materials useful in both orthopaedic and dental applications to prevent post-surgical infections.

Growth Factors: Incorporating growth factors such as bone morphogenetic proteins (BMPs) into bioactive glasses enhances their osteoinductive properties. BMPs stimulate the differentiation of mesenchymal stem cells into osteoblasts, promoting bone formation and accelerating the healing process. This approach is particularly beneficial in bone grafts and spinal fusion procedures.

Anti-inflammatory Compounds: Adding anti-inflammatory agents to bioactive glass can help reduce inflammation at the site of implantation, improving patient comfort and promoting faster healing. Compounds such as non-steroidal anti-inflammatory drugs (NSAIDs) can be incorporated to provide localized, sustained release of anti-inflammatory medication.

10.3.4.2 Applications in Clinical Settings

The versatility and therapeutic potential of bioactive glasses have led to their application across a broad range of clinical settings, particularly in orthopaedics, dentistry, and wound care.

1. **Orthopaedics**

   Bone Grafts: Bioactive glasses are extensively used in bone grafting procedures due to their osteoconductive and osteoinductive properties. Their ability to bond with bone tissue and promote new bone growth makes them ideal for repairing bone defects and fractures.

   Spinal Fusion: In spinal fusion procedures, bioactive glass promotes the fusion of vertebrae by facilitating bone growth and integration. This application leverages the material's ability to form a strong bond with existing bone and stimulate the formation of new bone tissue, ensuring stability and support for the spine.

2. **Dentistry**

   Periodontal Repair: Bioactive glass-containing composites and cements are used to repair periodontal defects. These materials support the regeneration of bone and periodontal tissues, improving the structural integrity of teeth and surrounding tissues.

   Dental Implants: The use of bioactive glass in dental implants enhances osseointegration, the process by which the implant becomes firmly anchored to the jawbone. This increases the longevity and stability of the implants, reducing the likelihood of implant failure.

3. **Wound Care**

   Antimicrobial Properties: Bioactive glasses with antimicrobial properties are increasingly utilized in wound care to prevent infections and promote healing. These materials can release antimicrobial ions, such as silver or zinc, which help eliminate pathogenic bacteria at the wound site.

   Angiogenesis Promotion: Bioactive glasses can also promote angiogenesis, the formation of new blood vessels, which is crucial for wound healing. The release of bioactive ions from the glass stimulates endothelial cell proliferation and migration, enhancing blood supply to the wound and accelerating the healing process.

The continued relevance and effectiveness of bioactive glasses in clinical settings are assured by the ongoing innovation and optimization of these materials. As research progresses, the scope of bioactive glass applications is expected to expand further, offering new solutions for a variety of medical conditions. The dynamic interplay between scientific research, regulatory support, and commercial development ensures that bioactive glasses will remain at the forefront of biomaterials science, contributing to improved patient outcomes and advancing the field of regenerative medicine.

10.4 TISSUE REGENERATION

10.4.1 Mechanisms of Tissue Regeneration

Bioactive glasses contribute significantly to tissue regeneration through their unique properties and interactions with biological systems [8]. The mechanisms underlying tissue regeneration with bioactive glasses involve several key processes:

- **Stimulation of Osteogenesis**: Bioactive glasses have the ability to stimulate osteogenesis, the formation of new bone tissue. This stimulation occurs through the release of ions, such as silicon, calcium, and phosphate, from the glass structure. These ions act as signalling molecules, promoting the differentiation and activity of osteoblasts, the cells responsible for bone formation.

10.4.1.1 Mechanisms of Osteogenic Stimulation

10.4.1.1.1 Ionic Dissolution and Release

Silicon (Si^{4+}) Ions: Silicon ions released from bioactive glasses play a crucial role in osteogenesis. Silicon is essential for the synthesis of collagen, a major component of the bone extracellular matrix (ECM). Silicon ions enhance the proliferation and differentiation of osteoblasts and increase the expression of osteogenic markers such as alkaline phosphatase (ALP) and osteocalcin.

Calcium (Ca^{2+}) Ions: Calcium ions are fundamental to bone metabolism. They are involved in the mineralization process, where they contribute to the formation of HA ($Ca_{10}(PO_4)_6(OH)_2$), the mineral phase of bone. Calcium ions also promote osteoblast differentiation and function, supporting the deposition of bone matrix.

Phosphate (PO_4^{3-}) Ions: Phosphate ions are critical for the mineralization of the bone matrix. They combine with calcium ions to form HA, providing the necessary structural rigidity to bone tissue. Phosphate ions also stimulate osteoblast activity and matrix production.

Cellular Responses: Osteoblast Differentiation: The release of silicon, calcium, and phosphate ions from bioactive glasses promotes the differentiation of mesenchymal stem cells (MSCs) into osteoblasts. These ions activate signalling pathways and transcription factors involved in osteogenesis, such as RUNX2 and osterix.

Osteoblast Activity: Bioactive ions enhance the metabolic activity of osteoblasts, increasing the production of bone matrix proteins like collagen and non-collagenous proteins such as osteopontin and bone sialoprotein. This leads to enhanced matrix mineralization and the formation of new bone tissue.

10.4.1.1.2 Activation of Signalling Pathways

Wnt/β-catenin Pathway: Silicon and calcium ions can activate the Wnt/β-catenin signalling pathway, which is crucial for osteoblast proliferation and differentiation. Activation of this pathway leads to increased expression of osteogenic genes and promotes bone formation.

MAPK Pathway: The Mitogen-Activated Protein Kinase (MAPK) pathway, including ERK, JNK, and p38 MAPK, is activated by bioactive glass-derived ions. This pathway regulates cell proliferation, differentiation, and survival, contributing to osteogenesis.

BMP/Smad Pathway: Bioactive glasses can also influence the Bone Morphogenetic Protein (BMP) signalling pathway. BMPs are potent osteogenic factors that bind to their receptors on osteoblasts, activating the Smad signalling cascade. This enhances the expression of genes involved in osteoblast differentiation and bone matrix production.

10.4.1.1.3 Hydroxyapatite Formation

Surface Reactions: The formation of a HA layer on the surface of bioactive glasses when in contact with physiological fluids is a key factor in their osteogenic potential. This layer mimics the natural bone mineral, providing a conducive environment for osteoblast attachment and proliferation. The HA layer serves as a template for new bone formation and integration with the host tissue.

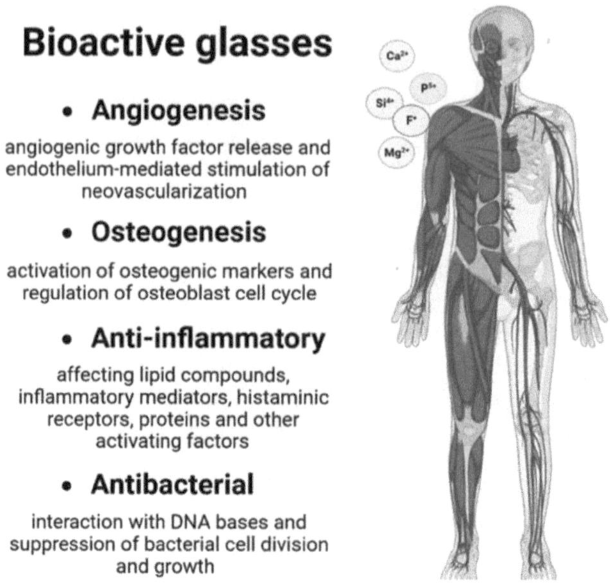

FIGURE 10.2 Applications of bioactive glasses in angiogenesis, osteogenesis, anti-inflammatory and anti-bacterial activities [9]

- **Angiogenic Effects**: Bioactive glasses also exhibit angiogenic properties, promoting the formation of new blood vessels. This is crucial for supplying nutrients and oxygen to regenerating tissues, facilitating their growth and integration into the surrounding biological environment.

The angiogenic properties of bioactive glasses make them invaluable in applications such as wound healing, bone regeneration, and tissue engineering, contributing significantly to their effectiveness in clinical settings (Figure 10.2).

10.4.2 Applications in Tissue Regeneration

The regenerative capabilities of bioactive glasses have led to their widespread use in tissue engineering applications. In tissue engineering, bioactive glasses serve as scaffolds or matrices that support the growth and organization of cells into functional tissues [10, 11]. Key applications include:

- **Bone Tissue Engineering**: Bioactive glasses are used as scaffolds for bone tissue engineering due to their ability to promote osteogenesis and integrate with existing bone. They provide a 3D structure for cell attachment, proliferation, and differentiation, leading to the formation of new bone tissue [12].
- **Cartilage Regeneration**: Bioactive glasses have shown promise in promoting the regeneration of cartilage tissue. They support chondrogenic cell differentiation and ECM production, facilitating the repair of cartilage defects caused by injury or degenerative conditions [13, 14, 15].

- **Dermal and Skin Regeneration**: In dermal and skin tissue engineering, bioactive glasses can be used to enhance wound healing and promote the regeneration of skin tissues. They support the migration and proliferation of dermal fibroblasts and keratinocytes, leading to improved tissue repair and reduced scarring [16].

10.4.3 Clinical Applications and Success Stories

Bioactive glasses have been successfully applied in clinical settings for tissue regeneration across various medical specialties. For instance:

In orthopaedic surgery, bioactive glass scaffolds have been used to repair bone defects and promote bone fusion in spinal fusion procedures. In dentistry, bioactive glass-based materials have been employed for guided bone regeneration in implant dentistry and the treatment of periodontal defects. In plastic and reconstructive surgery, bioactive glasses have been used to support soft tissue regeneration and wound healing in cases of trauma or surgical interventions. The success stories of bioactive glasses in tissue regeneration highlight their potential to revolutionize regenerative medicine and address a wide range of clinical needs. Ongoing research continues to explore novel applications and optimize the properties of bioactive glasses for enhanced tissue regeneration outcomes.

10.5 INNOVATION IN BIOACTIVE GLASSES

10.5.1 Development of Advanced Compositions

The evolution of bioactive glasses has seen significant advancements in the development of novel compositions tailored to specific applications and performance requirements [17]. Researchers and industry experts have focused on optimizing the chemical composition, structure, and properties of bioactive glasses to enhance their bioactivity, mechanical strength, and degradation kinetics.

Researchers have extensively explored variations in the elemental composition of bioactive glasses to fine-tune their properties and enhance their functionality for specific applications. This involves adjusting the ratios of key components such as silica (SiO_2), calcium (CaO), sodium (Na_2O), and phosphorus (P_2O_5), as well as incorporating additional elements like magnesium (Mg), strontium (Sr), and zinc (Zn) to impart specific biological and mechanical properties.

1. **Silica (SiO_2)**

   Structural Integrity: Silica is the primary network former in bioactive glasses, providing the structural backbone of the glass matrix. Adjusting the silica content can influence the glass's mechanical properties and degradation rate.

   Bioactivity: Silica plays a crucial role in forming a bioactive HA layer on the glass surface, which is essential for bonding with bone tissue. Silica also contributes to the stimulation of osteoblast proliferation and differentiation.

2. **Calcium (CaO)**

   Osteoconductivity: Calcium is vital for bone regeneration due to its role in forming HA ($Ca_{10}(PO_4)_6(OH)_2$), the mineral phase of bone. Higher calcium content enhances the osteoconductive properties of bioactive glasses.

   Ionic Release: The release of calcium ions during glass degradation promotes cellular activities related to bone formation and repair, including the activation of osteoblasts.

3. **Sodium (Na_2O)**

   Glass Formation and Stability: Sodium acts as a network modifier, reducing the viscosity of the glass melt and facilitating the formation of the glass structure. However, high sodium content can increase the degradation rate, which needs to be carefully balanced.

   Ionic Exchange: Sodium ions participate in ionic exchange processes at the glass surface, which can influence the formation of the bioactive HA layer.

4. **Phosphorus (P_2O_5)**

   Bone Regeneration: Phosphorus is a crucial component of the bioactive glass network and is essential for bone regeneration. It contributes to the formation of HA and enhances the bioactivity of the glass.

   Degradation Control: The phosphorus content affects the solubility and degradation rate of the glass. Higher phosphorus levels can lead to faster degradation, releasing therapeutic ions more quickly.

10.5.1.1 Incorporation of Additional Elements

1. **Magnesium (Mg)**

   Bone Health: Magnesium is essential for bone health, influencing the activity of osteoblasts and osteoclasts. Incorporating magnesium into bioactive glasses enhances their bioactivity and promotes bone cell adhesion and proliferation.

   Mechanical Properties: Magnesium can improve the mechanical strength and fracture toughness of bioactive glasses, making them more suitable for load-bearing applications.
2. **Strontium (Sr)**

   Dual Role: Strontium plays a dual role in bone regeneration by stimulating osteoblast activity while inhibiting osteoclast-mediated bone resorption. This makes strontium-doped bioactive glasses particularly effective in treating osteoporosis.

   Enhanced Bioactivity: The incorporation of strontium enhances the bioactivity of the glass, promoting faster formation of the HA layer and improving bone bonding.
3. **Zinc (Zn)**

   Antibacterial Properties: Zinc exhibits antibacterial properties, which can help prevent infections in clinical applications. Zinc-doped bioactive glasses can reduce the risk of bacterial colonization and biofilm formation.

Enzyme Activation: Zinc is a cofactor for various enzymes involved in cellular processes, including DNA synthesis and cell proliferation. Zinc incorporation can enhance cell attachment and proliferation, supporting tissue regeneration (Figure 10.3).

- **Multifunctional Glasses**: Advanced bioactive glasses are designed to exhibit multifunctional properties, combining bioactivity with antimicrobial activity, drug delivery capabilities, and controlled release of therapeutic agents. These glasses can serve as versatile platforms for addressing complex medical challenges, such as infection control, localized drug delivery, and tissue regeneration.

The development of multifunctional bioactive glasses represents a significant advancement in biomaterials science, offering a versatile platform for addressing complex medical challenges. By combining bioactivity with antimicrobial properties, drug delivery capabilities, and controlled release of therapeutic agents, these glasses provide comprehensive solutions for infection control, localized therapy, and tissue regeneration. Ongoing research and innovation in this field continue to expand the potential applications of multifunctional bioactive glasses, contributing to improved patient outcomes and advancing the field of regenerative medicine.

- **Composite and Hybrid Materials**: Innovations in bioactive glass composites and hybrid materials have expanded their applicability and performance. Combining bioactive glasses with polymers, ceramics, metals, or other biomaterials creates synergistic effects, enhancing mechanical properties, biocompatibility, and overall functionality [18, 19].

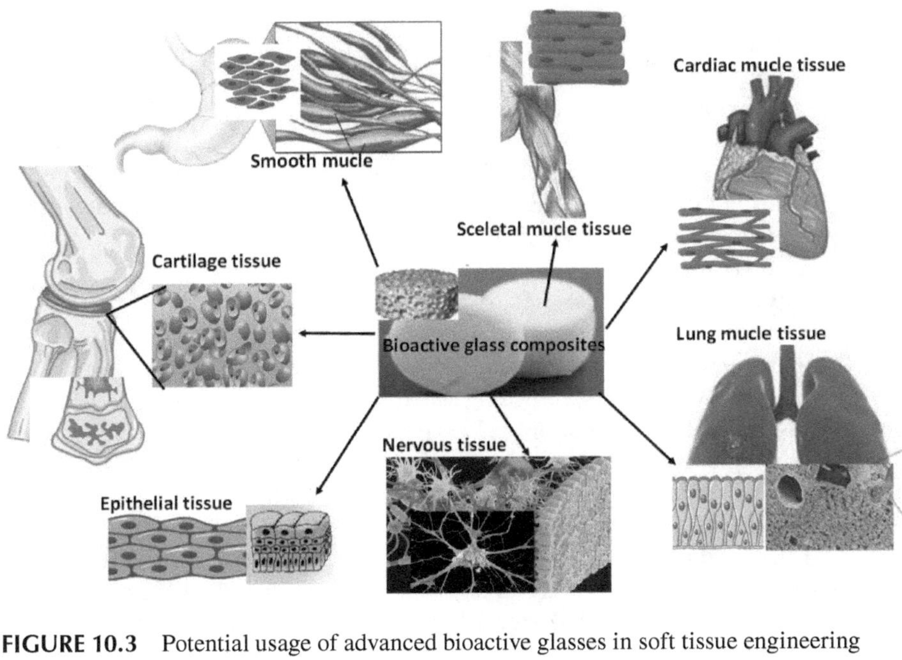

FIGURE 10.3 Potential usage of advanced bioactive glasses in soft tissue engineering

Innovations in bioactive glass composites and hybrid materials have significantly expanded their applicability and performance in biomedical applications. By combining bioactive glasses with polymers, ceramics, metals, or other biomaterials, researchers have created materials that exhibit synergistic effects, resulting in enhanced mechanical properties, biocompatibility, and overall functionality.

10.5.2 Future Research Directions

The future of bioactive glasses lies in ongoing research efforts aimed at pushing the boundaries of their capabilities and exploring new frontiers. Key research directions include:

Advanced Manufacturing Techniques: Innovations in manufacturing technologies, such as additive manufacturing (3D printing), electrospinning, and sol-gel processing, enable the fabrication of complex structures and customized implants with precise control over material properties.

- **Applications of Advanced Manufacturing Techniques**

1. **Orthopaedics**

   Patient-Specific Implants: 3D printing enables the production of customized implants that fit precisely into the patient's bone defects, improving surgical outcomes and reducing recovery times. These implants can be designed to match the mechanical properties of natural bone.

   Bone Tissue Engineering: Electrospun nanofibre scaffolds with embedded bioactive glass particles promote osteogenesis and angiogenesis, making them ideal for bone tissue engineering applications. Sol-gel-derived bioactive glass scaffolds can also be used to support bone regeneration.
2. **Dentistry**

   Dental Restorations: 3D printing allows for the fabrication of intricate dental restorations, such as crowns, bridges, and inlays, with high precision. These restorations can incorporate bioactive glass to enhance their bioactivity and durability.

   Periodontal Regeneration: Electrospun scaffolds with bioactive glass particles are used to regenerate periodontal tissues, supporting the healing of gums and bone around teeth and dental implants.
3. **Wound Healing**

   Advanced Dressings: Electrospun nanofibre dressings containing bioactive glass promote wound healing by releasing therapeutic ions that stimulate tissue repair and prevent infections. These dressings can be tailored to degrade at specific rates, providing sustained therapeutic effects.

   Topical Applications: Sol-gel-derived bioactive glass powders can be used in topical formulations to treat chronic wounds and burns, accelerating the healing process and reducing the risk of infection.
4. **Drug Delivery Systems**

   Localized Delivery: 3D printed and electrospun devices can be designed to deliver drugs locally to the target site, providing controlled and sustained release. This approach enhances therapeutic efficacy and minimizes systemic side effects.

Multifunctional Devices: Advanced manufacturing techniques enable the creation of multifunctional devices that combine structural support with drug delivery capabilities, offering comprehensive treatment solutions for complex medical conditions.

- **Bioactive Glass Nanocomposites**: Nanotechnology is increasingly being integrated into bioactive glasses to create nanocomposites with enhanced bioactivity, mechanical strength, and surface properties [20]. Nanoscale modifications offer opportunities for targeted drug delivery, cell signalling modulation, and tissue-specific regeneration [21].

1. **Enhanced Bioactivity**

   Increased Surface Area: The incorporation of nanoparticles into bioactive glass matrices increases the surface area, enhancing the interaction with biological tissues. This leads to faster and more efficient formation of the HA layer, which is crucial for bonding with bone tissue.

   Bioactive Ion Release: Nanocomposites can be engineered to release bioactive ions, such as calcium, silicon, and phosphate, at controlled rates. These ions stimulate cellular activities that promote bone formation, angiogenesis, and tissue regeneration.
2. **Improved Mechanical Strength**

   Reinforcement with Nanoparticles: Adding nanoparticles, such as carbon nanotubes, graphene oxide, or nanoclay, to bioactive glasses improves their mechanical properties, including tensile strength, fracture toughness, and elasticity. This makes the nanocomposites suitable for load-bearing applications.

   Homogeneous Distribution: Nanoscale dispersion of reinforcing particles ensures a homogeneous distribution within the glass matrix, reducing the likelihood of stress concentration points and improving the overall mechanical integrity of the material.
3. **Superior Surface Properties**

   Nanotopography: Modifying the surface of bioactive glasses at the nanoscale creates a unique nanotopography that enhances cell adhesion, proliferation, and differentiation. This is particularly beneficial for applications in bone and soft tissue engineering.

   Antimicrobial Surface: Nanocomposites can incorporate nanoparticles with intrinsic antimicrobial properties, such as silver or zinc oxide, to create surfaces that prevent bacterial adhesion and biofilm formation, reducing the risk of infection.

- **Applications of Bioactive Glass Nanocomposites**

1. **Targeted Drug Delivery**

   Nanoscale Carriers: Bioactive glass nanocomposites can be engineered to serve as carriers for targeted drug delivery. These carriers can be designed to release therapeutic agents in response to specific physiological conditions or stimuli, ensuring precise delivery to the target site.

Controlled Release Systems: The nanoscale modifications allow for controlled and sustained release of drugs, reducing the frequency of administration and improving patient compliance. This is particularly useful for localized treatment of infections, inflammation, and cancer.

2. **Modulation of Cell Signalling**

   Bioactive Ion Modulation: The release of bioactive ions from nanocomposites can modulate cellular signalling pathways involved in tissue regeneration. For example, silicon ions can enhance the expression of genes related to osteogenesis and angiogenesis, promoting bone and blood vessel formation.

   Surface Functionalization: Nanocomposites can be functionalized with bioactive molecules, such as peptides, growth factors, or antibodies, to modulate cell behaviour and improve tissue integration.

3. **Tissue-Specific Regeneration**

   Bone Regeneration: Bioactive glass nanocomposites are highly effective in bone regeneration applications due to their enhanced bioactivity and mechanical properties. They can be used to create scaffolds that support the growth and differentiation of osteoblasts, promoting rapid bone healing.

   Soft Tissue Repair: The unique surface properties of nanocomposites, such as nanotopography and bioactive coatings, make them suitable for soft tissue engineering. They can be used to repair tissues such as skin, cartilage, and ligaments, supporting cell attachment and proliferation.

- **Bioactive Glasses for Non-Skeletal Applications**: While bioactive glasses have primarily been used in orthopaedics and dentistry, future research aims to explore their potential in non-skeletal applications, such as cardiovascular implants, wound healing dressings, and neural tissue regeneration.

10.5.3 Potential Non-Skeletal Applications of Bioactive Glasses

10.5.3.1 Cardiovascular Implants

Vascular Stents: Bioactive glass coatings on vascular stents can enhance their biocompatibility and reduce the risk of restenosis (re-narrowing of the artery). The release of therapeutic ions from the bioactive glass can promote endothelial cell proliferation and inhibit smooth muscle cell proliferation, reducing the likelihood of stent occlusion.

Heart Valve Prostheses: Bioactive glass materials can be used to create or coat heart valve prostheses to improve their integration with surrounding tissues and reduce the risk of calcification and thrombus formation. Their bioactivity can promote the formation of a stable endothelial layer on the valve surface, enhancing its durability and function.

10.5.3.2 Wound Healing Dressings

Antimicrobial Properties: Bioactive glass-based wound dressings can provide antimicrobial protection, preventing infections in chronic and acute wounds. The release of bioactive ions such as silver or zinc can create an antimicrobial environment, aiding in faster wound healing.

Enhanced Healing: Bioactive glass dressings promote angiogenesis and the formation of granulation tissue, accelerating the wound healing process. The ions released from the glass can stimulate cellular activities that are crucial for tissue repair and regeneration.

Moisture Control: These dressings can help maintain an optimal moisture balance at the wound site, which is critical for effective healing. The bioactive glass components can also absorb wound exudates while keeping the wound environment moist.

10.5.3.3 Neural Tissue Regeneration

Nerve Conduits: Bioactive glass can be incorporated into nerve conduits to support nerve regeneration in cases of peripheral nerve injuries. The bioactive ions released can stimulate neural cell growth and differentiation, promoting the repair of damaged nerves.

Scaffolds for Neural Tissue: Bioactive glass scaffolds can provide a supportive environment for the growth of neural tissues. The bioactivity of the glass can enhance cell attachment and proliferation, aiding in the regeneration of neural networks.

Drug Delivery Systems: Bioactive glasses can be used to deliver neurotrophic factors and other therapeutic agents directly to the site of neural injury. Controlled release from the bioactive glass matrix ensures sustained therapeutic effects, promoting nerve regeneration and functional recovery.

- **Biomimetic Design Strategies**: Drawing inspiration from biological systems, biomimetic design approaches aim to mimic the hierarchical structure and functionalities of natural tissues. Bioactive glasses designed using biomimetic principles can better integrate with host tissues, promote cellular responses, and support tissue regeneration [22].

10.5.3.4 Key Biomimetic Design Approaches

10.5.3.4.1 Hierarchical Structure

Nanostructure Mimicry: Biomimetic bioactive glasses are engineered to replicate the nanoscale features of the ECM, such as fibrillar collagen networks and mineralized matrices found in bone tissue. This involves the creation of hierarchical structures with well-defined nanotopography and porosity, which promote cell adhesion, proliferation, and differentiation.

Surface Functionalization: The surface of biomimetic bioactive glasses is modified to mimic the bioactive cues present in the ECM, such as cell-adhesive peptides and growth factors. These biomolecules enhance cellular interactions with the material, facilitating tissue regeneration processes.

10.5.3.4.2 Functionalization with Biologics

Cell-Responsive Signals: Biomimetic bioactive glasses are functionalized with biologics, such as growth factors, cytokines, and ECM proteins, to provide cell-responsive signals that regulate cellular behaviour. These signals mimic the natural microenvironment of tissues, promoting specific cellular responses, such as migration, proliferation, and differentiation.

Mimicking Cell-Matrix Interactions: By mimicking the interactions between cells and the ECM, biomimetic bioactive glasses create an environment conducive to tissue regeneration. This involves presenting bioactive ligands on the material surface that bind to cell receptors, initiating intracellular signalling pathways that drive tissue repair processes.

10.5.3.4.3 Dynamic Response to Environmental Stimuli

pH and Ion Sensitivity: Biomimetic bioactive glasses are designed to respond dynamically to changes in pH and ion concentrations, mimicking the physiological conditions of the tissue microenvironment. This responsiveness allows the material to release bioactive ions and therapeutic agents in a controlled manner, modulating cellular activities and promoting tissue regeneration.

Adaptive Degradation Kinetics: Biomimetic bioactive glasses exhibit adaptive degradation kinetics, wherein the material degrades at rates that match the rate of tissue regeneration. This ensures that the scaffold provides structural support during the early stages of healing and gradually resorbs as new tissue forms, minimizing the risk of implant rejection.

10.5.4 Applications of Biomimetic Bioactive Glasses

10.5.4.1 Bone Regeneration

Osteoconductive Scaffolds: Biomimetic bioactive glasses serve as osteoconductive scaffolds for bone regeneration, providing a biomimetic microenvironment that supports the growth and differentiation of osteoblasts. The hierarchical structure and surface functionalization promote cell adhesion and mineralization, facilitating new bone formation.

Angiogenic Stimulation: By mimicking the natural cues present in the bone microenvironment, biomimetic bioactive glasses promote angiogenesis, enhancing vascularization and nutrient delivery to regenerating tissues.

10.5.4.2 Dental Applications

Periodontal Regeneration: Biomimetic bioactive glasses are used in periodontal regeneration to support the growth of periodontal ligament cells and promote the formation of new cementum and alveolar bone. The surface functionalization with bioactive cues enhances the attachment and differentiation of periodontal progenitor cells.

Dental Implants: Biomimetic bioactive glasses improve the integration of dental implants with surrounding tissues, reducing the risk of peri-implantitis and implant failure. The dynamic response to environmental stimuli ensures optimal osseointegration and long-term stability of the implant.

10.5.4.3 Soft Tissue Engineering

Skin Regeneration: Biomimetic bioactive glasses are used in wound dressings and skin substitutes to promote the regeneration of skin tissue. The surface functionalization with cell-adhesive peptides enhances the attachment and migration of keratinocytes and fibroblasts, facilitating wound closure and tissue repair.

Cartilage and Ligament Repair: Biomimetic bioactive glasses support the regeneration of cartilage and ligaments by providing a scaffold that mimics the native tissue microenvironment. The dynamic response to environmental stimuli promotes the differentiation of mesenchymal stem cells into chondrocytes and tenocytes, facilitating tissue remodelling and repair.

As advancements in bioactive glass technologies continue to evolve, ensuring regulatory compliance and standardization becomes increasingly critical. Collaborative efforts among researchers, manufacturers, and regulatory agencies are essential to establish guidelines, standards, and quality control measures for the safe and effective use of advanced bioactive glass products. By adhering to regulatory requirements and implementing standardized practices, stakeholders can mitigate risks, facilitate product development, and enhance patient safety in biomedical applications.

Patient Safety Assurance: Compliance with regulatory standards ensures that bioactive glass products meet stringent safety and efficacy requirements, minimizing the risk of adverse effects and ensuring patient well-being. Regulatory oversight helps to identify and address potential hazards associated with the use of bioactive glasses in medical devices and implants.

Market Access and Global Trade: Regulatory compliance enables manufacturers to obtain necessary approvals for market access, facilitating the commercialization and global distribution of bioactive glass products. Adherence to international standards promotes harmonization of regulatory frameworks, streamlining trade and enhancing market competitiveness.

Quality Assurance: Regulatory guidelines establish quality control measures and manufacturing practices to ensure consistency, reliability, and reproducibility of bioactive glass products. Compliance with quality standards fosters confidence among healthcare professionals and patients regarding the safety and efficacy of these materials.

10.5.4.4 Collaborative Efforts for Standardization

Research and Development Collaboration: Collaborative initiatives between academia, industry, and regulatory bodies promote the development of standardized testing methods, characterization techniques, and preclinical evaluation protocols for bioactive glass materials. Shared resources and expertise facilitate the translation of research findings into clinically viable products.

Industry Standards Development: Industry organizations play a pivotal role in developing voluntary consensus standards for bioactive glass products, encompassing material specifications, manufacturing processes, and performance criteria. These standards serve as benchmarks for quality assurance and regulatory compliance within the industry.

Regulatory Harmonization: Regulatory agencies collaborate with international counterparts to harmonize standards and regulations governing bioactive glass products, ensuring alignment with global requirements. Harmonization efforts facilitate market access, reduce regulatory burdens, and promote innovation while safeguarding public health.

10.5.4.5 Implementation of Quality Management Systems

ISO Certification: Adoption of ISO 13485 certification, specifically tailored for medical device quality management systems, demonstrates a manufacturer's commitment to regulatory compliance and product quality in bioactive glass production. Compliance with ISO standards fosters continuous improvement and regulatory alignment.

Good Manufacturing Practices (GMP): Adherence to GMP principles ensures the consistency and traceability of manufacturing processes for bioactive glass products, from raw material procurement to final product distribution. GMP compliance mitigates risks of contamination, batch variability, and product non-conformities.

Post-Market Surveillance: Implementation of post-market surveillance systems enables ongoing monitoring of bioactive glass products' safety and performance in clinical use. Timely reporting and analysis of adverse events facilitate risk management and product optimization through feedback-driven improvements.

By exploring these research directions and fostering collaboration across disciplines, the future of bioactive glasses holds tremendous potential for addressing healthcare challenges, advancing regenerative medicine, and improving patient outcomes.

10.6 INDUSTRIAL COMPLIANCE

10.6.1 Regulatory Frameworks

The development and commercialization of bioactive glasses require adherence to stringent regulatory frameworks to ensure their safety, efficacy, and quality. Regulatory bodies such as the U.S. Food and Drug Administration (FDA), the European Medicines Agency (EMA), and other national regulatory authorities set standards and guidelines for the approval and marketing of medical devices and biomaterials. Key aspects of regulatory compliance for bioactive glasses include:

- **Classification and Registration**: Bioactive glasses are classified as medical devices or biomaterials, depending on their intended use and mode of action. Manufacturers must register their products and obtain regulatory approvals before marketing them for clinical use.

10.6.1.1 Classification as Medical Devices or Biomaterials

10.6.1.1.1 Medical Devices

Bioactive glasses intended for use in medical applications, such as orthopaedic implants, dental materials, or wound dressings, are classified as medical devices. These products undergo rigorous evaluation to assess their safety, performance, and effectiveness in treating specific medical conditions.

Biomaterials: Bioactive glasses used as research tools or components in biomaterial formulations may be classified as biomaterials. While not always subject to the same regulatory requirements as medical devices, biomaterials must still meet quality and safety standards to ensure compatibility with biological systems.

- **Biocompatibility Testing**: Regulatory agencies require comprehensive biocompatibility testing to assess the interactions between bioactive glasses and biological systems. This includes evaluations of cytotoxicity, genotoxicity, immunogenicity, and hemocompatibility to ensure the safety of the materials.

10.6.1.2 Cytotoxicity Testing

10.6.1.2.1 Cell Viability Assays

Bioactive glass extracts or direct contact with cells are evaluated using cell viability assays such as MTT, XTT, or AlamarBlue. These assays assess the metabolic activity and proliferation of cells exposed to bioactive glass materials.

Lactate Dehydrogenase (LDH) Release Assay: The LDH release assay measures the leakage of cytoplasmic LDH enzyme from damaged cells, indicating cytotoxic effects of bioactive glass materials. Increased LDH release suggests cellular damage or membrane disruption.

10.6.1.2.2 Genotoxicity Testing

Ames Test: The Ames test assesses the mutagenic potential of bioactive glass materials by exposing bacterial strains to material extracts. Mutagenicity is determined based on the induction of reverse mutations in the bacteria.

Micronucleus Assay: In vitro micronucleus assays evaluate the potential of bioactive glass materials to induce chromosomal damage or genomic instability in cultured cells. The presence of micronuclei in cells indicates genotoxic effects.

10.6.1.2.3 Immunogenicity Testing

Lymphocyte Proliferation Assay: Bioactive glass extracts are incubated with lymphocytes to evaluate their immunostimulatory or immunosuppressive effects. Increased lymphocyte proliferation may indicate an immune response to the material.

Cytokine Release Assay: The release of pro-inflammatory or anti-inflammatory cytokines from immune cells exposed to bioactive glass materials is measured to assess their immunomodulatory properties. Altered cytokine levels may indicate immune activation or suppression.

10.6.1.2.4 Hemocompatibility Testing

Hemolysis Assay: Bioactive glass materials are evaluated for their potential to cause hemolysis, the disruption of red blood cells, using a hemolysis assay. Hemolytic activity is quantified by measuring the release of haemoglobin from lysed red blood cells.

Platelet Adhesion and Activation Assay: Platelet adhesion and activation on bioactive glass surfaces are assessed to evaluate their thrombogenic potential. Platelet activation markers, such as P-selectin expression and release of thromboxane A2, are measured to determine platelet reactivity.

10.6.2 Quality Control and Standardization

Key aspects of quality control and standardization include:

- **Material Characterization**: Thorough characterization of bioactive glass materials is essential to understand their properties, composition, and performance. Techniques such as X-ray diffraction (XRD), scanning electron microscopy (SEM), Fourier-transform infrared spectroscopy (FTIR), and thermal analysis are used for material characterization.
- **Batch-to-Batch Consistency**: Manufacturers must implement stringent controls to ensure batch-to-batch consistency in bioactive glass production. This includes monitoring raw material quality, process parameters, and product specifications to minimize variations and ensure uniformity in product performance.

Achieving batch-to-batch consistency in bioactive glass production is a complex but crucial endeavour. By meticulously controlling the quality of raw materials, rigorously managing process parameters, and ensuring the uniformity of product specifications, manufacturers can produce bioactive glasses that consistently meet the high standards required for medical applications. Such rigorous quality control not only enhances the reliability and safety of bioactive glass products but also fosters confidence among healthcare providers and patients in their therapeutic efficacy.

- **Validation and Verification**: Validation and verification processes are conducted to confirm that bioactive glass products meet predefined specifications and performance criteria. This includes validation of manufacturing processes, sterilization methods, packaging, and labelling to ensure product integrity and efficacy.

Validation and verification are fundamental to the production of bioactive glass products, ensuring that each product meets stringent specifications and performs reliably in clinical settings. Through the meticulous validation of manufacturing processes, sterilization methods, packaging, and labelling, manufacturers can maintain the integrity and efficacy of their products. Furthermore, thorough verification of product performance ensures that bioactive glasses can fulfil their intended therapeutic roles effectively. These comprehensive quality control measures are vital for delivering safe, effective, and reliable bioactive glass products for medical use.

- **Post-Market Surveillance**: Continuous post-market surveillance is essential to monitor the safety and performance of bioactive glass products once they are in clinical use. Manufacturers are required to collect and analyse data on adverse events, device failures, and patient outcomes to identify potential risks and implement corrective actions as needed.

Post-market surveillance is a critical process in the lifecycle of bioactive glass products, providing essential insights into their real-world performance and safety. Through systematic data collection and analysis, risk identification, and timely corrective actions, manufacturers can enhance product reliability and patient outcomes. Compliance with regulatory requirements and a commitment to continuous improvement ensure that bioactive glass products remain safe and effective for their intended medical applications. This ongoing vigilance is crucial for sustaining the therapeutic benefits of bioactive glass materials in clinical practice and fostering confidence among healthcare providers and patients.

International harmonization and collaboration are critical for the effective regulation and commercialization of bioactive glass products. Programmes like Medical Device Single Audit Programme (MDSAP) and mutual recognition agreements (MRAs) simplify regulatory processes and enhance global market access, while alignment with international standards and robust quality control measures ensure product compliance and safety. Collaborative efforts among regulatory agencies, industry stakeholders, and research institutions foster innovation and streamline the path to market for bioactive glass technologies. Through these concerted efforts, manufacturers can deliver safe, effective, and high-quality bioactive glass products to meet the diverse needs of the global healthcare market.

10.6.3 International Harmonization and Collaboration

International harmonization efforts and collaboration among regulatory agencies, industry stakeholders, and research institutions are key strategies to facilitate industrial compliance and streamline regulatory processes for bioactive glasses. Initiatives such as MDSAP and MRAs aim to harmonize regulatory requirements across different jurisdictions and promote global market access for medical devices and biomaterials. By aligning with regulatory standards, implementing robust quality control measures, and fostering collaboration, manufacturers of bioactive glasses can ensure industrial compliance, meet regulatory expectations, and deliver safe and effective products for clinical use.

10.7 LIFE CYCLE ANALYSIS

10.7.1 Methodology of Life Cycle Analysis

Life cycle analysis (LCA) is a comprehensive approach used to assess the environmental impact of bioactive glasses throughout their entire life cycle, from raw material extraction and production to use and disposal. The methodology of LCA involves several key steps:

- **Goal and Scope Definition**: The first step in LCA is defining the goal and scope of the analysis. This includes identifying the functional unit (e.g., per unit of bioactive glass produced or per patient treated), setting boundaries for the study (e.g., cradle-to-gate, cradle-to-grave), and determining the environmental impact categories to be assessed (e.g., greenhouse gas emissions, energy consumption, waste generation).
- **Inventory Analysis**: The inventory analysis involves compiling data on the inputs (e.g., raw materials, energy, water) and outputs (e.g., emissions, waste) associated with the production and use of bioactive glasses. This

includes collecting data from suppliers, manufacturing facilities, transportation activities, and end-of-life disposal processes.

- **Impact Assessment**: The impact assessment phase evaluates the environmental impacts identified in the inventory analysis. Impact categories such as global warming potential, acidification, eutrophication, and resource depletion are quantified and analysed using impact assessment methods and characterization factors.
- **Interpretation**: The final step in LCA is interpreting the results and drawing conclusions based on the environmental performance of bioactive glasses. This includes identifying hotspots (e.g., processes with significant environmental impacts), conducting sensitivity analyses, and comparing alternative scenarios or product designs to identify opportunities for improvement.

10.7.2 Environmental Impact and Sustainability

The environmental impact of bioactive glasses is influenced by various factors throughout their life cycle. Key aspects of environmental impact and sustainability considerations include:

- **Raw Material Sourcing**: The extraction and processing of raw materials for bioactive glasses can have environmental implications, including land use, energy consumption, water usage, and emissions of pollutants. Sustainable sourcing practices, such as using recycled materials or optimizing material efficiency, can reduce environmental impacts.

10.7.2.1 Challenges and Opportunities

Implementing sustainable sourcing practices for bioactive glasses presents several challenges. One of the main obstacles is the availability and cost of high-quality recycled materials. While the use of recycled glass can reduce environmental impacts, ensuring consistent quality and supply can be challenging. Moreover, the market for recycled materials may not always meet the specific purity and composition requirements needed for bioactive glass production.

Another challenge is the integration of sustainable practices within existing supply chains. Many raw material suppliers may not currently prioritize environmental sustainability, and transitioning to more sustainable sources may require significant changes in procurement strategies and partnerships.

- **Manufacturing Processes**: The energy consumption, emissions, waste generation, and use of chemicals during the manufacturing of bioactive glasses contribute to their environmental footprint. Implementing energy-efficient processes, reducing waste generation, and using eco-friendly materials and technologies can improve sustainability.
- **Product Use Phase**: During the use phase, bioactive glasses contribute positively to sustainability by promoting tissue regeneration, reducing the need for repeated interventions, and improving patient outcomes. However,

factors such as device longevity, maintenance requirements, and end-of-life considerations can influence their overall environmental performance.

- **End-of-Life Disposal**: Proper disposal and recycling of bioactive glasses at the end of their life cycle are critical for minimizing environmental impact. Options such as recycling glass waste, using biodegradable packaging, or implementing take-back programmes can enhance sustainability and circular economy principles.

10.7.3 Sustainable Practices and Continuous Improvement

To enhance the environmental sustainability of bioactive glasses, manufacturers and stakeholders can adopt sustainable practices and continuous improvement strategies:

- **Green Manufacturing**: Implementing green manufacturing practices, such as renewable energy use, waste reduction, and pollution prevention, can minimize the environmental footprint of bioactive glass production.
- **Life Cycle Optimization**: Conducting life cycle optimization studies and incorporating eco-design principles into product development can identify opportunities to reduce environmental impacts across the entire life cycle of bioactive glasses.
- **Environmental Certification**: Seeking environmental certifications, such as ISO 14001 (Environmental Management Systems), demonstrates a commitment to environmental responsibility and can enhance market competitiveness.
- **Stakeholder Engagement**: Engaging with stakeholders, including regulatory agencies, customers, suppliers, and the community, fosters transparency, accountability, and collaboration in sustainable practices.

10.8 CHALLENGES AND SOLUTIONS

10.8.1 Overcoming Regulatory Hurdles

One of the primary challenges in the industrial compliance and LCA of bioactive glasses is navigating complex regulatory frameworks. Regulatory approvals for medical devices and biomaterials require rigorous testing, documentation, and adherence to standards to ensure safety and efficacy. Some key challenges in regulatory compliance include:

- **Stringent Testing Requirements**: Regulatory agencies require extensive testing to assess the biocompatibility, safety, and performance of bioactive glasses. This includes preclinical studies, clinical trials, and post-market surveillance, which can be time-consuming and costly.
- **Global Harmonization**: Differences in regulatory requirements across regions and countries can pose challenges for manufacturers seeking international market access. Harmonizing standards, mutual recognition agreements, and collaboration among regulatory bodies can facilitate regulatory compliance and market acceptance.

- **Emerging Technologies**: The rapid pace of technological advancements in biomaterials and medical devices presents challenges in keeping up with evolving regulatory expectations. Continuous education, engagement with regulatory agencies, and proactive compliance strategies are essential to address these challenges.
- **Comprehensive Documentation**: Maintaining thorough documentation of product specifications, testing protocols, quality control measures, and regulatory submissions is crucial for demonstrating compliance and expediting regulatory reviews.
- **Collaboration and Advocacy**: Collaborating with industry associations, regulatory consultants, and advocacy groups can provide insights, resources, and support in navigating regulatory challenges and advocating for favourable regulatory policies.
- **Continuous Compliance Monitoring**: Establishing robust compliance monitoring systems, conducting internal audits, and staying updated on regulatory updates and industry best practices ensure ongoing compliance and readiness for regulatory inspections.

10.8.2 Enhancing Industrial Processes

Another challenge in the industrial compliance and LCA of bioactive glasses is optimizing industrial processes to improve efficiency, sustainability, and quality. Key challenges in industrial processes include:

- **Resource Efficiency**: Minimizing resource consumption, waste generation, and energy usage in bioactive glass production processes is essential for sustainability and cost-effectiveness.
- **Quality Assurance**: Ensuring consistent product quality, batch-to-batch uniformity, and adherence to specifications require robust quality control measures, process validation, and continuous improvement initiatives.
- **Supply Chain Management**: Managing supply chain complexities, sourcing raw materials responsibly, and ensuring supply chain resilience are critical for uninterrupted production and delivery of bioactive glass products.

Solutions to enhance industrial processes include:

- **Lean Manufacturing**: Implementing lean manufacturing principles, process optimization strategies, and continuous improvement methodologies such as Six Sigma can streamline operations, reduce waste, and enhance productivity.
- **Green Technologies**: Adopting environmentally friendly technologies, renewable energy sources, and eco-friendly materials in manufacturing processes can reduce environmental impact and align with sustainability goals.

- **Quality Management Systems**: Implementing ISO 13485-compliant quality management systems, good manufacturing practices (GMP), and quality assurance protocols ensure product quality, regulatory compliance, and customer satisfaction.
- **Supplier Collaboration**: Collaborating closely with suppliers, establishing long-term partnerships, and conducting supplier audits and evaluations promote supply chain transparency, reliability, and resilience.

10.8.3 Addressing Environmental Concerns

Environmental sustainability is a growing concern in the production and use of bioactive glasses. Challenges related to environmental concerns include:

- **Resource Depletion**: Extraction of raw materials, energy-intensive processes, and waste generation contribute to resource depletion and environmental degradation.
- **Pollution and Emissions**: Production processes may result in air and water pollution, greenhouse gas emissions, and waste disposal challenges, impacting ecosystems and public health.
- **Circular Economy**: Promoting circular economy principles, waste reduction, recycling, and responsible end-of-life disposal practices are essential for minimizing environmental impact and promoting sustainability.

Solutions to address environmental concerns include:

- **Sustainable Sourcing**: Using sustainably sourced raw materials, recycled materials, and renewable resources reduces environmental footprint and supports responsible resource management.
- **Green Technologies**: Investing in green technologies, clean production methods, and pollution control measures mitigate environmental impacts and improve eco-efficiency.
- **Waste Management**: Implementing waste reduction strategies, recycling programmes, and waste-to-energy initiatives minimize waste generation and promote circularity in material utilization.
- **Environmental Impact Assessments**: Conducting comprehensive environmental impact assessments, life cycle analyses, and sustainability audits guide decision-making, identify areas for improvement, and demonstrate environmental stewardship.

By addressing these challenges and implementing sustainable solutions, stakeholders in the bioactive glass industry can promote industrial compliance, enhance environmental sustainability, and contribute to a greener and more responsible healthcare sector [23].

10.9 FUTURE OUTLOOK AND INNOVATION

10.9.1 Advancements in Material Science

The future of bioactive glasses and their industrial compliance and LCA is intertwined with ongoing advancements in material science, biomaterials engineering, and healthcare technologies. Key areas of innovation and future outlook include:

- **Advanced Composition Design**: Continued research into novel compositions of bioactive glasses, including the incorporation of bioactive ions, nanomaterials, and functional additives, aims to enhance bioactivity, mechanical properties, and therapeutic functionalities.
- **Smart and Responsive Materials**: Development of smart bioactive glasses with responsive properties, such as controlled drug release, stimuli-responsive behaviour, and bioresponsive surfaces, opens new avenues for targeted therapies, personalized medicine, and regenerative treatments.
- **Biocompatibility and Immunomodulation**: Advances in understanding the immune response to biomaterials, surface modifications for improved biocompatibility, and immunomodulatory properties of bioactive glasses pave the way for immune-informed design strategies and enhanced tissue integration.

10.9.2 Sustainable Manufacturing Practices

The future of bioactive glasses also emphasizes sustainable manufacturing practices, environmental stewardship, and circular economy principles. Key trends and initiatives include:

- **Green Chemistry and Process Innovation**: Integration of green chemistry principles, eco-friendly processing methods, and sustainable manufacturing practices minimize environmental impact, reduce resource consumption, and promote eco-efficiency.
- **Circular Economy Models**: Adoption of circular economy models, waste valorization strategies, and closed-loop material cycles transform waste into valuable resources, promote material reuse, and support sustainable production and consumption patterns.
- **Lifecycle Assessment and Environmental Footprinting**: Advancements in lifecycle assessment methodologies, environmental footprinting tools, and sustainability metrics enable comprehensive analysis of environmental impacts, resource efficiency, and carbon footprint across the entire value chain.

10.9.3 Digitalization and Industry 4.0 Integration

The digital transformation and integration of Industry 4.0 technologies in bioactive glass manufacturing and compliance processes are key drivers of future innovation and efficiency gains:

- **Digital Twin and Simulation**: Utilization of digital twin models, simulation tools, and virtual prototyping techniques optimize product design, process validation, and performance prediction, accelerating time-to-market and reducing development costs.
- **Data Analytics and Predictive Maintenance**: Harnessing big data analytics, machine learning algorithms, and predictive maintenance strategies improve process control, quality assurance, and equipment reliability, enhancing productivity and regulatory compliance.
- **Supply Chain Visibility and Traceability**: Blockchain technology, IoT sensors, and supply chain management systems provide real-time visibility, transparency, and traceability across supply chains, ensuring product quality, regulatory compliance, and risk mitigation.

10.9.4 Collaboration and Interdisciplinary Research

Collaboration among academia, industry, healthcare providers, and regulatory agencies is essential for driving innovation, addressing complex challenges, and translating research discoveries into clinical applications:

- **Interdisciplinary Research Consortia**: Formation of interdisciplinary research consortia, collaborative partnerships, and innovation hubs foster knowledge exchange, cross-disciplinary collaborations, and technology transfer, accelerating innovation and commercialization.
- **Regulatory Science and Policy Development**: Engagement with regulatory agencies, participation in standardization initiatives, and advocacy for science-based policies promote regulatory harmonization, facilitate market access, and ensure patient safety and efficacy of bioactive glass products.
- **Global Health Initiatives**: Alignment with global health initiatives, sustainable development goals, and patient-centred healthcare models drive innovation toward affordable, accessible, and equitable healthcare solutions, addressing unmet medical needs and improving healthcare outcomes worldwide.

In conclusion, the future of bioactive glasses is characterized by continuous innovation, sustainability, digitalization, and collaborative partnerships, shaping a transformative landscape for healthcare technologies, biomaterials engineering, and patient-centred care.

Continuous innovation in bioactive glass research and development will lead to the creation of novel compositions, enhanced properties, and expanded functionalities, unlocking new possibilities for medical applications. Sustainability will play a crucial role, with a focus on minimizing environmental impact, optimizing resource usage, and adopting eco-friendly production processes. Digitalization will revolutionize the field through the adoption of technologies such as digital twins, data analytics, and predictive modelling, enabling more efficient product design, manufacturing processes, and healthcare delivery.

Collaborative partnerships will foster cross-disciplinary collaborations, knowledge exchange, and technology transfer, accelerating the translation of research findings into practical applications and commercial products. These partnerships will bring together expertise from diverse fields, including materials science, biology, medicine, engineering, and digital technology, to address complex healthcare challenges and improve patient outcomes.

10.10 CONCLUSION AND RECOMMENDATIONS

10.10.1 Key Takeaways

The exploration of challenges in industrial compliance and LCA of bioactive glasses has revealed significant opportunities for innovation, sustainability, and collaboration in the healthcare and biomaterials sectors. Key takeaways from this analysis include:

- **Regulatory Navigation**: Navigating complex regulatory frameworks requires early engagement, comprehensive documentation, and collaboration with regulatory agencies and industry partners to ensure compliance and market access.
- **Sustainability Imperative**: Embracing sustainable manufacturing practices, circular economy principles, and environmental stewardship is crucial for minimizing environmental impact, enhancing resource efficiency, and meeting global sustainability goals.
- **Technological Advancements**: Leveraging advancements in material science, digitalization, and Industry 4.0 technologies drives innovation, efficiency gains, and quality improvements in bioactive glass manufacturing and compliance processes.
- **Interdisciplinary Collaboration**: Fostered collaboration among academia, industry, healthcare providers, and regulatory agencies is essential for driving innovation, addressing complex challenges, and translating research discoveries into clinical applications.

10.10.2 Recommendations for Future Action

Based on the insights gained, the following recommendations are proposed to advance the field of bioactive glasses and ensure sustainable growth and compliance:

- **Investment in Research and Development**: Allocate resources and funding for research and development initiatives focused on novel compositions, smart materials, sustainable manufacturing processes, and regulatory science to drive innovation and competitiveness.
- **Education and Training**: Provide education, training, and capacity-building programmes for industry professionals, researchers, and regulatory experts to enhance knowledge, skills, and best practices in industrial compliance, sustainability, and technology adoption.

- **Collaborative Networks**: Foster collaborative networks, research consortia, and public-private partnerships to facilitate knowledge exchange, interdisciplinary collaborations, and technology transfer, accelerating the translation of research into commercial products and clinical solutions.
- **Regulatory Harmonization**: Advocate for regulatory harmonization, alignment with international standards, and science-based policies to streamline regulatory pathways, promote market access, and ensure patient safety and efficacy of bioactive glass products.
- **Sustainability Integration**: Integrate sustainability principles, environmental impact assessments, and life cycle analyses into product development, manufacturing processes, and supply chain management to promote environmental responsibility, resource efficiency, and circular economy practices.
- **Digital Transformation**: Embrace digital transformation, data analytics, and Industry 4.0 technologies to optimize manufacturing operations, enhance quality control, and improve regulatory compliance through real-time monitoring, predictive analytics, and automation.

By implementing these recommendations, stakeholders in the bioactive glass industry can foster innovation, sustainability, and compliance excellence, paving the way for transformative advancements in healthcare, biomaterials engineering, and patient care.

Through investment in research and development initiatives, stakeholders can drive innovation in bioactive glass materials, enabling the development of novel compositions, smart materials, and sustainable manufacturing processes. By integrating sustainability principles into product development, manufacturing operations, and supply chain management, stakeholders can minimize environmental impact, conserve resources, and promote circular economy practices, contributing to a more sustainable and resilient bioeconomy.

Furthermore, by embracing digital transformation, data analytics, and Industry 4.0 technologies, stakeholders can optimize manufacturing operations, enhance quality control, and improve regulatory compliance through real-time monitoring, predictive analytics, and automation. These digital initiatives enable stakeholders to leverage data-driven insights and advanced technologies to streamline processes, reduce costs, and ensure consistency and reproducibility in manufacturing operations, ultimately driving efficiency and competitiveness in the bioactive glass industry.

Overall, by adopting a comprehensive approach that encompasses innovation, sustainability, and compliance excellence, stakeholders in the bioactive glass industry can unlock new opportunities for growth, differentiation, and impact. Through collaborative partnerships, interdisciplinary collaboration, and a commitment to continuous improvement, stakeholders can collectively drive transformative advancements that benefit patients, healthcare providers, and society as a whole, ultimately advancing the field of healthcare, biomaterials engineering, and patient care.

REFERENCES

1. L. L. Hench, "The story of Bioglass®," *J Mater Sci Mater Med*, vol. 17, no. 11, pp. 967–978, Nov. 2006, doi: 10.1007/s10856-006-0432-z.
2. M. Montazerian and E. Dutra Zanotto, "History and trends of bioactive glass-ceramics," *J Biomed Mater Res A*, vol. 104, no. 5, pp. 1231–1249, May 2016, doi: 10.1002/jbm.a.35639.
3. A. Shearer, M. Montazerian, J. J. Sly, R. G. Hill, and J. C. Mauro, "Trends and perspectives on the commercialization of bioactive glasses," *Acta Biomater*, vol. 160, pp. 14–31, 2023, doi: 10.1016/J.ACTBIO.2023.02.020.
4. F. Baino, "Bioactive glasses and glass-ceramics," *Ency Mater Tech Ceram Glass*, vol. 3, no. 2, pp. V3-614–V3-623, 2021, doi: 10.1016/B978-0-12-803581-8.12088-0.
5. H. R. Fernandes, A. Gaddam, A. Rebelo, D. Brazete, G. E. Stan, and J. M. F. Ferreira, "Bioactive glasses and glass-ceramics for healthcare applications in bone regeneration and tissue engineering.," *Materials (Basel)*, vol. 11, no. 12, 2018, doi: 10.3390/ma11122530.
6. A. C. Profeta and C. Huppa, "Bioactive-glass in oral and maxillofacial surgery," *Craniomaxillofac Trauma Reconstr*, vol. 9, no. 1, pp. 1–14, 2016, doi: 10.1055/s-0035-1551543.
7. "Global bioactive glass market analysis | size & forecasts." Accessed: May 22, 2024. [Online]. Available: https://www.globalmarketestimates.com/market-report/bioactive-glass-market-3489
8. M. Rizwan, M. Hamdi, and W. J. Basirun, "Bioglass® 45S5-based composites for bone tissue engineering and functional applications," *J Biomed Mater Res A*, vol. 105, no. 11, pp. 3197–3223, 2017, doi: 10.1002/jbm.a.36156.
9. N. Al-Harbi *et al.*, "Silica-based bioactive glasses and their applications in hard tissue regeneration: a review," *Pharmaceuticals*, vol. 14, no. 2, pp. 1–20, 2021, doi: 10.3390/PH14020075.
10. H. Yu, J. Peng, Y. Xu, J. Chang, and H. Li, "Bioglass activated skin tissue engineering constructs for wound healing," *ACS Appl Mater Interfaces*, vol. 8, no. 1, pp. 703–715, 2016, doi: 10.1021/acsami.5b09853.
11. D. Vukajlovic, J. Parker, O. Bretcanu, and K. Novakovic, "Chitosan based polymer/bioglass composites for tissue engineering applications," *Mater Sci Eng C*, vol. 96, pp. 955–967, 2019, doi: 10.1016/j.msec.2018.12.026.
12. N. A. P. Van Gestel, J. Geurts, D. J. W. Hulsen, B. Van Rietbergen, S. Hofmann, and J. J. Arts, "Clinical applications of S53P4 bioactive glass in bone healing and osteomyelitic treatment: a literature review," *Biomed Res Int*, vol. 2015, p. 684826. 2015, doi: 10.1155/2015/684826.
13. M. T. Souza, S. Tansaz, E. D. Zanotto, and A. R. Boccaccini, "Bioactive glass fiber-reinforced PGS matrix composites for cartilage regeneration," *Materials (Basel)*, vol. 10, no. 1, p. 83. 2017, doi: 10.3390/ma10010083.
14. R. Lin *et al.*, "Copper-incorporated bioactive glass-ceramics inducing anti-inflammatory phenotype and regeneration of cartilage/bone interface," *Theranostics*, vol. 9, no. 21, pp. 6300–6313, 2019, doi: 10.7150/thno.36120.
15. J. Zhou *et al.*, "In vivo and in vitro studies of borate based glass micro-fibers for dermal repairing," *Mater Sci Eng C*, vol. 60, pp. 437–445, 2016, doi: 10.1016/j.msec.2015.11.068.
16. M. H. Kaou, M. Furkó, K. Balázsi, and C. Balázsi, "Advanced bioactive glasses: the newest achievements and breakthroughs in the area," *Nanomaterials*, vol. 13, no. 16, p. 2287, Aug. 2023, doi: 10.3390/NANO13162287.
17. C. H. Kong, C. Steffi, Z. Shi, and W. Wang, "Development of mesoporous bioactive glass nanoparticles and its use in bone tissue engineering," *J Biomed Mater Res B Appl Biomater*, vol. 106, no. 8, pp. 2878–2887, 2018, doi: 10.1002/jbm.b.34143.

18. S. Lee, A. Matsugaki, T. Kasuga, and T. Nakano, "Development of bifunctional oriented bioactive glass/poly(lactic acid) composite scaffolds to control osteoblast alignment and proliferation," *J Biomed Mater Res A*, vol. 107, no. 5, pp. 1031–1041, 2019, doi: 10.1002/jbm.a.36619.
19. Y. Li *et al.*, "Bioactive antibacterial silica-based nanocomposites hydrogel scaffolds with high angiogenesis for promoting diabetic wound healing and skin repair," *Theranostics*, vol. 10, no. 11, pp. 4929–4943, 2020, doi: 10.7150/thno.41839.
20. N. Dey, F. P. Mohny, G. Betsy Reshma, D. Rao, M. Ganguli, and D. Santhiya, "Bioinspired synthesis of bioactive glass nanocomposites for hyaluronic acid delivery to bone and skin," *Int J Biol Macromol*, vol. 253, p. 127262.2023, doi: 10.1016/j.ijbiomac.2023.127262.
21. X. Zhou, N. Sahai, L. Qi, S. Mankoci, and W. Zhao, "Biomimetic and nanostructured hybrid bioactive glass," *Biomaterials*, vol. 50, no. 1, pp. 1–9, 2015, doi: 10.1016/j.biomaterials.2015.01.024.
22. Bos, G., 2018. ISO 13485: 2003/2016—medical devices—quality management systems—requirements for regulatory purposes. In *Handbook of Medical Device Regulatory Affairs in Asia* (pp. 153–174). Jenny Stanford Publishing.
23. A. E. Lottes *et al.*, "Navigating the regulatory pathway for medical devices-a conversation with the FDA, clinicians, researchers, and industry experts," *J Cardiovasc Transl Res*, vol. 15, no. 5, pp. 927–943, 2022, doi: 10.1007/S12265-022-10232-1.

Index

Kolibri 360 GmbH
Ferdinand-Jühlke-Straße 7
99095 Erfurt, Deutschland
produktsicherheit@kolibri360.de